CROOKED

ALSO BY CATHRYN JAKOBSON RAMIN

Carved in Sand: When Attention Fails and Memory Fades in Midlife

CROOKED

OUTWITTING THE BACK PAIN INDUSTRY

AND GETTING ON THE ROAD TO RECOVERY

CATHRYN
JAKOBSON
RAMIN

HARPER

An Imprint of HarperCollinsPublishers

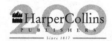

HarperCollins books may be purchased for educational, business, or sales promotional use. For information, please e-mail the Special Markets Department at SPsales@harpercollins.com.

FIRST EDITION

Designed by Fritz Metsch

Library of Congress Cataloging-in-Publication Data has been applied for.

ISBN 978-0-06-264178-6

17 18 19 20 21   LSC   10 9 8 7 6 5 4 3

Author's Note

THIS BOOK IS a work of investigative journalism. The scientific and factual material herein is complementary to the narrative and should be used to supplement rather than replace the advice of your physician or another trained health professional. If you know or suspect you have a health problem, I recommend that you consult your physician before embarking on any medical program, treatment, or exercise regimen. Both the publisher and I disclaim liability for any medical outcomes that may occur as a result of applying the methods suggested in this book.

All efforts have been made to ensure the accuracy of the information contained herein as of the date of publication. I researched this book for over five years, with extensive help from medical practitioners, scientists, and experts in many fields, conducting hundreds of hours of interviews. In addition, the book was rigorously and thoroughly checked by three professional fact-checkers. However, any errors, misattributions, inaccuracies, or other defects that remain are of my own making and are my responsibility alone.

This book is dedicated to my late father, who taught me that my reach should always exceed my grasp; and to my late mother, who did not believe in giving up.

Contents

CROOKED

Introduction: A Terrible Affliction

WHEN I WENT LOOKING FOR A SOLUTION, I FOUND A MUCH BIGGER PROBLEM

THE NOTE IN my calendar, put there on April 14, 2008, says, "Find a spine surgeon." For decades, I'd sought to avoid open warfare with my back, but on that date, the truce officially ended.

Over the years, I'd spent a fortune on chiropractic care, acupuncture, physical therapy, and massage. I'd signed up for Pilates, yoga, Tai Chi, and strength training, but instead of abating, my pain intensified. By 2007, I could not sit or walk comfortably for more than a few minutes. My hip ached and my right leg was on fire. There seemed to be no escaping the pain. Like a rat in a lab experiment, without a prayer of avoiding the offending stimulus, I felt anxious, angry, and trapped. When my dear friend Stacey asked me to join her on a hiking trip in the Peruvian Andes, I told her I could not manage it. My anatomy was holding me hostage; instead of climbing mountains, I would be going under the knife.

I thought fixing my back would be as straightforward as fixing a broken wrist. I'd find a surgeon and get it done. But as I made my way through overwhelming amounts of material on the Internet, I saw that I was wrong. As an ordinary patient, I risked drowning in a sinkhole of hype.

However, as an investigative reporter with three decades of experience in digging for the facts, I recognized that I'd arrived on the scene at the ideal moment. Back pain treatment was a microcosm of everything that was wrong with the health care system. Back trouble, in all its permutations, costs the United States roughly $100 billion a year, more than is spent annually to treat cancer, coronary artery disease, and AIDS (acquired immunodeficiency syndrome) combined. On a per capita basis, other nations—chief among them, the United Kingdom, Australia, Canada, Germany, Sweden, Denmark, the Netherlands, China, and South Korea—also pay hefty bills.

When I did my first Internet search, I had no idea that I'd spend six years studying this topic. Nor did I realize that in the interim, procedures that, for decades, had been upheld as the gold standard in spine care would be relegated to the dusty and crowded shelves of misguided medicine. Spine surgeons' go-to procedure—lumbar spinal fusion—would be discredited, primary care doctors would find that they'd launched a prescription opioid epidemic, and interventional pain physicians—those who perform epidural spinal injections—would be faced with evidence that their shots didn't work. Federal prosecutors would punish device manufacturers for selling spinal instrumentation that was inadequately tested. Painkiller manufacturers and the U.S. Food and Drug Administration would be found tucked into bed with each other, working the drug approval process without regard to patients' best interests. As the story evolved, the journalist in me relished each appalling revelation. As a patient, however, I felt as if I'd barely avoided stepping off the curb in front of a bus. Many people, I realized, were not so lucky: They got caught in a relentless loop, and were commonly harmed in the process. As one mother, whose most recent episode of back pain commenced when she bent forward to hand her toddler a lollipop, wrote in an e-mail, "In an effort to resolve my back problems, I've had a host of ridiculous medical encounters over the last few years, some confusing, some offensive, some harmful—and I feel completely upside down and unclear about how to best find help."

My goal with *Crooked* is to set the back pain industry's offerings in their proper context, so that patients have the information they need to make good decisions; to know what works sometimes, what works rarely, and what can cause harm. With luck, I will spare you the side effects of "optimism bias": the very human proclivity to seek out information that supports your own views, while ignoring that which does not. Patients have a tendency to overestimate the benefits of treatments, while underestimating the downside, especially when in the presence of a health care provider who would prefer not to admit that he doesn't know. Whether he or she wears a white coat, hospital scrubs, or workout gear; cracks your back; cossets you with heating pads; sticks you with needles; or hands you a set of free weights (and then ignores you in favor of his Twitter feed); remember that *every stakeholder wants and needs your business.*

Epidemiologist and internist Richard Deyo, a keen thinker about these issues, and the Kaiser-Permanente Endowed Professor of Evidence-Based Medicine at Oregon Health and Science University, summarized the problem: "There's this very mechanical view of the human body," he said, "one that suggests that you can find out what's broken and replace it or fix it.

"These expectations did not arise in a vacuum," he emphasized, eyebrows lifting slightly above the black frames of his glasses. "Those of us in the medical profession are probably guilty of creating them. We seem to be doing more and more, but there's no evidence that people are getting better pain relief. [Industry players] are just making money hand over fist from back pain patients who are desperate for something that will help them. They're very easy targets. Anyone who says he has something that might help can set up a practice and hang out a shingle without an iota of proof, and make a pretty good living off of it."

It is fair to say that all professions—in medicine, commerce, finance, or government—harbor many who are ethical and well intentioned, as well as some who are greedy and unscrupulous. It is not always easy to tell one from the other in advance, or even in retrospect. And it is remarkably easy, as so many patients have discovered, to undergo a series of treatments and procedures that are both unnecessary and terribly destructive.

YOU CAN APPROACH this book in the conventional way—starting with part I, where I examine what the scientific evidence says doesn't work and why, before moving to part II, where I tell you what experts say you need to know in order to get on the road to recovery. Or, as I suspect will be the preference of many long-suffering chronic back pain patients, you can reverse that plan and dive right into part II, jump-starting your return to function before heading back to read part I.

Successful rehabilitation is never passive: It requires sweat, persistence, and a lifetime of hard work. Although it won't be easy or quick or painless, by the time you finish this book, you'll know how to avoid therapeutic dead ends. No matter what you've heard, back pain is not the unsolvable enigma of modern medicine. So stand by: You're about to learn what it takes to win this game.

PART I

PROBLEMS

1

Back Pain Nation

HOW WE GOT INTO THIS MESS

K EEPING TO MY plan, in the spring of 2008, I made an appointment to visit my primary care doctor, who suggested yet another
round of physical therapy. He offered to write me a prescription for
painkillers, to help me get through what he described as "this rough
patch." I'd already had three fruitless assignations with the local physical therapy clinic, I reminded him, and painkillers were out of the
question, because even a single Vicodin addled my brain. Sighing, as
if he had been through this routine too many times before, my doctor
scribbled out an order for magnetic resonance imaging (an MRI) and
the address of a private radiology clinic in the city rather than that of
the local hospital's department, a few blocks away.

Several days after I had the scan, the physician's assistant outlined
the contents of radiologist's report over the phone, mentioning two
herniated discs and a condition called "degenerative disc disease." In
a flash, my brain translated that diagnosis into "life in a wheelchair."
I should come in immediately, she said, so that we could plan my next
steps. In the interim, I should be careful of how I moved and what
I lifted. That evening, I babied my ostensibly fragile spine through
dinner and dishes. Then, I sat down next to my husband on the sofa
and told him the news.

A week later, my primary care doctor read the same radiology report to me in person. The intervertebral discs in my spine, he said,
had lost their resiliency. He did not explain that there was often no
correlation between flat or black discs, as seen on an MRI, and pain,

or that "degenerative disc disease" was a very controversial diagnosis.

It took a couple of weeks to get an appointment with an orthopedic surgeon, and no wonder: The reception area was jammed. The waiting crowd meant that the surgeon was tops, I assumed.

After an hour's delay, however, I learned that I wasn't going to see the surgeon. Instead, the physician's assistant would evaluate me. Although my more detailed spinal MRI was less than a month old, I'd need a fresh set of X-rays, done right in the office, as soon as she finished asking me some questions. The X-ray technician aimed the camera at my neck. The pain, I reminded him, was in my hip and my leg and my low back. "It's written right here that we need the cervical," he said, and fired away. By the time I was dressed again, the physician's assistant realized that she'd checked the wrong box. I stripped for yet another unnecessary dose of radiation.

On my next visit, I was sure I would see the surgeon. But the physiatrist, who scrutinized me as he darted around the exam room on a rolling stool, explained that the surgeon was booked three months out. In any event, slots in his schedule were reserved for patients who had already failed conservative treatment. (Physiatrists are often confused with podiatrists or psychiatrists, but they are MDs who specialize in physical medicine and rehabilitation. Those who work independently are worth their weight in gold, because they're expert anatomical sleuths and skilled in exercise physiology. Those who work for spine surgeons typically make a living performing spinal injections and other interventional pain management procedures, bolstering the surgeons' bottom line.)

After talking to me for less than five minutes, this particular physiatrist whipped out a prescription pad emblazoned with OxyContin's boxy logo. Then he scribbled down a list of options for conservative care. He could perform a series of epidural steroid injections, or order more physical therapy. He could destroy the spidery nerves that grow around the facet joints of the spine. He could send me off to the affiliated pain management practice, where I could get a prescription for opioids.

When I asked him what he would do, and what it would cost, he invoked the phrase "shared decision-making." Ideally, that term describes a very informed choice, made with the help of a physician who explains the risks and benefits of each option. Instead, this doctor said I should research my choices on the Web, and get back to him. If I wanted to talk about dollars, I should call my health insurance provider. He had a lot of weapons in his arsenal, he emphasized, and he was willing to try them all.

At that news, I grabbed my stuff and fled the exam room, with no plan to return. After a ten-minute wait, the receptionist handed me the films for two cervical and two lumbar X-rays, and a bill that included charges for both. She couldn't find my MRI, she said, but I was welcome to call in a week to see if the CD had turned up. To my dismay, I realized that a month had passed, with no discernible progress.

As I was leaving, I met an acquaintance who was parking the car after dropping off her barely mobile husband. I told her what I'd just turned down. After many of the same interventions, she said, her mate had opted for a two-level lumbar spinal fusion. At the six-month follow-up, the surgeon noted that the vertebral bones had grown together just as he'd anticipated. Perfect union or not, the pain had not abated, the ailing man's wife said. "He's still home on the couch, still totally miserable, and so stoned on painkillers he can't even take out the trash." They were considering another operation.

Searching for direction, that night I called an old friend, an internal medicine doc. I described my chronically aching hip, leg, and low back and told her I was contemplating spine surgery. She asked if I was familiar with the term "iatrogenic." I wasn't, so she defined it for me: It meant physician-induced damage, whether intentional or accidental. In the surgical treatment of low back pain conditions, she said, iatrogenic outcomes were far too common. There was evidence that recent-onset leg pain from a disc herniation could be alleviated with a simple nerve decompression procedure. But lumbar spinal fusion for chronic low back pain was an iffy proposition.

When I told her what was on my imaging—the herniated discs, the diagnosis of "degenerative disease," she acknowledged that ordering that first MRI scan was the medical equivalent "of launching a Scud missile; it was hard to control and capable of causing enormous destruction." Often, surgeons had investments in radiology clinics, so it was no surprise that the radiology report came back full of ominous-sounding things, panicking the patient, who insisted on his inviolable right to see the same local spine surgeon who had operated on his friends. Such "community spine surgeons" tended to be cavalier, she said, operating on everyone who came through the door. Surgeons with academic affiliations could also be under pressure from their university hospitals to keep the OR (operating room) schedule full. In short, it was pandemonium out there.

Six months later—and this was the worst part—the patient for whom she'd agreed to order the scan was back in her office, too often dependent on painkillers, overweight, and with the beginnings of type 2 diabetes and hypertension. "And from that moment," she said glumly, "taking care of him becomes my responsibility for the rest of his life."

AS I PLANNED my next move, I tuned in to what I would come to call the "Back Pain Channel": populated by those fellow sufferers I encountered daily. Much of the time, I carried a plastic tractor seat–shaped device called a BackJoy, a $36 lifesaver that allowed me to abide even the most unforgiving perches in restaurants and theaters and on airplanes. When I bought one in DayGlo orange, it attracted a lot of attention. Before one flight, as I handed my license and boarding pass to the TSA (Transportation Security Administration) agent, he grilled me about this object and then held up a long line of passengers so that he might rest his back a moment.

The Back Pain Channel never stopped broadcasting news. Many victims were young. Ethan, a literary agent in his early twenties, gave up a bookstore job for a much more promising one that chained him to his desk chair. He'd gone through two jumbo-size bottles of Advil in a few months. A friend requested that her daughter's buff thirty-year-old fiancé sit next to me at dinner, so he could fill me in on the details of his condition.

In midlife, people had just as many problems. Richard, an ad agency creative director, had taught his team to bring pillows to staff meetings, so that they could join him as he stretched out flat on the floor. Melanie, a writer, had bought and sold three used cars, but still had not found one she could bear to sit in for more than an hour. Roxie, an administrative assistant, had concluded that she and her partner "could stay home and eat ice cream, or have sex and go to the hospital." Jeannette, a middle school principal, admitted that she could not carry her own briefcase from the parking lot to her office. Simon reported that his back spasms had nearly caused him to skip his eldest son's bar mitzvah, while Pam said that on her long-awaited trip to the Vatican, she'd had to sit and wait in St. Peter's Basilica, while everyone else took the entire tour of the holy city. People in their seventies, eighties, and nineties cornered me with similar frequency, desperate to know what to do about the spinal stenosis that made it difficult to walk a block. "You start to design your life to fit your pain," said Barbara, who was extremely active until chronic back and leg pain made for agonizing days and nights. "It's a hellish way to live, and you can't put it out of your mind. It always wins."

Few people reported pain of recent onset, which is properly referred to as "acute" pain. For most, the problem had persisted for decades. That puzzled me, because early in my research I'd come upon what is known as "the 90/10 hypothesis," which held that 90 percent of the 31.4 million people each year who see U.S. physicians about back pain recover on their own within two to three months, while only 10 percent develop chronic conditions.

Epidemiologist Peter Croft, who directed Keele University's Primary Care Musculoskeletal Research Centre in the United Kingdom, made it clear that he did not trust the 90/10 hypothesis. In Croft's estimation, only a quarter of back pain patients recovered within a year. It was true that 90 percent of back pain patients did not return to their primary care doctors within three months of a back pain episode, he noted in the *British Medical Journal*, but this did not mean that they had resolved their problems. Instead, they'd abandoned primary care as a potentially helpful resource, and moved on to other types of practitioners and interventions.

University of North Carolina internist and epidemiologist Timothy S. Carey continued to dismantle the 90/10 hypothesis. In a paper published in the *Archives of Internal Medicine* in 2006, his team replicated a study of four thousand North Carolina residents that had been first performed fourteen years earlier. In 1992, roughly 4 percent of North Carolina's population had undergone lumbar spine surgery, but by the time the study was repeated, the number of spine procedures had leaped by 157 percent. In those fourteen years, the number of people who said they couldn't work or attend to daily activities more than doubled, while those who were enrolled in the Social Security Disability Insurance (SSDI) program increased by nearly 160 percent. These were "regular folks who happened to answer the phone," Carey explained. "They were a nice ethnic mix of urban, rural, rich, and poor, with a very high rate of chronic illness." This massive increase in back trouble and disability was not limited to North Carolina, Carey suspected.

The type of care patients received depended largely on the practitioners they saw. "If you went to a primary care doctor, you got lots of pain pills, and maybe a physical therapy referral," said Carey. (Historically, primary care doctors have prescribed about half of all opioid analgesics, and most initial MRIs. A patient who was scanned once had a 50 percent chance of having a second MRI in the same year.) A quarter of the patients underwent passive treatments like ultrasound, traction, and electrical stimulation, for which scientific evidence of effectiveness is weak or absent. If you went to a chiropractor, you would have spinal manipulation—and more than 25 percent of the patients Carey's team surveyed had been under chiropractic care, for an average of twenty-two office visits each. Although nearly half of the patients said they struggled with depression, very few had received any form of psychological counseling. More than half reported that their doctors had never recommended exercise (though some patients may have ignored such a prescription). Not one had been sent to intensive functional rehabilitation, combined with cognitive behavioral therapy, despite evidence that this approach produces superior results in chronic back pain patients.

Carey's team found that about a fifth of the patients acknowledged that they used opioid analgesics, mostly without a prescription, to treat their chronic back pain. The actual number who used painkillers was probably higher, he observed, but not all patients would be willing to admit to a researcher on the phone that "they were using Uncle Charlie's oxycodone." Carey learned that muscle relaxants, as well as benzodiazepines such as Ativan and Xanax, were often prescribed in combination with narcotics, increasing the risk of opioid poisoning, overdose, and death, although there's no clinical evidence for the use of these drugs in the treatment of chronic back pain.

CAREY'S TEAM UNEARTHED a great deal of valuable data. But for epidemiologists, the most unnerving statistic involved "occupational disability," a term that describes on-the-job injuries, work incapacity, and related loss of productivity.

Rheumatologist Nortin Hadler at the University of North Carolina, an expert on the subject of occupational medicine, is the author of *Stabbed in the Back*, a book with a title so trenchant that I wish I'd arrived at it first. "The system was designed with amputees and burn victims in mind," Hadler asserted. "Ever since, back 'injury' has hung like Damocles' sword over the resource-advantaged world, inside and outside the workplace, wreaking havoc on the lives of workers with disabling backache for whom workers' compensation insurance is designed to provide a remedy."

In any country where the government has adopted a liberal policy regarding back pain as an occupational disability, such claims are common. When U.S. legislators liberalized disability laws in 1984, the number who claimed "musculoskeletal disease" as their cause of disability first doubled and then almost tripled, with 6.5 million beneficiaries at this writing. Chronic back pain complaints (rather than, say, tendonitis) top the list of the costliest cases settled.

In the United States, the Social Security Administration supports the disability program, which spends $143 billion on medical care, about a third of which can be attributed to the cost of supporting back pain patients. Per capita, the United Kingdom spends more than twice as much as the United States on disability benefits. Australia and Scandinavia also struggle with exorbitant expenses related to occupational medicine. But as we will see, very few of these patients actually recover and go on to live productive lives.

In the United States, plaintiffs' attorneys—the lawyers who represent patients—usually receive about 40 percent of a patient's court settlement. The more aggressive and invasive the medical care a patient receives, the more the case is worth in court—and the more the case is worth, the more the attorney stands to gain. It's a sad truth that spinal fusion surgery, tremendously costly and not supported by scientific evidence, nets the largest possible settlement. The money flows into the coffers of workers' compensation underwriters, plaintiffs' attorneys who specialize in disability-related lawsuits, surgical hardware manufacturers, pharmaceutical companies, hospitals, and health care providers engaged in "occupational medicine."

THE IDEA THAT you should be compensated for being injured in the course of your daily toil can be traced to ancient Arab civilizations, where legal doctrine held, rather illogically, that the on-the-job loss of a penis would be recompensed based on the amount of length lost. In more recent centuries, employers were harsh: If the worker's injury was deemed to be a result of his own negligence, there was no payment. If the employer's equipment was damaged in the accident—say the worker lost an arm, gumming up the machinery—he or his surviving relatives were expected to make restitution.

That was the status quo until the start of the Industrial Revolution. In 1871, in a wily political move, the Prussian chancellor, Otto von Bismarck—a man not otherwise known for his generosity toward the working class—introduced "workers' accident insurance." In exchange for the promise of minimal compensation, the worker relinquished the right to sue his employer in the case of a casualty.

Von Bismarck's legislation won him both workers' and industrialists' support. Soon afterward, Britain's Parliament passed a similar law.

The idea caught on in North America in 1911, when the progressive state of Wisconsin passed a law requiring employers to pay mutilated workers what they would have earned if they stayed on the job. Pain without an inciting calamity was not considered a compensable injury.

Everything changed in 1934, at Massachusetts General Hospital in Boston. In an effort to resolve a male patient's back and leg pain, a neurosurgeon and an orthopedist successfully removed what they believed was a spinal tumor. The pain relented, but when the physicians examined the tissue, they realized that instead of cutting out a tumor, they had excised one of the twenty-three intervertebral discs that act as cushions between the bones of the human spine. The surgeons, William Jason Mixter and Joseph Barr, knew they were onto something. Barely able to contain their enthusiasm for the procedure, they described "diskal rupture," a condition nearly endemic among workers whose jobs included any kind of physical exertion.

ON THE BASIS of this invisible condition, which conveniently could be diagnosed in anyone with a backache, the Massachusetts surgeons built what would eventually become a moneymaking machine. It would take several decades—and the transformation of a physically active population, accustomed to chopping wood and hauling water, into a primarily chair-based one—for the spine business to reach maturity. That transition to a sedentary lifestyle would vastly exacerbate the prevalence of chronic pain.

In a world that is increasingly virtual and screen-based, the musculoskeletal system suffers. Today, the average U.S. adult spends almost nine hours a day in a seated position: watching television, working at a computer, or driving a car. As a result, the gluteal and postural muscles, essential for supporting the spine, rest idly and grow lax. Modern societies, observed Australian researchers Brigid Lynch and Neville Owen, "are engineered, physically and socially, to be sitting-centric."

Too much sitting and too little exercise make for a potent combination. The way that most people arrange themselves in chairs—with curved spine, collapsed pelvis, jutting chin, and slumped shoulders—overworks ligaments and joints, and restricts the oxygen supply to spinal nerves and discs. When circulation is inadequate, muscles turn to fatty tissue, resulting in weakness and deconditioning.

In the United States in 2014, roughly a quarter of the population reported having done no physical activity whatsoever in the previous thirty days. The rest of the resource-advantaged world doesn't do much better. The World Health Organization reports that more than a third of the global population does not come close to meeting the recommendation of 150 minutes a week of exercise.

Today, a third of all kids are obese. Kids in general get less exercise than any generation of children in history. The Centers for Disease Control and Prevention found that public schools in only two states—Illinois and Massachusetts—meet the recommendation for 150 minutes or more per week of exercise at the elementary school level. In high school, it's worse: The 2011 National Youth Risk Behavior Survey of U.S. high school students found that 48 percent did not attend a physical education class in the course of the school week, while 32 percent watched TV for three or more hours and spent three or more hours per day on the computer. Since many parents today feel that children are safest when left to their digital devices, murdering virtual enemies instead of climbing trees and throwing baseballs, it's not surprising that young people in their teens and twenties are the fastest-growing cohort of back pain patients.

New science in the field of "inactivity physiology" (yes, that discipline is flourishing) suggests that chronic back pain, as costly and pernicious as it is, barely ranks as a problem, compared with other disorders attributable to sedentary lifestyles. Researchers have found an independent relationship between long sitting and cardiovascular disease, and breast, colon, colorectal, endometrial, and ovarian cancers, as well as type 2 diabetes. The World Health Organization says that the lack of physical activity is one of the top four leading causes of preventable death worldwide, ahead of high cholesterol, alcohol, and drug abuse. Sitting around for most of the day has become as deadly as smoking or obesity, the medical journal *Lancet* reported: While 5.1 million cigarette smokers die each year, about 5.3 million individuals succumb as a result of inactivity.

"Sitting too much is not the same as exercising too little," said University of Houston microbiologist Marc Hamilton, who studies inactivity and sedentary behavior. When you're sitting, your legs hang lifelessly below you, he explained in a *Businessweek* interview. If you don't stand for a sufficient amount of time, utilizing the specialized leg muscles known as the "deep red quadriceps," there is a rapid and dramatic loss of an enzyme known as LPL (lipoprotein lipase) in the bloodstream. That enzyme, Hamilton said, "grabs fat and cholesterol from the blood, burning the fat into energy while shifting the cholesterol from LDL (the bad kind) to HDL (the healthy kind)." When a person sits for long periods of time, he observed, "the muscles are relaxed and enzyme activity drops by 90 to 95 percent, leaving fat to camp out in the bloodstream."

Although researchers have yet to track down a specific correlation between obesity and back pain, obesity increases the mechanical load on the spine, and twice as many overweight patients complain of back pain as people of normal weight. The repercussions go beyond that: Obesity is associated with systemic chronic inflammation, a condition that may be the foundation of at least one type of persistent pain.

Bone mass loss is another feature of inactivity. Older adults—nearly a third of whom never engage in physical activity—are particularly vulnerable to what is known as "bone remodeling," reflecting the body's effort to maintain spinal stability at any cost. They develop bone spurs inside the spinal canal and in the openings in the vertebrae through which the nerve roots exit. When those tiny daggerlike impediments meet tender spinal nerves, the result may be painful spinal stenosis.

When the *British Medical Journal* published a study that followed almost 170,000 respondents for more than nine years, the lead investigators found that if adults reduced their time spent sitting to less than three hours a day (admittedly tricky, if you're at work, and have to get there and back), life expectancy in the United States would increase by *two years*. Even reducing TV viewing to less than two hours a day increased life expectancy by almost a year and a half. How such a change in lifestyle would alter the prevalence of back pain remains an open question. But it's something to consider.

Although it would be helpful, moving around more wouldn't resolve the public health crisis, especially not as the year 2016 came to a close, a new president prepared to assume office, and this book went to the printer. As we will see in chapters to come, back pain is as much an emotional problem as it is a physiological one. In terms of its ability to generate stress-related ailments, the upcoming year was likely to be a corker. In ever-increasing numbers, people would suffer from migraines or abdominal pain, insomnia or clinical depression. But for others, in an uncertain and challenging political environment, unmanageable emotions such as dread, fear, and hopelessness would assert themselves in the vulnerable region between the rib cage and hips. The misery would send an unprecedented number of people to their primary care doctors with back pain complaints, generating orders for millions of scans, injections, and surgical plans. With so much at stake, the pain was going to get worse before it got better. It was tempting to hoist the white flag and take to the couch with a heating pad, but that would solve nothing. As a patient, it was more essential than ever to understand what you were being offered, and what it was actually worth.

IN THE CHAPTERS that follow, we'll take a close look at the alternatives that are available to back pain patients, tackling these options in roughly the same order that patients undertake them. Frequently, the first stop on that journey involves nonsurgical "conservative treatment." That's a term that encompasses many interventions. But it often begins with a visit to a chiropractor or physical therapist— and, several months and thousands of dollars later, leaves patients no better off than they were when they started.

2

A Tale of Two Tables

WHY BACK PATIENTS "FAIL" CHIROPRACTIC
TREATMENT AND PHYSICAL THERAPY

ALONG MY TOWN'S main boulevard, I counted twenty-three signs for chiropractors' offices and nearly as many for physical therapy practices. It seemed as if everyone I knew was seeing a chiropractor, a PT, or both. More than thirty-five million Americans visit chiropractors each year, at a cost of roughly $7 billion. About nine million see PTs, at a cost of $13.5 billion. Much of that treatment is for back pain. But what are patients actually getting for their money?

Both physical therapy and chiropractic are described as "manual therapy," but the philosophies and techniques that underlie them are different. Chiropractors vary in how they practice (some don't ever perform spinal adjustments, and have adopted other approaches), but "straight" (i.e., traditional) chiropractors apply a high-velocity, low-amplitude thrust to a specific intervertebral joint, thereby manipulating that joint beyond its normal range of motion. By manipulating the joints of the spine and relieving what they call "vertebral subluxations," traditional chiropractors say they can cure many types of physical dysfunction. Rather than practicing manipulation, physical therapists—or "physiotherapists," as they are referred to in Europe and Australia—practice "mobilization," exerting gentle pressure on a joint in order to expand the existing range of motion.

The Cochrane Collaboration is a reliable international network of physicians and scientists, established to review and summarize the medical literature with the least bias possible. (In the pages to come, we'll hear from them often. It's always a good idea to check on what they have to say about the scientific evidence regarding the management of any condition.)

Although chiropractors often tell patients that long-term treatment is essential, there is no evidence that *ongoing* chiropractic care of back pain (or any other symptom or disorder) is effective. The Cochrane Collaboration makes it very clear that the only evidence for chiropractic in the treatment of back pain is in cases where the pain is of a very recent onset. In such cases, one or two sessions of chiropractic manipulation may be helpful. (And it should be noted that at this stage, the problem often resolves by itself.) But if two sessions don't do the trick, there's no reason to expect any benefit from further visits, nor is there any evidence that "maintenance" treatments are effective. If that news surprises you, you're not alone: People typically pay for year after year of treatment, certain that this is the way to stave off future problems.

In the early 1990s, the mother of one of my young son's friends sent me to my first chiropractor. After taking X-rays, conducting a physical exam, and having me hold small glass vials, which would allow him to "test my muscle strength" and "assess organ dysfunction," he reported that beyond the "vertebral subluxations" he'd already detected, I suffered from weak adrenal glands and poor kidney and liver function. The good news was that with a year's worth of twice-a-week adjustments, which my health care plan would pay for, I'd be fine. As a mother of an infant and a four-year-old, on call 24/7 for heavy lifting at awkward angles, I signed on, agreeing to have my back and neck cracked on Tuesdays and Fridays. I figured that it couldn't hurt. Immediately after each treatment, I experienced a modicum of relief. But by the time I got home, the pain was as bad as ever.

I NEVER THOUGHT to ask questions about those subluxations, but if I had, I would have learned that they were unidentifiable on X-rays, in hands-on examination, or by any other methods. The premise that the spinal joints can freely slip into and out of position is false; such dislocations do occur, but only in the event of serious trauma, the kind that takes you to a hospital's emergency department rather than a chiropractor's office. One study showed that, even when they were presented with identical copies of a patient's X-rays, a group of experienced chiropractors could not muster consensus about where in the spine the subluxations occurred or what the proper course of treatment should be.

Like most people, I assumed that chiropractic treatment was safe. But most of the troubles that send patients to a chiropractor in the first place are included on the World Health Organization's list of contraindications to chiropractic adjustment: disc herniation, severe or painful disc pathology, leg pain, dislocation of a vertebra, the presence of spinal hardware from fusion surgery, hypermobile joints, vertebral instability, inflammatory arthritis, osteoporosis, or a history of long-term glucocorticoid treatment, which can make bones fragile, especially in older people.

When chiropractors treat pain that is caused by undetected malignancies, the outcome can be catastrophic. Two women who were interviewed for this book visited chiropractors for many sessions, to treat what they assumed was ordinary neck and back pain. When they finally had CT scans at the behest of their MDs, both had spinal tumors, as well as advanced lung, liver, and brain cancer. Neither one survived.

In *Trick or Treatment*, a must-read book about fallacies in alternative medicine, science reporter Simon Singh and his coauthor, scientist Edzard Ernst, describe an experiment conducted by psychiatrist Stephen Barrett, one of the most fervent naysayers regarding chiropractic. To see what they might advise, Barrett arranged for a twenty-nine-year-old woman to make four visits to different chiropractors. The first chiropractor "diagnosed 'atlas subluxation' [an improperly situated vertebra at the top of the spine] and predicted 'paralysis in 15 years' if the problem was not treated. The second practitioner found not just one, but many vertebrae 'out of alignment' and one hip 'higher' than the other. The third said that the woman's neck was 'tight.' The fourth said that misaligned vertebrae indicated the presence of 'stomach problems.'"

Despite the disparity in diagnosis, all four recommended long-term regular adjustments. These high-velocity low-amplitude thrusts would elicit the chiropractor's trademark popping or cracking noise, referred to as "cavitation." Chiropractic patients have been brainwashed into believing that cavitation conveys some benefit, but, says retired chiropractor Samuel Homola, the author of *Inside Chiropractic: A Patient's Guide*, all that the popping or cracking noise means is that a bubble of oxygen has been released from the lubricating synovial fluid in the spine's butterfly-shaped facet joints, reducing pressure on tiny, infiltrating nerve endings. Within a few hours of cavitation, as synovial fluid pressure is restored, the facet joints return to their original position—and the pain comes back, until the joint pops again. Some patients develop what is called "chiropractic neurosis," the compulsion to have the joint pop many times a day (or an hour), and they start to self-adjust, twisting sharply in an effort to summon that sound.

Too-frequent adjustments may lead to joint irritation and "over-manipulation syndrome," in which spinal ligaments, meant to be taut as guitar strings, become weak and overstretched, developing microscopic tears. Overstretching the ligaments is a special risk for women of childbearing age, whose robust estrogen levels make their pelvic ligaments especially relaxed.

In a chronic chiropractic patient's later years, overstretched ligaments may contribute to spinal instability. Pain, numbness, or even the loss of motor control of the feet can be the result. Surgeons often use a diagnosis of spinal instability as a reason to order spinal fusion surgery.

Studies show that, at any age, roughly half of all chiropractic patients experience temporary adverse side effects after treatment, including pain, numbness, stiffness, dizziness, and headaches. But these are minor in comparison with a more serious threat: the possibility that a cervical (neck) adjustment may result in a chiropractic stroke.

Here's how it happens: The vertebral arteries, which run roughly parallel to the cervical spine, make a sharp turn around the uppermost cervical vertebrae, just before those arteries travel into the brain. At the top cervical vertebrae, they form a harmless kink—until a chiropractor performs a "tug and twist" adjustment that violently rotates the neck. That movement can tear the delicate walls of one or more arteries, producing a blood clot or swelling that cuts off the blood supply to the brain. The resulting stroke may lead to permanent brain damage or death.

Chiropractors downplay the risk of such a stroke as insignificant, but on Google, I found too many reports of people who had gone in for a simple adjustment and been damaged for life. The statistic that's usually cited is that there are 1.46 strokes for every million necks cracked. But some papers describe chiropractic stroke prevalence at between three strokes per million and sixty strokes per million. Given that one million chiropractic adjustments are made in the United States each day, it is possible that someone has a chiropractic stroke every twenty-four minutes.

Because chiropractic strokes don't usually happen immediately—they may occur several days after an adjustment—both physicians and patients may fail to make the connection, meaning that the majority of these incidents are never reported. Symptoms immediately prior to the stroke include headaches, neck pain, and visual impairment, and therefore may be mistaken for drunkenness, drug overdose, or the flu. A person who feels dizzy or nauseated after a neck adjustment should be alert to the possibility that the artery has been damaged. In recent years, the American Heart Association and the National Stroke Association have both recommended that before a chiropractor adjusts a patient's neck, he or she should inform the patient of the statistical association between cervical artery dissection and manipulation therapy.

I'd never heard of chiropractic stroke until a colleague introduced me to Kelley Lowery. When she was twenty-nine, Lowery, who was working as a bartender, struggled with low back pain. That made it very difficult to meet the demands of her job, which included bending, lifting, squatting, and stretching. In the last week of December, just before the New Year's Eve rush, she dropped in to see her newly licensed chiropractor, who adjusted her neck. Lowery left his office with a raging headache. When she called him that evening, he asked her to come in again the following morning.

The next adjustment really hurt. Afterward, Lowery slept for twelve hours. When she awoke, her head still throbbed, and she couldn't hear well through her left ear. A friend rushed her to the hospital, but Lowery had her first stroke while she was still in the car. By the time her friend got her to the emergency department's check-in desk in a wheelchair, her speech was slurred and her signature was unrecognizable. She was on the phone with her mother, trying to explain her situation, when another stroke rendered her unconscious.

The MRI showed two torn regions in the vertebral artery. With a breathing tube in her trachea, she went by ambulance to Stanford University Medical Center, for more advanced brain imaging. Lowery remained in a coma for two months. When she emerged, she learned that the chiropractor had dropped by her hospital room to ask why her family had retained a personal injury lawyer. Then he left town and moved to another state, where, as far as Lowery is aware, he continues to practice.

The brain damage from the strokes left her paralyzed on her left side. Six years later, she still walked with a cane, spoke haltingly, and could not depend on her left hand, which meant that bartending was no longer an option. She was interviewing for other jobs, but she had only recently begun to drive again. Her favorite physical therapist charged $250 a session, so she saw him rarely. In an effort to increase awareness of chiropractic stroke, she had started an advocacy group. On the group's website, there were multiple tales of adjustments gone wrong—and nearly all the victims were young or middle-aged.

Soon after I met Lowery, I noticed that a chiropractic clinic in my area had posted an advertisement in its street-front window, listing the conditions that chiropractic could purportedly resolve. On that roster, in addition to back pain, neck pain, headaches, and menstrual complaints, were disorders such as erectile dysfunction and tonsillitis. On the clinic's website, I learned that the chiropractor-owner did his magic by "removing the interference in the upper part of the neck where the Brainstem [*sic*] sits, with one simple adjustment." The content advised that "by simply removing the interference that blocks the communication in the body, health is maintained along with preventing conditions which can occur later in life." I wondered how many people I knew had drifted by that window and dropped in to make an appointment.

A SELF-PROCLAIMED HEALER born in 1845 near Toronto, Daniel David Palmer was the father of chiropractic. He began as a revival tent mesmerist and entertainer who could make people fall asleep, dance wildly, or tumble into convulsions. Later, he described a "vitalistic force" or "innate intelligence" that existed in the spine; it could organize, maintain, and heal the body. But vertebral subluxations could derail that energy, with dire physiological consequences.

In 1924, when most states began to license chiropractors, *Baltimore Sun* journalist, essayist, and social critic H. L. Mencken, famous for his attacks on any aspect of life that struck him as absurd, unleashed a vitriolic critique. A "hearty blacksmith or ice-wagon driver, [might be] turned into a chiropractor in six months, often by correspondence," he observed, advising that "the backwoods swarm with chiropractors, and in most States they have been able to exert enough pressure on the rural politicians to get themselves licensed." Mencken advocated for scientific inquiry, recommending that chiropractic be studied "under rigid test conditions, by a committee of men learned in the architecture and plumbing of the body, and of a high and incorruptible sagacity. Let a thousand patients be selected, let a gang of selected chiropractors examine their backbones and determine what is the matter with them, and then let these diagnoses be checked up by the exact methods of scientific medicine. Then let the same chiropractors essay to cure the patients whose maladies have been determined. My guess is that the chiropractors' errors in diagnosis will run to at least 95% and that their failures in treatment will push 99%. But I am willing to be convinced."

In 1963, after many years of seeking to contain chiropractic's expansion, the American Medical Association established the Committee on Quackery. In a meeting of the Michigan State Medical Society, chairman and physician Joseph Sabatier observed that "rabid dogs and chiropractors fit into about the same category." The AMA asked physicians to lobby to end federal recognition of chiropractic education and to recommend that health care plans and Medicare stop their reimbursement for chiropractic care. Five years later, the U.S. Department of Health, Education, and Welfare announced that chiropractic professionals would need to adhere to the standards of modern medicine, and stop discussing subluxations, if they were to be allowed to continue to practice.

The government's antipathy should have checked chiropractic's popularity, but in the early 1970s, under intense pressure from chiropractic lobbying organizations, Congress ordered Medicare to pay for spinal manipulation. To be reimbursed by Medicare, the chiropractor needed to show that a subluxation existed on an X-ray. That should have imposed an impossible hurdle, because as we've established, subluxations are not visible on X-rays or, for that matter, in any form of imaging.

Undeterred by that detail, chiropractors installed X-ray machines in their clinics and adopted the now-standard practice of taking a complete series of spinal images, and doing so repeatedly over the course of treatment, thus exposing patients to unnecessary radiation. Financially, this was a boon, allowing chiropractors to collect payments for both X-rays and treatment. In the nine years that followed, Medicare payments to chiropractors jumped nearly 20 percent annually. In synchrony, the number of chiropractors grew, tripling between 1970 and 1990.

In 1976, an anonymous source within the American Medical Association (referred to as "Sore Throat," in homage to "Deep Throat," the mysterious background source in the infamous Watergate scandal) leaked material that revealed details of the extent of the AMA's campaign against chiropractors. In response, Chicago chiropractor Chester Wilk filed an antitrust lawsuit against the AMA. An eleven-year court battle ensued, concluding only when a U.S. district court judge found the AMA and its codefendants guilty of violating the Sherman Antitrust Act. In her comments, Judge Susan Getzendanner described the AMA's decision to "destroy a competitor" while the organization attempted to "contain and eliminate chiropractic as a profession." The AMA, said Getzendanner, should notify all 275,000 of its members that no further disparagement of the chiropractic profession would be permissible; from that moment on, from a professional standpoint, chiropractors were to have the same standing as physicians. As the result of this ruling, in some states, chiropractors (who were most assuredly not trained in surgical methods) were permitted to admit patients and treat them at ambulatory surgery centers.

In the state of California, chiropractors teamed up with anesthesiologists, so that they could perform a procedure called "manipulation under anesthesia," or MUA, on sedated patients. It was a pot of gold: As part of occupational medicine, workers' compensation insurers reimbursed chiropractors up to $20,000 for three successive days of such treatment, in addition to the charges levied by the ambulatory surgery center. Especially when the chiropractor was part owner of the surgery center, it made for a handsome payday.

In 1990, the *British Medical Journal* described spinal manipulative therapy as "seven percent more effective" than standard hospital physical therapy, without acknowledging that physical therapy was notoriously ineffective as a treatment for low back pain patients. Some viewed the sampling as unreliable: Bewilderingly, even before outcomes were established, three-quarters of the chiropractic participants had dropped out of the study.

Saying that chiropractic was 7 percent better than an ineffective protocol was faint praise, indeed. Instead of claiming an increase of 7 percent, the General Chiropractic Council in Britain employed the figure 70 percent. That number showed up on many chiropractors' websites. When the mistake was discovered, the Chiropractic Council chalked it up to a typo. But by then, based on the oversight, the United Kingdom's National Institute for Health and Care Excellence (NICE) had opted to support the British National Health Service's plan to endorse chiropractic as an approved therapy for low back pain.

When he found out about the prospective government endorsement, just before it became official, journalist Simon Singh (the co-author of *Trick or Treatment*) published an editorial in the *Guardian*. In that British newspaper, he admonished NICE for having endorsed "bogus treatments," mocking its "promotion of chiropractic to treat all sorts of conditions for which it is utterly useless." In response, the British Chiropractic Association (BCA) sued Singh for libel. In assembling his costly defense in the British court system, he drew the support of those who believed that individuals should be permitted to criticize the way the crown spent taxpayers' money.

When Royal Court judges ruled against him, Singh appealed. In April 2010, the court held that the BCA had misinterpreted what Singh had written. The chiropractors' organization withdrew the suit, but within twenty-four hours of the judge's ruling, medical groups and individuals had filed more than five hundred allegations of false advertising against British chiropractors. The British Chiropractic Association ordered members to take down their websites in self-preservation, before their businesses and reputations were damaged. Within months, one in four British chiropractors was under investigation for profiteering, misleading marketing, and advertising excesses.

In the United States, in light of this news and amid increased concern that chiropractors were taking patients for a ride on the government's dime, Medicare altered its confusing stance—"show subluxations in an X-ray, and then we'll pay for treatment"—instead ordering chiropractors to restrict their Medicare billings to "active therapy" rather than "maintenance services." Quickly, chiropractors altered the way they described their treatments so that they could code every session as "active therapy."

Medicare inspectors didn't take notice, but eventually the U.S. Office of the Inspector General did, estimating that, in 2001, Medicare had paid chiropractors some $285 million for improperly billed (and mostly unnecessary) chiropractic services. In the future, the OIG pronounced, any chiropractor who billed improperly would be fined

$2,000. But that did not stem the billing frenzy: In 2014 alone, Medicare reported that it spent $496 million on chiropractic care.

IN RECENT DECADES, chiropractors have divided over philosophical issues. Those who cling to Palmer's metaphysical and nonscientific theories are known as "straights." Others, called "mixers," acknowledge the existence of bacteria, viruses, and other scientific nuts and bolts, but still adhere to most of Palmer's tenets. Although they call themselves "chiropractic physicians" and employ the honorific "Dr.," practitioners who entered chiropractic college before 1974, when the rules changed, may have gone directly from high school to practice after only eighteen months of training.

Currently, after a minimum of two years of college, chiropractic training takes roughly thirty-two months, or four thousand hours of study. That training includes instruction in such nonmedical métiers as nerve palpitation, nerve tracing, and spinal adjustment, as well as guidance in how to perform and analyze X-rays, normally the bailiwick of a radiologist with highly specialized training. There are high-speed classes in anatomy, physiology, symptomatology and diagnosis, hygiene and sanitation, chemistry, histology, and pathology. Much time is spent training students in "practice-building," that is, the art of convincing a patient to seek regular and long-term treatment.

While they're in school, chiropractic students typically perform two hundred spinal adjustments, twenty physical exams, and twenty-five blood and urine analyses. (In contrast, medical students perform about four thousand examinations.) The chiropractor checkups are often performed on family and friends rather than on sick people. There's a licensing exam, but some chiropractic schools leave copies of old tests lying around the classrooms. Year to year, the questions are the same.

Because older chiropractors (who were trained by yet older chiropractors) serve as faculty, teachers are not necessarily well informed. In 2011, the Council on Chiropractic Education, the sole accrediting agency for U.S. chiropractic institutions, acknowledged to the U.S. Department of Education that thousands of chiropractors had graduated from accredited programs that did not meet minimum requirements. Subsequently, enrollment at some chiropractic colleges saw a 46 percent decline, and for most of the last decade, a number of well-known chiropractic college programs in the United States have struggled financially.

Still, there is no shortage of chiropractors, or people who want to be treated by them. A recent widely publicized Gallup poll—one that the Palmer College of Chiropractic commissioned, thereby ensuring bias—found that two-thirds of individuals who took the survey believed that chiropractic treatment was effective for back and neck pain, and that the same percentage were in accord with the ambiguous statement that "chiropractors have patients' best interests in mind." In the United States, about sixty thousand chiropractors treat thirty-five million Americans. But most health insurance providers are no longer willing to cut checks for "active" treatment that continues longer than a few months. To stay in business, many chiropractors bill themselves as "family physicians," offering cradle-to-grave care, while others have invented new treatment specialties, focusing on complex endocrine and neurological disorders for which it is an understatement to say they are inadequately trained. In several states, before the risks of opioid prescription were identified, chiropractic groups lobbied for permission for members to prescribe painkillers. As I write, the Texas Board of Chiropractic Examiners has proposed recognition of a specialty in "chiropractic neurology." Some Texas chiropractors have already begun advertising to attract patients with neurological problems.

Medical doctors, annoyed by policy changes that limit their freedom, while chiropractors do pretty much what they want, are no longer abiding by Judge Getzendanner's mandate. In 2011, two medical journals, the *Archives of Internal Medicine* and *American Family Physician*, rejected advertisements that promoted chiropractic's role in serving as a patient's "medical home."

For chiropractors who have come to question the relevance of their profession—and I met many—there are options. I spent a training weekend with Craig Liebenson, DC, who is the director of the International Society of Clinical Rehab Specialists, which retrains chiropractors, physical therapists, physicians, and sports medicine specialists. Liebenson practices what he preaches at L.A. Sports and Spine, a West Los Angeles clinic, but the training session I attended was held in the Bay Area, where he held court for three dozen chiropractors, each intent on a new career path. The author of two insightful books and two DVDs, Liebenson maintains the "DC" behind his name, but says he decided while in school that chiropractic founder Palmer's theories were hogwash. Hands-on adjustment is what patients want, he explained, but it is not what they need. "Repeat after me," he intoned to the group: "We refrain from the laying on of hands."

Instead of being made to feel good, said Liebenson, back pain patients needed "graded exposure to feared stimuli," which translated as intensive exercise meant to build ability, strength, and confidence. "We need to focus on function, not on pain and scans and symptoms, because all these poison the minds of patients," he told his audience. The chiropractors nodded at his words, and scribbled down notes.

IN THE EARLY 1900s, B. J. Palmer, Daniel David Palmer's son, took over his father's chiropractor training business. Hunting for a way to actually identify a subluxation, he invented a device that made him a rich man. The "neurocalometer" was priced at a heady $1,500, and according to Palmer's doctrine, every chiropractor needed one. Later, the "E-meter" became indispensable. In theory (but not in practice), it detected subluxations as a patient held two electrical contacts, using a quivering needle that moved across a scale.

In recent decades, chiropractors embraced an even larger and more expensive device: the "disc decompression table." This contemporary electric equivalent of the Hippocratic bench, circa 400 BCE, is divided into two sections. A harness on the lower end of the therapeutic table anchors the patient's hips and lower body, while the upper end of the table glides back and forth, elongating the trunk. For about forty minutes, this process separates or "distracts" the vertebrae, before allowing the spinal segments to return to their original positions. Sadly, there's no scientific evidence that this treatment is more effective than a brief dangle from a pull-up bar. But for several thousand dollars, payable in advance, chiropractors who own or lease such machines offer treatment packages of sixteen to twenty-four sessions.

When the FDA approved the first modern spinal decompression unit in 1989, it did so on the basis of clinical trial data citing an 86 percent success rate. A company called Axiom Worldwide quickly produced a copycat device. Axiom promised that the clinical studies were so good that chiropractors who leased or bought the machines for $100,000 were going to be reimbursed by health insurance providers and Medicare for years into the future. To kick things off, Axiom provided glossy patient brochures, full of unsubstantiated claims, and a selection of similar print-ready ads.

By 1995, chiropractors had one thousand spinal decompression machines in their clinics. For more than a decade, just as Axiom had promised, health insurance providers and Medicare picked up the bill. But when the federal Agency for Healthcare Research and Quality reanalyzed the data that had elicited the FDA's original thumbs-up, officials learned that, out of seven clinical trials that were conducted, only one trial showed that patients who were treated on the machine showed an improvement in pain, leaving them better off than patients who did not undergo the treatment.

With that news, in 2007 the FDA rescinded its approval, and health care plans and Medicare stopped paying for the procedure. Still responsible for the cost of these machines, chiropractors made promises meant to attract patients who would pay out of pocket.

To this end, in a full-page ad in the *San Francisco Chronicle*, one chiropractor promised to conduct a "free 19-point 'squashed disk' [*sic*] qualifying assessment," which would evaluate whether a patient was "a candidate for this revolutionary new therapy." Some chiropractors substituted the CPT code for surgical disc decompression performed in the operating room for the one corresponding to mechanical disc decompression on the machine. They collected handsomely, in the process defrauding Medicare of millions of dollars. When Blue Cross and Blue Shield of Georgia caught on, the insurance provider went after the perpetrators, who wound up in prison, while insurers in other states also endeavored to collect.

Three years after the FDA reversed its decision on the spinal decompression unit, there was still one humming away in a chiropractic clinic near me. Hoping to sell me on the procedure, the chiropractor offered to let me observe a session. In a back room, HIPAA requirements notwithstanding, he presented me to a young woman, a sidelined ballerina, who was strapped into place on the table. Then he pushed the "on" button and left us alone. As her spine was alternately "distracted" and "relaxed," the patient explained that for a year and a half, she hadn't been able to rehearse or perform. Compared with her normal practice routine, the gentle exercises assigned in PT were a joke. After hearing from her father's friend, who'd had some success with his own spinal decompression treatment, she'd signed up, but today marked her nineteenth session, without noticeable improvement. "My dad loaned me the two thousand dollars to pay for this," she said. "And I have no idea of how I will pay him back." As the machine clicked off, the chiropractor returned. "Looks like you're cooked," he said. With a tear rolling down her cheek, she tried to smile.

NOT EVERY LOW-BACK-PAIN patient sees a chiropractor, but a prescription for physical therapy is practically a given. In 2004, Chris Livingston, a carpenter with a small construction business, stood up after a couple of hours of pounding nails into a subfloor and heard a loud pop. He was no stranger to back pain after a long workday, but this time, he couldn't straighten up. The searing leg pain came on a little later.

His buddy recommended his longtime chiropractor, who, for the next month, adjusted his spine twice weekly. Three weeks in, when he started to stumble over his own foot, his primary care doctor sent him to a physical therapy clinic, one that was conveniently in network with his health care plan. "I didn't have to pay much for it," Livingston said, "and that was important. I wouldn't have known how to tell good PT from bad PT. I was looking for convenience and price."

After the facility's head therapist did a quick evaluation, a young assistant took charge of his care. Her priority, it seemed to Livingston, was to avoid screwing up. "I'd say that I had pain and tingling down my leg," Livingston said, "and she'd tell me to stop for the day." After several weeks of no progress, the head PT told Livingston that he'd used up his sessions, and should see a spine surgeon.

He followed this advice. After a couple of unsuccessful lumbar discectomies, the surgeon sent him to a pain management doctor. Under the influence of strong opioids, he couldn't find the motivation to get back to work. "I let the business go, and the house, too," he said. "The pain was too great, and I couldn't handle it, and to be honest, the drugs made me not really care."

Unsurprisingly, Livingston didn't realize that in the presence of a herniated disc, chiropractic treatment is contraindicated. Nor was he aware that in the acute phase—within a couple of weeks after the injury—the McKenzie Method of Mechanical Diagnosis and Therapy (MDT), also known as the McKenzie Method, could have put him back on his feet.

The late Robin McKenzie, a Wellington, New Zealand, physiotherapist who died in 2013, loved to tell the story of how, quite by accident, he developed his technique. Because he was occupied with another patient at that moment, he sent his next appointment, a patient who suffered from a disc herniation—and associated back and leg pain—into a room, to wait. He told him to lie on his stomach on the examination table, in preparation for the standard ultrasound and heat therapy. But McKenzie did not know that his colleague, who used that room last, had left one end of the table elevated like the backrest of a chair, at nearly a ninety-degree angle.

Given the awkward configuration, the patient evidently did his best, configuring his spine in an awkward backbend. Upon entering the room, McKenzie was horrified—until, the patient explained that the pain had finally relented.

McKenzie realized that he had placed the patient's spine in "extension," thus eliminating the disc herniation's pressure on the spinal nerve root. But spinal extension, he would learn, did not always end acute pain. Depending on how the protruding disc made contact with the spinal nerve root, a forward bend that put the spine in "flexion" could be just the ticket. When treatment was appropriately delivered, recovery from an acute episode could take only a few days. (Note, yet again, that many people recover from an acute episode without any professional assistance.) Once a patient knew what worked, he could rescue himself if he was in a crisis.

Starting in the late 1950s, McKenzie taught this method to PTs who came from all over the world to study at his clinic in Wellington. Two decades later, he started the McKenzie Institute and spelled out his teaching methods, transforming an error made in a small clinic's treatment room into one of the few therapeutic approaches with well-quantified outcomes. There are thirty-six hundred MDT practitioners in the United States and seventy-two hundred worldwide, as far afield as Brazil and Saudi Arabia. Overall, the technique gets a very high approval rating.

That's an encouraging story, but a less auspicious one plays out at thousands of corporate physical therapy facilities, like the one Chris Livingston visited, which order the same "cookie-cutter" routine for most low-back-pain patients, ensuring that many won't get better. Patients who "fail physical therapy," especially several times in succession, often use that information as evidence that the obvious next step is surgery. "They don't recognize that cookie-cutter physical therapy is a pseudo-intervention," said John D. Childs, director of the physical therapy program at U.S. Army–Baylor University, "or that PT serves as a holding tank for patients who are not quite ready to get on the gravy train of scans and tests and injections and surgery and pain management."

To get on the right road, Childs explained, a patient with debilitating low back pain—whether it is persistent or episodic—needs a custom exercise-based rehabilitation program. The best way to find such treatment is to locate a doctorate-level PT (DPT) who is also an orthopedic clinical specialist (OCS). DPTs and OCSs spend three to four postgrad years in training, followed by an orthopedics-focused residency. They are rarely in network with health care plans, and they charge up to $125 a session. Sometimes, insurance providers pick up a fifth of the tab.

YOU MAY HAVE wondered why it's often necessary to get a physician's "prescription" for PT, when that's not required for chiropractic or for other interventions like therapeutic massage or biofeedback or exercise. The answer lies in the hierarchical relationship between physicians and PTs. The latter have traditionally served as support staff rather than independent operators. "At the end of the day, physician lobbying groups don't want PTs to gain direct access," said John Childs, the Baylor therapist. "If you talk to a physician over a few beers, he will tell you that if you go to an excellent PT to treat a musculoskeletal condition, you will not need drugs, or imaging. You will not need a surgeon." Therefore, remarked Childs, physicians have a vested interest in keeping patients under their own care.

That relationship is changing, slowly: As of this writing, eighteen states allow unlimited direct access to PTs; others will allow thirty days of treatment before requiring a physician's prescription; and seven states insist on a prescription before treatment begins. Insurance providers are even more restrictive, refusing to reimburse for any part of a PT session without a doctor's prescription, while Medicare limits treatment without a prescription to thirty days.

Unlike chiropractic, which has American roots and has barely made inroads into the rest of the world (the United Kingdom is an exception, with thirty-one hundred chiropractors), physical therapy is a Scandinavian and central European export, with the most important center at the Prague School of Rehabilitation and Manual Medicine, in the Czech Republic. Shortly after the start of World War I, the first U.S. school of physical therapy opened at Walter Reed Hospital, on the outskirts of Washington, D.C. Before she arrived in the capital, Mary McMillan had been director of orthopedic rehabilitation for

Great Britain's military. At Walter Reed, she trained women in ther-apeutic massage and then shipped them overseas to military hospi-tals, where they would serve as "reconstruction aides." When the war ended, McMillan started the American Women's Physical Therapeu-tic Association, training women as physical therapy technicians, to work with polio victims, always under the treating doctors' direction. The organization's name was changed to the American Physiother-apy Association in 1922, and men were admitted as well.

That stratified relationship remained unchallenged until the 1980s, when a new business model appeared. Large, multi-facility physical therapy practices that employed a fast food–style model with a healthy profit margin became the norm. They negotiated contracts with health care plans, relying on high volume and standardized pro-tocols. With the support of minimally compensated assistants and aides, a PT could see thirty-five patients in a day rather than the stan-dard nine.

Physical therapy aides, paid even less than assistants, provided what are called "shake and bake" treatments, which could be billed as "add-ons," thus boosting profit margins. These included ultrasound (deep heating, to make muscles more pliable), cold and hot packs, electrical muscle stimulation (high-pulsed galvanic current, to reduce muscle spasms and swelling), and low-level laser therapy. There was no scientific evidence for any of it, but patients liked it, and they kept coming back.

From a spine surgeon's perspective, however, the corporate PT model had a major shortcoming: If he sent a patient to a corporate PT facility, she might ask questions, learn of another spine surgeon, and take her business there. The Stark Law prevented surgeons from referring to external PT practices that they owned, but a loophole in the law did not stop them from staffing their own offices with phys-ical therapists, who were on their payrolls and thereby under their thumbs. That was problematic, noted John Childs. "When physicians hire physical therapists for their own practices," he said, "you can bet your bottom dollar that they will end up profiting from their own referrals. In general, the kind of PT who will work for a physician is not a high-end quality PT, and you tend to get suboptimal outcomes, where patients don't recover."

The American Physical Therapy Association's guidelines state that a PT protocol must incorporate an individualized exercise program. Still, most patients expect passive therapy, and they get it. As recently as 2013, in an episode of television's *The Dr. Oz Show* called "Cutting-Edge Solutions for Back Pain," the physical therapist who chatted with Dr. Oz described ultrasound, Tiger Balm patches, and a massage ball as the main treatment components, but she never mentioned exercise. "What was demonstrated," said John Childs, "showed the worst of what PT has to offer—the absolute worst. You have a patient lying there on a plinth, receiving ultrasound and other passive treatments which, when coupled together, encourage more passivity and result in a patient not participating in her own recovery. Based on the antiquated techniques that PT discussed, she could have been working in the 1970s. We have very good scientific data about the benefits of active care." This misinterpretation of standard practice outraged the APTA. Members sent a nasty letter to Oz, noting that he'd done his viewers a great disservice.

PHYSIATRIST HEIDI PRATHER, chief of the Physical Medicine and Rehabilitation Department at Washington University School of Medicine in St. Louis, blamed many of physical therapy's failures on the confusion of physicians, who, in their referrals, were supposed to specifically describe the nature, extent, and duration of the problem and how they wanted the PT to treat it. That was rare, because in medical school, physicians underwent just three or four hours of training in how to handle musculoskeletal disorders. Typically, said Prather, physicians just scrawl "diagnose and treat" on their prescription pads and leave it at that. They rarely follow up, said Prather.

The term for this nonchalant approach is "rocket launching," Prather said. "It's hoping the PT knows what he's doing, and sending the patient into space with no tether and no supervision." When she sends patients to PT, she observed, "I say, 'This is what I saw in my evaluation, and this is what I think should be done.' If there's something I missed, I expect the PT to tell me about it." The follow-up is just as important, notes Prather: "When the patient returns to see me, if what she's been doing with the therapist in terms of exercise has nothing to do with the prescription I wrote—if she's telling me she's mostly had hot packs and muscle stimulation, and she's seen five different people in that office, and no one has taken ownership of the case and developed a relationship with her—then she's out of there, and I won't send anyone else to that facility."

At Rush University Medical Center in Chicago, physiatrist Sheila A. Dugan also sets firm guidelines. It helps that she worked as a physical therapist before getting her medical degree. "If the therapist has ten people going at the same time, and she's walking from table to table, forget it," she said. "As a patient, you want to find a provider who will spend time with you. They are not a dime a dozen. They are not punching clocks or working for peanuts. If you can find someone who eats, drinks, and sleeps spine care, that's the person you want."

EVERYONE WHO GOES to PT is assigned home exercises, but very few people do them. For an exercise to work, you not only have to do it but must do it correctly. For the patient left to his own devices, that's unlikely. As the late Karel Lewit, who led the Prague School of Rehabilitation, was famous for saying: "The capacity of the patient to alter his prescribed exercise knows no bounds."

In January 2009, when I was about three months out of spine surgery (no, you did not miss that episode; we'll be getting to it soon), I went hunting for a talented independent PT with an orthopedic clinical specialty certification. Post-surgery, the pain in my leg was less clamorous, but my back felt weak and sore, and my neck ached badly. I worried that I'd exchanged one set of problems for another.

The colleague who referred me to Brian Beaudoin assured me that the $125 per session he charged was worth it. He used no modalities. He had no assistants. He'd tell me what he thought and, at no additional charge, he'd give me the skinny on what was right and wrong in the world of physical therapy.

At my first appointment, Beaudoin peered at me over half-height horn-rimmed glasses, his brow furrowed in concern. He asked me to tell him about any trauma I'd had, starting from birth. I enumerated the skiing, biking, and ice-skating dustups, as well as one spectacular tumble down the stairs, when my right foot lost track of what it was doing. But that paled in comparison with the horseback riding wrack-up I'd had at sixteen, when, moving at high speed, I flew from the saddle and landed squarely on my right hip. I was training horses that summer, and couldn't afford any time off, so I dragged my nonfunctional right leg around for a couple of weeks and never saw a doctor. Beaudoin winced when he heard that, as if it hurt him, too.

With my bio of trauma in hand, he checked my range of motion, posture, and muscle strength. He palpated every one of my joints. He asked me to walk back and forth, and stand on one bare foot, which I could not manage for more than a couple of seconds. I had poor balance, no control of my core, terrible posture, and bad proprioception, Beaudoin said. In short, I suffered from what was called "sensory-motor amnesia."

From an economic perspective, this news was distressing. For a full year in advance of my surgery—in the hope of avoiding it—I'd trained twice a week at the local gym, under the supervision of a certified personal trainer. We did standard stuff, making the rounds of the glossy machines that filled the gym floor. At session's end, I got my reward. As I lay on my back on a big therapy table set in the middle of the room, the personal trainer bent my right leg at the knee and pressed it toward my chin. For a few wonderful minutes, that stretch relieved the pain in my glutes and low back, and my leg felt better. When I told Brian Beaudoin about this maneuver, his face flushed in irritation. "Never let anyone do that to you again," he said. "She was stretching an already hot sciatic nerve, which only makes it worse."

Certified personal trainers, he explained, could get their "degrees" after a weekend online course. And recently, some had begun to abbreviate the CPT to "PT," in this case standing for "personal trainer."

This suggested expertise and education that they did not possess. "They tend to treat an out-of-shape middle-aged person such as yourself as if she is a fit twenty-five-year-old," Beaudoin said. "And they injure people all the time. I make a very good living taking care of the people they have hurt."

When I told him how much time I'd spent on the leg press machine, he said that unless the goal was to push something really heavy uphill with my feet, the isolation of any group of muscles meant nothing to my motor cortex. What I needed was functional training, to develop the skills I'd use daily. "We have six hundred muscles in our bodies, and when we pick up the laundry or empty the dishwasher, hundreds are engaged at once," Beaudoin explained. "You need functional training for the things you do all the time."

When he asked about other exercise, I said I took yoga classes. My spine was actually very flexible, so I excelled at spinal twists, especially when the teacher helped. Beaudoin looked disgusted. "You're not flexible. You're weak and hypermobile, which is a dangerous combination. Every time you put yourself in one of those twists, you're stretching out your ligaments further, imperiling your spine."

After flopping me this way and that on the treatment table for fifteen minutes, he offered his conclusions. My pelvis was rotated to the right; I had slight functional scoliosis; my facet joints were thick and bulky. "Your right hip is boggy and arthritic," he said. "Your scalene and levator scapulae are very tight on both sides, and you have a slight disc bulge at C7-T1—that's the big vertebrae at the base of your neck. Don't ever think about doing a yoga headstand."

None of this was good, Beaudoin said. But my real problem was self-inflicted when I agreed to have spine surgery. Blood vessels that deliver oxygen and nutrients to muscles and bone had been disrupted, as had the feathery multifidi muscles that extend in five separate segments along both sides of the spine from coccyx to atlas. When the multifidi work properly, they absorb the load and torque on connective tissues, thus reducing the strain on other soft tissues. The surgery had put an end to all that: My multifidi, he supposed, were moth-eaten, asymmetrical, atrophied, and infiltrated with fatty tissue.

"Patients almost always tell me that their surgeons never discussed what would be required for rehabilitation. They expect to get up and go the morning after the procedure, but even if they do everything right, it can take months to recover," and many patients never regained their previous level of function. "They do not realize that if they'd preserved the integrity of the spine and its musculature," he said, "and instead worked with a good PT and an exercise specialist, with actual training, they could have avoided a lot of pain and disappointment."

Such an exercise specialist would be essential to my recovery. On a scrap of paper, he scribbled Diana Williams's name and phone number. "She knows her stuff," he said, "and most important, she will know how not to hurt you. She and I are going to communicate. And believe me when I tell you that what she says will matter to me. If she says you are not trying, I won't be happy about treating you."

He led me to an exercise mat and showed me a squishy, red, grapefruit-sized plastic ball filled with liquid, a blue plastic disc about the size of a buffet plate, and a foam roller. These he referred to as "your new toys." When I lowered my weight onto the ball, the resulting pressure would drive blood and oxygen into starved muscle fibers. I'd use the blue disc, placed under my backside, to perform a "pelvic clock," an exercise in which I shifted my hips diagonally; first toward two o'clock, then toward seven o'clock, and so on. The foam roller would go just under my shoulder blades. From there, I could roll down to the bottom of my rib cage, but I should be sure not to roll onto the bones of my lumbar spine, which were delicate. I could also place the foam roller vertically, allowing the triangular bones of my shoulder girdle, which jutted out like bird wings, to drop into a better position. No distractions were allowed when I did the exercises; I was to pay careful attention to form. "You've got to get the motor cortex involved," Beaudoin said, adding that unless I recruited the precise muscle groups that needed strengthening, in exactly the way he described, I'd be wasting my time yet again.

"You are going to do these exercises three times a day. I will be able to tell if you don't do them," he said. The goal was to make me independent. In his eyes, a patient who was reliant on him, who showed up week after week, was not a success.

Before that week ended, I would have my first workout with Diana Williams. (A lot more about that later.) After six PT sessions, Beaudoin told me that I was doing well and that henceforth he would leave me in Williams's hands. I could come back anytime for a tune-up.

No longer in treatment, but very interested in his thoughts, I asked Beaudoin to breakfast. What had stopped him from following his colleagues into a corporate physical therapy model? "I made a decision, years ago, about what my time was worth and how I was going to spend it," Beaudoin told me as we made our way to a table in a local café.

At corporate PT facilities, Beaudoin said, the paradigm, "is 'treat 'em more but don't treat 'em well, and try to get as much money out of them as you can.'" "Shake and bake," where patients receive identical protocols, and "bells and blinkers," where they are hooked up to all kinds of machinery, meant that the PT did not actually have to spend his valuable time with the patient. "These facilities do whatever might scrape out a few more dollars from the insurance company," he said, "despite the fact that there is no evidence whatsoever that 'shake and bake' or 'bells and blinkers' works."

The good news was that "shake and bake" might be in its final days, Beaudoin said. In several states, new legislation makes it illegal for anyone other than the PT to assume primary responsibility for a clinic's patients. "The health insurance providers have just about figured out that electric stimulation therapy and ultrasound and heat and ice are a total waste of time and money," Beaudoin said. "They've also learned that if a patient seems to be stuck forever in boomerang PT, going back time after time with the same complaint, something is not working right."

There are always patients, Beaudoin said, who really don't want to recover. "They'll show up because the mobilization I do makes them feel temporarily better. But if the patient gets the idea that the therapist is the one who regulates his pain, that's a disservice. The worst thing you can do as a practitioner is to allow the patient to believe that a passive approach to recovery—something I do to you, or for you—is plausible, because it isn't. There is nothing I can do for people who are not willing to maintain their gains with regular, specific exercises meant to strengthen their particular weaknesses."

Beaudoin prepared to return to his office, where he had a patient scheduled in every clinical hour until dinnertime. But he had one thing to add: "After thirty years in practice, I have seen every type of orthopedic patient there is. The bottom line is that to be considered a candidate for elective spine surgery, you must have undergone and failed conservative care, of which PT is a major part. If everyone came through PT with flying colors, there would be a lot less work for spine surgeons. When a patient reports that he has failed PT—even though he only went twice before he quit—that patient is one step closer to getting on the surgery schedule."

3

Hazardous Images

WHY YOU DO NOT NEED—
OR WANT—TO HAVE AN MRI

*Who among us can look at an image of our own spine and not feel
disquiet as we come to realize how many discs have degenerated,
how many facet joints have spurs, how peculiar is the alignment.*
—Nortin Hadler, in *Stabbed in the Back*

I PAID A HANDSOME health insurance premium every month.
Surely that meant that I had the right to take my turn inside the
MRI scanner. I had no doubt that the imaging would reveal the source
of my pain and give a surgeon the information he needed to make it
go away. (I use the pronoun "he" here and elsewhere because out of
almost thirty thousand orthopedic surgeons in the U.S. fewer than
fourteen hundred of them are female, and only a handful of those are
spine surgeons.)

Hearing that I suffered from degenerative disc disease had been
unnerving, but when I saw the evidence—when the scan was slapped
up on a surgeon's light box—my heart sank. In black, white, and gray,
my spine appeared sunbaked and ancient, on the verge of returning,
as we all must, to dust.

By the time I left his office, that image—the dinged-up discs, the
proliferation of bone spurs—had been seared into my brain. Like so
many other patients, I thought that I finally knew what was wrong.
And no medical professional I would see over the next six months
would say anything that would change my mind.

I'd fallen into the same trap that had ensnared so many others. But it would be a long time before I understood that.

IN THE MID-1980S, Richard Deyo, the epidemiologist, was just starting to make a name for himself as an expert in public health. Magnetic resonance imaging was on the cusp of becoming widely available, and he was worried. Deyo thought that ordering X-rays for low back pain sent the wrong message, initiating a cascade of unnecessary, expensive, and detrimental interventions. Telling a patient he needed a scan, contended Deyo, was enough to convince him that he must suffer from a serious medical condition. Once he saw what was on that scan, he would become "overwhelmingly preoccupied" with his bulging discs and unable to accept the fact that what appeared on that scan was perfectly normal and existed in a large part of the population.

Although several studies in the medical community supported Rick Deyo's findings, his concerns were mostly ignored. Then, in 1990, in a study of sixty-seven patients who did not suffer from back pain, orthopedic surgeon and spine researcher Scott Boden showed that more than 90 percent had degenerated or bulging discs, while a third had herniated discs, and a fifth showed evidence of spinal stenosis. "A diagnosis that is based on magnetic resonance imaging, in the absence of objective clinical findings," Boden wrote, "may not be the cause of the patient's pain, and an attempt at operative correction could be the first step towards disaster." It was, he said, "the beginning of a dangerous thought process."

The party should have ended right there, but it did not. A 2009 study showed that nearly 30 percent of back pain patients underwent some form of imaging within four weeks of onset. Six years hence, Medicare and private health care plans would spend about $300 million annually on spinal imaging that rarely revealed useful answers.

UNTIL THE 1930S, unless you'd suffered a calamity or developed spinal tuberculosis, ordinary low back trouble was viewed as a normal artifact of aging or the expected consequence of hard manual labor. Often describing the complaint as "lumbago," physicians in the Victorian era sought to eliminate the "buildup of rheumatic phlegm" in the muscles. That perspective could be traced to the ancient Greeks, who held that "rheum," a watery discharge or evil humor, brought on by cold or damp, flowed from the brain to cause pain in the joints or other parts of the body. Sciatica, that searing leg pain, was believed to be the result of excessive or ill-considered sexual activity; in Shakespeare's plays, characters who suffer from it are also assumed to have syphilis.

The treatment for either lumbago or sciatica, beyond a large dose of laxatives, involved the application of turpentine directly to the skin or onto a plaster, to create skin lesions that would draw out the poison. The same inflammatory treatment is employed today, in the form of a sticky patch saturated with counterirritants, such as Salonpas, an inexpensive product available over the counter in most pharmacies.

The invention of the X-ray or "radiograph" in 1895 allowed physicians to detect structural abnormalities in the bones of the spine, but the state of the soft tissue, including the intervertebral discs, remained a mystery. Nor were physicians certain of the significance of what they saw in the imaging. "The confusion about lumbago is increasing," wrote one bewildered doctor of the period. "The single most striking chaos in the whole field of medicine is a disease that is the most common."

That confusion would prevail for decades. Spine surgery was anything but elective: The surgical notes from the late nineteenth and early twentieth centuries drip with blood and gore, and frequently end with the observation that the patient died on the gurney. Even when the Massachusetts General Hospital surgeons realized, after their initially mistaken ID, that the tissue of the intervertebral disc could be surgically excised, it was optimistic to hope for a normal life after the operation. Without the disc to anchor them, the vertebral bones slid back and forth over each other like bricks without mortar, leaving patients in excruciating pain and with profound neurological deficits, including paralysis.

In 1964, the Swedish orthopedic surgeon Alf Nachemson, on his way to becoming the most prominent spine researcher of the twentieth century, confirmed Mixter and Barr's earlier assertion that the damaged intervertebral disc caused lumbar back pain. There was no turning back. Forty-two years later, when spine surgery was minting money for doctors, hospitals, workers' compensation insurers, and device manufacturers, the much-revered surgeon publicly recanted. "Our knowledge of back pain causation remains poor," Nachemson told a group of orthopedists. "We still do not have diagnostic techniques that can link the structural abnormalities to symptoms with any accuracy."

Just as Rick Deyo had forecast, MRI scans became the go-to diagnostic tool for back pain. Unlike CT (computerized tomography) scans and X-rays, MRI scans carried no radiation burden; a physician could order them as often as he liked, without risking patients' safety. Very quickly, physicians forgot that MRI was not a stand-alone diagnostic tool but instead, was properly used to supplement objective clinical findings. Doctors, especially primary care physicians, began to regard hands-on examinations, which required both time and skill, as barely relevant since the right notes on a radiologist's report satisfied health insurance providers' and Medicare's requirements for reimbursement for further interventions.

The financial implications were considerable. It cost about a million dollars to buy an MRI unit (and many facilities leased them), but once in place, that machine was a cash cow. Scan ten patients a day, and you could bring in more than half a million dollars a year in income. The temptation was great: Primary care practitioners and spine surgeons set up radiology clinics, to which they referred legions of their own back pain patients.

"You'd get a fast-talking salesman in your office, telling you why you ought to have your own MRI machine," said Brian Nelson, who began his career as an orthopedic surgeon but later built a therapeutic program based on exercise at Physicians Neck and Back Center in Minneapolis. "He'd tell you, 'Here's what the lease payments will be, but you'll do a lot of scans, and it will be so much more convenient for your patients.'"

BY 1994, WHEN the *New England Journal of Medicine* published the results of an imaging study performed at a California hospital, there was no doubt that the excessive use of MRI in the early stages of back pain was a mistake. It was clear, just as it had been from Scott Boden's study, that such spinal abnormalities as bulging, herniated, and degenerated discs were commonplace in asymptomatic individuals— people who did not suffer from low back pain. Rick Deyo supplied an astringent commentary in the *NEJM*: "I hope this study is very influential," he wrote. "Many doctors routinely use MRIs to diagnose back pain. Misuse of this imaging method is a bigger problem than physicians and patients realize. The opportunity to be misled is substantial."

When the Agency for Health Care Policy and Research, a branch of the United States Public Health Service, asked Deyo and colleagues to establish treatment guidelines for acute low back pain—that is, lumbar back pain of recent onset—they concluded that doctors and other health care providers should refrain from using imaging tests like X-rays, CT scans, and magnetic resonance imaging in the early stages of a back pain episode. The orthopedic spine surgery community responded furiously, setting up letter-writing committees and insisting that Congress do something. It worked: AHCPR's budget vanished, the spine care panel was disbanded, and its well-considered guidelines, which, had they been followed, would have saved billions of dollars in the United States, wound up in the dustbin.

In the meantime, between 2000 and 2005, the number of MRI machines in hospitals and private radiology centers more than tripled. By 2012, the United States had nearly four times more scanners per capita than were operating in Canada. As the number of machines grew, so did the slots in the schedule that needed to be filled in order to make them profitable. The number of MRI facilities grew so rapidly, according to Maggie Mahar, the author of *Money-Driven Medicine*, that one Toledo, Ohio, surgeon said that he expected the cars rolling down the main boulevard to swerve toward the many "magnets" (doctor jargon for an MRI machine) that were inside the medical buildings lining one side of the street.

In the first month that new machines were in place, observed a paper published in the journal *Health Affairs*, orthopedists ordered 38 percent more scans, and they maintained that increase for as long as they kept the machines.

Thousands of new diagnostic radiologists were required to read all those scans. Many were employed by spine surgeons, which meant that they could be relied on to find something both nasty and operable to put in the report. One former radiologist told me that the spine surgeons who employed him for years at their imaging facility expected him to find an operable skeletal abnormality on every scan. If he didn't include an indication for surgery in his notes, his boss revised the report.

TELLING A PERSON that there is an anomaly in his spinal column can cause panic. But, saying there is nothing to worry about also affects behavior. In an experiment, neuroradiologist Jeffrey G. Jarvik included a message in a third of the spine radiology reports issuing from his department at the University of Washington. At the bottom of each of those reports, patients found this statement: "The following findings are so common in people without low back pain that while we report their presence, they must be interpreted with caution, and in the context of the clinical situation."

"We were surprised at the magnitude of the effect," Jarvik observed. Results showed that patients whose imaging reports contained his message were less likely to undergo other medical evaluations, or to have repeated imaging, or to get prescriptions for narcotics at follow-up visits, or even to schedule such follow-up visits. Once they understood that their discomfort did not reflect dangerous pathology, they felt secure enough to pursue exercise and other rehabilitative strategies. Doctors at the University of Washington's medical facility were in favor of including the message, said Jarvik, because it meant that they could spend less time explaining things to their patients. But despite its simplicity and low cost, Jarvik's approach, which was bad for business, failed to catch on.

Finally, in a policy statement issued in 2011, the American College of Physicians announced that routine spinal imaging should be eliminated from modern back pain treatment. The identification of asymptomatic spinal abnormalities, the statement said, led to an expensive onslaught of unnecessary referrals, diagnostic interventions, nonsurgical treatments, interventional pain management procedures, and surgery.

That recommendation to eliminate imaging is not what appears in most current guidelines, which generally ask physicians to wait at least six to eight weeks into a back pain episode before ordering advanced imaging. Even in the presence of sciatica, which occurs when disc material impinges on a tender spinal nerve root, sending lightning bolts of pain down the leg to the foot, imaging is of questionable benefit because it often leads to unwarranted surgery. Although disc surgery often speeds recovery from sciatica in the very short term, there are risks (later, we'll examine what happened to Golden State Warriors head coach Steve Kerr) and, to avoid a recurrence, there is a need for lengthy post-op rehab. Randomized controlled trials show that, in the treatment of sciatica, long-term outcomes of surgical and nonsurgical care are similar.

Some would suggest that the problem doesn't start with the scanner; instead, it begins when a patient first sets foot in his primary care physician's office. In *Annals of Internal Medicine*, physician Roger Chou, one of the most respected thinkers in the field, who practices at the Oregon Health and Science University, suggested that people suffering an acute bout of low back pain avoid the doctor's office entirely for two to three weeks, unless: the pain runs down the leg below the knee; the leg, foot, groin, or rectal area feels numb; there is fever, nausea, vomiting, stomachache, weakness, or sweating; bowel or bladder control is lost; the pain was caused by an injury; or it is impossible to move around.

Based on the presence of such symptoms, early imaging may be required. Numbness in the groin or rectal area, coupled with incontinence, may signify cauda equina syndrome, which calls for immediate imaging, and usually a trip to the OR. "Progressive neurologic deficit," diagnosed over a period of days after a specialist's evaluation that produces specific findings of "dropped foot" (one that does not properly flex toward the shin) and diminished reflexes, also demands an MRI. Fever or vomiting in conjunction with severe low back pain may require imaging to rule out a spinal infection. After an accident, imaging may be used to detect the presence of a vertebral fracture. And because the spine is the most common site of secondary cancer in the human skeleton, cancer patients or those in remission who develop back pain are routinely sent to the scanner.

The same year that the American College of Physicians came out against imaging, Francisco Kovacs, a Spanish orthopedic surgeon and researcher and opponent of overuse of imaging and other interventions, obtained MRIs from fifty-three back pain patients and asked five senior radiologists to interpret them. A few weeks later, when Kovacs returned the scans, with different patient ID labels attached, to the same experienced radiologists, the images had not changed, but the radiologists' interpretations had. In the subsequent review, spinal abnormalities identified in the first round were found to have vanished or to have mysteriously moved to different locations.

The bad news kept coming: Anywhere that people fancy high technology—South Korea is a good example—MRI units were humming and spine surgery was booming. In 2014 at the Mayo Clinic, researchers found, yet again, that disc degeneration was normal at all ages; it was present in more than a third of asymptomatic twenty-year-old subjects, and in 96 percent of eighty-year-olds. "Black" discs, often employed as one of the indications for a diagnosis of degenerative disc disease, were found in more than half of these normal subjects over forty—and in nearly 90 percent of those over sixty. Those bone spurs I'd picked out on my scan were common in pain-free subjects as well. Mayo Clinic scientists concluded that such changes were not "part of a pathologic process requiring intervention."

Although only 40 percent of family practice and 13 percent of internal medicine physicians report ordering routine diagnostic imaging for acute low back pain, common sense suggests that the actual numbers are much higher. The most recent data available, published in *JAMA Internal Medicine* in 2013, assessed how often advanced imaging was ordered in nearly twenty-five thousand physician visits. The proportion of patients who left their doctors' appointments with orders for MRIs increased from 7.2 percent in 1999 to 11.3 percent in 2010. As a result of this increase in imaging, the percentage of patients who were directed to spine specialists for interventional procedures and surgery more than doubled, rising from 6.9 percent to 14 percent in the same period. In 2015, orders were still creeping upward. A significant number of practitioners acknowledged that they ordered all those scans defensively, in an effort to avoid malpractice liability.

Orthopedist John Bruno Jr. explained that primary care practitioners and spine surgeons often give their rapt attention to "incidentalomas" on MRI reports but manage to overlook the presence of other serious disorders that may be causing back pain. (Bruno, who practices in Alexandria, Virginia, stopped doing spine surgery ten years ago, in favor of running a rehabilitation-based practice.)

"There's not enough diagnostic talent afoot," he says. "Spine surgeons are myopic. The back pain that they so readily attribute to a herniated disc could in fact stem from an aortic aneurysm, or kidney stones, or endometriosis, or pancreatitis, or gallbladder disease, or ovarian cysts, or a dozen other diseases. Serious pathologies go unrecognized, even when there are objective clinical findings, or they show up clearly on the scan."

Anti-MRI sentiment is growing, albeit slowly: When the National Physicians Alliance published its top five list of unnecessary procedures in 2011, ordering spinal imaging within the first six weeks of a back pain episode made the top slot.

More than a quarter century has passed since Richard Deyo first tried to put a stop to unnecessary imaging. For him, the recent resolutions are bittersweet—a matter of too little, too late. It's impossible to know how many people have been fast-tracked straight from MRI into procedures that have hurt more than they have helped. When he and I talked, he acknowledged that, yes, he'd seen the future, but sadly, he hadn't been able to stop it from arriving.

4

Needle Jockeys

HOW EPIDURAL STEROID INJECTIONS
CAN GO WRONG

N EAR MY OFFICE, there's a breakfast-and-lunch joint where strangers sit down at shared tables. When Joseph, an attorney in his early seventies, heard that I was writing a book about the back pain industry, he started asking questions.

That afternoon, he was scheduled to have the first of three epidural spinal injections, meant to relieve the symptoms of spinal stenosis, a condition in which the spinal canal narrows to the point where it squeezes the nerves. The weakness and cramping in his legs were so bad that he couldn't walk a long city block without stopping to recover.

The injections were his best hope, he said, making it even harder for me to break the news. A few months earlier, in a 2015 review of the medical literature, the Agency for Healthcare Research and Quality had found no evidence that epidural steroid injections were effective in treating symptoms of spinal stenosis or typical low back pain. Even in the presence of a recent disc herniation and ensuing sciatica, the benefits of injections were small and not sustained over time. That news followed on the heels of an FDA statement warning that injection of the active medication in these shots, glucocorticoids—a class of corticosteroids—into the epidural space of the spine could result in rare but serious neurological problems, including loss of vision, stroke, paralysis, and death. Based on those and other findings, the *Journal of the American Medical Association* (*JAMA*) advised physicians to refrain from recommending injection therapy to patients with any kind of chronic back pain.

That news did not go over well with the doctors known as "interventional pain physicians," who make a living performing such procedures. In the United States, more than ten million epidural steroid injections are delivered each year, a number that makes them the bread and butter of interventional pain management practices.

I was not surprised that my lunch partner didn't have the facts. Primary care physicians who ordered the shots were rarely informed about the lack of evidence and the risks of treatment. Even young, healthy people, explained anesthesiologist James Rathmell, the chair of the Department of Anesthesiology, Perioperative and Pain Medicine at Boston's Brigham and Women's Hospital, could go in with manageable low-back-pain symptoms and come out with catastrophic neurological injuries. "The bottom line," said Rathmell, "is that if you come into my clinic with chronic axial back pain, you're not going to get epidural steroid injections—because they don't work.

"People should get the best evidence-based treatment they can," he added. "As a rule of thumb, if you pay practitioners to do stuff, they will do more stuff. Frankly, what's happened in interventional pain management is just a microcosm of what's happened in all of medicine."

AS I EXPLAINED these things to Joseph, he paled. Why would his doctor advise him to undergo a worthless and risky procedure?

Three decades ago, anesthesiologists had no trouble getting jobs in hospital ORs. On a busy morning, they could run five cases at once, and get paid for them all, while depending on registered nurses to keep an eye on individual patients. Starting in the early 1990s, cost-conscious health management organizations (HMOs) realized that the nurses could manage without supervision, and they stopped paying fees to doctors who at best were marginally present. Many anesthesiologists found themselves underemployed. They knew little about treating musculoskeletal disorders or how to address the feelings of depression, anger, and isolation that often afflict back pain patients, but when they retooled, they set up pain management practices.

Torpedoed into entrepreneurship, the most successful interventional pain physicians offered an ever-expanding menu of injections, including facet and sacroiliac joint blocks, selective nerve blocks, discography, needle electromyography, radiofrequency and thermal facet ablations, botulinum toxin, and trigger point injections. They implanted intrathecal drug delivery pumps and spinal cord stimulators, and cemented together vertebral compression fractures. They used medical lasers to heat, shave, and slice soft tissue. By the turn of the new millennium, interventional pain management, which a decade before had barely existed, had become one of the most profitable aspects of spine care.

THERE ARE INDEED people who undergo one perfectly targeted epidural steroid injection and hit the golf course the next morning, completely cured. In the more typical scenario, however, the first injection—if in fact it provides any relief at all—is only briefly effective. Then the numbing medicine and the anti-inflammatory effect of the glucocorticoid wear off, and the pain returns.

Generally, the shots are ordered in a series of three, although no expert I asked could say why, and the American Society of Anesthesiologists' guidelines do not advise the administration of a specific number. "You always do three, even if the first two do no good at all," wisecracked neurosurgeon Charles Burton, who publicly questioned the safety and effectiveness of the procedure, long before *JAMA* and the FDA got on board. Some doctors construed the "rule of three" to mean that, in a single visit, they could give three shots at each affected vertebral level, thereby exposing a patient to a colossal dose of glucocorticoid. In fact, when Colorado researchers mined an insurance company's database, they found that one doctor had billed a single patient for fifty-one such injections in one year. The same database showed that a New Jersey patient had received thirteen shots in a five-month period and had subsequently developed kidney failure.

The FDA had been issuing cautionary statements about epidural steroid injections since 1981. But in 2014, the agency took a further step, compelling pharmaceutical manufacturers that produced the injectable glucocorticoids to clearly state the risks on every vial's label, advising that "serious neurologic events, some resulting in death, have been reported with epidural injection" and that the "safety and effectiveness of epidural administration of corticosteroids have not been established." The FDA stopped short of requiring manufacturers to notify physicians or their purchasing departments that things had changed, and most did not notice. One pain physician, Cleveland Clinic's Richard Rosenquist, told *Bloomberg* reporter David Armstrong that because he'd used such drugs for his entire career, unless he was alerted to do so, he was "unlikely to go back and spend time reading the package insert."

The implications were significant: Properly "consented," a patient who was about to receive an epidural steroid injection would hear about specific risks, including damage to the dura mater (the sturdy sleeve surrounding the spinal cord), nerve root injury, elevated cholesterol levels, vertebral fractures, the death of muscle and bone tissue, staph infection, epidural abscess, immune system deficits, stroke, and death. But in reality, if this information was conveyed at all, it was in boilerplate format, which the patient signed after only a cursory glance.

There are two dominant techniques for administering epidural steroid injections. In the first, known as "interlaminar," the needle is directed into the epidural space, around the spinal nerves. In the second approach, referred to as "transforaminal," the needle is inserted at an angle, which places it closer to the targeted nerve but also in the vicinity of vessels and arteries. Incorrectly placed, the needle can sever an artery or deliver medication into the blood vessels, clogging them and preventing adequate blood flow to the brain. The result, in either case, may be stroke or paralysis.

Whether the approach is transforaminal or interlaminar, research shows that a quarter of epidural steroid injections miss their targets. In "blind" injections, performed without fluoroscopic guidance, the needle is incorrectly placed in up to half of epidural steroid procedures.

In roughly 6 percent of epidural steroid injections (a number that sounds small but is not, because thousands of injections are delivered every day), the needle nicks the dura mater, the sturdy sleeve surrounding the spinal cord, allowing cerebrospinal fluid to leak out. Typically, this is not terribly serious. It results in a severe headache, which goes away after the patient lies flat for a couple of days. Sometimes, another procedure, known as a "blood patch," is used to stop the leak of cerebrospinal fluid.

But when the needle actually punctures the dura mater, it's a different story. Then the payload of glucocorticoid and anesthetic may be delivered into a region of fragile nerve tissue called the subarachnoid space. From there, the cerebrospinal fluid, bearing its toxic load, circulates to the brain, where the cortisone solution efficiently strips the insulating (and essential) myelin layer off neurons. One result is "adhesive arachnoiditis," a condition so grossly debilitating that neurologist Dewey Nelson described it as akin to "having a blowtorch up your rectum. It binds the nerves, like gunky cooked spaghetti, and the result is unrelenting pain that may last for a lifetime."

IN 2009 THE FDA required the companies that manufactured the drugs used in epidural steroid injections to collect and report on associated adverse events. Aggregating this information can be onerous. It would also open the door to lawsuits. In response, large pharmaceutical companies slashed their output or stopped production. Seeing a chance to profit, smaller companies jumped in—and increased long-standing wholesale prices by almost 40 percent.

Faced with a sudden shortage of cheap glucocorticoid solution, purchasing departments in interventional pain clinics, hospitals, and ambulatory surgery centers found alternatives. "Sterile bulk compounders" were overseen by state pharmacy boards. They were not regulated by the FDA, nor were they required to report adverse events or open their records to federal inspectors. They existed in the shadows.

In Framingham, Massachusetts, New England Compounding Center (NECC) offered quantities of methylprednisolone acetate, a generic glucocorticoid solution, at an excellent price. "From the practitioners' point of view, and perhaps naively, doctors and hospitals thought what they were selling was equal to what was coming from the pharmaceutical industry," observed James Rathmell, the Brigham and Women's Hospital pain physician. "There was nothing to tell us it was riskier, or that maybe we should have been more suspect of what their standards were."

Between May and September 2012, when the FDA finally closed it down, NECC shipped nearly eighteen thousand vials of methylprednisolone acetate to hospitals and pain clinics in twenty-three states. NECC was required by law to attach a patient's name to the label of each vial of methylprednisolone before it left its facility. Since the drug was sold in bulk, and no such names existed, NECC's purchase orders included made-up prescriptions for Big Baby Jesus, Donald Trump, Calvin Klein, Jimmy Carter, David Letterman, Robert Redford, and Chris Rock.

A few weeks later, when health officials discovered that these and other vials were contaminated with a deadly fungal mold identified as *Exserohilum rostratum*, pain clinics could not identify which patients had received the tainted medication. By spring of 2013, 751 patients in twenty states had fallen ill with fungal meningitis, and sixty-four people had died. A wave of fungal infections in back pain patients who had received injections spread rapidly across the country, hitting hardest in Tennessee, Virginia, and Michigan. When the Centers for Disease Control and Prevention (CDC) published a list of clinics and hospitals that used NECC as a vendor, patients and their families searched it anxiously, hoping the name of the facility they'd visited would not be on the list.

As news of the crisis spread, a colleague e-mailed me. After her adult daughter's lumbar fusion surgery failed to relieve her pain, she elected to have a series of three epidural steroid injections. The third syringe, it seemed, had come from the tainted batch. My friend was watching her only child anxiously, but it was hard to separate symptoms of impending mortal illness from those of the flu, which was also going around. Patients who developed symptoms were immediately put on intensive antifungal drug therapy, but there were serious side effects, including kidney damage.

Doctors continued to diagnose cases of fungal meningitis for months after the recall. The CDC expected the toll of death and illness to trickle to a halt, but instead, throughout the spring and well into the summer of 2013, patients continued to develop epidural abscesses, inflamed intervertebral discs, bone infections, and the early stages of adhesive arachnoiditis.

Public health experts questioned why it was that some patients suffered catastrophic neurological trauma and death, while others never developed symptoms. The initial hypothesis—that those who fell sick had a weak immune system, or were elderly and infirm—was wrong. Many otherwise healthy, younger people were among the victims, while older people did not necessarily get sick. Experts suspected that physician accuracy, rather than patient age, was the issue. When spinal injections pierced the dura, they flooded the subarachnoid space with tainted glucocorticoid solution, which entered the cerebrospinal fluid and went straight to the brain. The prevalence of illness in Tennessee, Virginia, and Michigan suggested that some pain interventionists in those states pierced the dura more often than they hit their mark.

Within weeks of NECC's closure in September, there were hundreds of lawsuits. Personal injury attorneys pursued several other businesses held under the same ownership. In December 2012, NECC filed for bankruptcy. Although the presiding judge in the case told NECC's executives and owners not to even think about moving their money, the company's majority shareholders transferred $33.3 million in eighteen separate transactions, according to a government indictment.

The wheels of justice turned slowly over the next two years. Then, in a series of predawn raids, law enforcement arrested and charged fourteen of NECC's executives and staffers, including the co-owner and head pharmacist, Barry Cadden; and the corner-cutting supervisory pharmacist, Glenn Chin. Both were charged with twenty-five acts of second-degree murder, in seven states. In court, in response to every question, Cadden invoked the Fifth Amendment. Other NECC employees were charged with mail fraud, racketeering, conspiracy, and contempt. After being delayed several times, Cadden and Chin's jury trial was scheduled for January 2017.

In the wake of the fungal meningitis crisis, I spoke with back pain patients who had decided to cancel their epidural steroid injections, at least until their absolute safety could be ensured. They knew nothing of the FDA's long-standing concerns. So, just as soon as people stopped dying, interventional pain management doctors were back at work, delivering injections in spite of negligible benefits and considerable risks.

IN THE SPRING of 2015, by the time I sat down to have breakfast with Joseph, the attorney who was slated to have an epidural injection that afternoon, the public's memory of the meningitis scourge had faded. Once again, with their physicians' encouragement, people submitted to the procedure.

I was grabbing a snack in a tiny café when a fit-looking middle-aged woman in a wheelchair rolled by, steered by her husband. Once I was settled on the only available stool, the three of us started to chat. She was in real estate, or at least she had been, she said. I told her that I was an investigative reporter in the midst of writing a book about the back pain industry. "This," she said, pointing to the wheelchair, "is the result of an epidural steroid injection gone wrong."

Then they described a nightmare.

Years earlier, Carol* (hereafter * will indicate pseudonyms), as we'll call her, had an epidural steroid injection that helped a lot; it got her through an acute episode of sciatica. For a long time, she was fine. To stay in shape, she did Pilates and also walked—some days, for five

miles. The previous autumn, when the pain returned, she got a referral to a top spine surgeon at a major academic medical center.

The surgeon identified some instability in her spine and recommended lumbar fusion, advising her to have the operation while she
was still young enough to have a good prognosis for recovery. Carol
said she'd prefer to have another injection. Christmas was coming
and, with it, a visit from the couple's young grandchildren. "My motivation," she said, "was to feel a little better over the holidays. I saw
it as something like getting a shot of Botox." A few days later, an
interventional pain management doctor at the same medical center
examined her and asked her to return for the injection in the afternoon.

"As soon as he gave me the shot," Carol said, "I knew something
had happened. Out loud, I said, 'Oh, no, this is not good.' I've had
babies. I'm not a weenie. When that needle went in, I had sharp, deep
pain—terrible pain, a pain I'd never felt before. It went all the way
down my legs. It was in my buttocks." Within seconds, Carol realized
that she had no feeling from the waist down. "I couldn't control any
muscles or feel the floor," she said. "And I was incontinent, immediately."

She remembers being transferred to an ambulance and admitted
through the emergency department. Fluid was accumulating in her
brain; in days, her spinal canal grew sludgy with the sticky scar tissue that is the hallmark of adhesive arachnoiditis. The spine surgeon
whose offer of spinal fusion she'd already turned down performed
exactly that procedure, not only in her lumbar spine but also in the
region between her shoulder blades. Later, said Carol, he claimed that
he'd "saved the day," though it wasn't clear to her why he felt such a
surgery was needed or how it was expected to resolve her weakness
and absence of sensation.

After three weeks in the hospital, Carol was still wheelchair bound
and incontinent. She and her husband had retained a personal injury
attorney and gathered her medical records. To their surprise, there
was nothing on the physician's note about the trauma or her trip in
the ambulance. It was as if it had never happened.

They wanted me to use their story as a way of warning others, Carol and her husband said. As we sat together in their living room, where I'd been invited to join them after our initial meeting in the café, I asked if I might check in with their attorney, just to confirm some details. They gave me his mobile number. For a month, I called it repeatedly, leaving many messages.

When the personal injury lawyer finally called back, it was only to say that he would not speak to me. And because talking to me might damage their chances of getting a good settlement, he'd ordered Carol and her husband to stay clear of all reporters. He did not want his client's name made public, nor did he want the pain management doctor's name revealed. When I asked why, he explained that this was part and parcel of how he did business: He kept everything nice and quiet for the doctor and the hospital. In return, as long as they played the game right and signed a nondisclosure agreement, he'd get his clients what they deserved. (He didn't mention it, but he'd also get his contingency fee, about a third of the total.) The next time a personal injury case arose, the hospital would "work with him." For a man who had, at the outset of the call, said he would not talk to me, this personal injury attorney had said a lot. When we hung up, I reported the details of this conversation to Carol. She didn't want to talk further. No one was to know the specifics of what had happened to her, or where. What other choice did she have?

This irked me, of course. This doctor, who happened to be a media darling, was going to walk away with his reputation unscathed. He was not required by law to report the event to the FDA. Several months later, I checked in, just to see how things were going. The day Carol was due to give her deposition, she could not. She was in the hospital, after suffering a spinal cord infarction—essentially, a stroke within the spinal cord or the arteries that supply it—that left her legs, which since the injection had been very weak, now entirely paralyzed. She was seeking new legal counsel and had new doctors, affiliated with a different hospital. She'd undergone dozens of tests and scans. Everything took a lot of time; she was no closer to a resolution than she'd been when we met. And she wanted to be sure that I would tell her story, as long as she retained her anonymity.

I promised that I would. Meanwhile, interventional pain management doctors were fighting the FDA's recently imposed labeling requirement, insisting that such neurological events were so rare as not to require any special advisory.

EARLY IN MY research, a slightly older friend called to tell me that she'd "broken her spine" while slamming the hatch on her SUV. In fact, she'd suffered a couple of vertebral compression fractures, crushing the tiny bones at two levels. Four times a year, for the past decade, her interventional pain physician had administered lumbar epidural steroid injections. But he'd never explained that glucocorticoids could make her bones fragile. There was an easy fix, he'd told her: He could repair the damage with a procedure called "kyphoplasty."

Systemic glucocorticoid treatment in tablet form has long been recognized as a factor in bone mass loss, as well as a harbinger of increased risk of bone fracture. Although the FDA does not recommend oral steroids (methyl prednisolone, prednisolone, and prednisone) for the treatment of any type of low back pain or sciatica, epidural steroid injections, which involve the same class of medication, have conventionally escaped scrutiny.

At least that was true until 2012, when scientists at Michigan's Henry Ford Health System, led by internal medicine specialist Shlomo Mandel, investigated the implications for bone health among women over the age of sixty-five who underwent epidural steroid injections. For *each* epidural steroid injection administered, the study found, the risk of suffering a vertebral compression fracture increased by 21 percent. Injected glucocorticoids adversely affected bone strength by diminishing new bone formation and increasing bone breakdown, in much the same way that the tablets did. In both cases, the end result was bone destruction.

Nor was the spine the only part of the anatomy in jeopardy. After a single epidural injection, bone density loss in the hip was six times more profound than it was in women who did not have these shots. And the more shots a patient received, the more likely she was to have a painful vertebral compression fracture.

As painful as her back felt, my friend wasn't too worried. "They're going to put a balloon in my spine and fill it with cement," she reported, "and I'll be as good as new." Her doctor had not told her that when researchers studied the procedure he recommended, they'd found it to be, at best, of only marginal benefit.

THE HISTORY OF vertebroplasty, and its close relative, kyphoplasty, was long and checkered. In 1993, two radiologists at the University of Virginia Health System, Mary E. Jensen and Jacques E. Dion, first injected polymethylmethacrylate—a bone cement that is chemically identical to the adhesive that bonds the glass in an aquarium—into the crumbling spine of a woman whose breast cancer had spread to her vertebrae. The patient's pain abated, and this encouraged Jensen and Dion to perform the same procedure on patients with osteoporotic fractures. For four years, they worked with a biomedical engineer to produce the ideal cement mixture. When Medicare agreed to pay for the vertebroplasty procedure, Jensen and Dion started to train other physicians in the technique.

Although no one ran a randomized controlled trial of vertebroplasty to identify how well it worked, by 2001 surgeons and interventional pain physicians were doing fourteen thousand such procedures each year. There were problems: When the bone cement filled the vertebral cavity, it altered the spine's biomechanics in such a way that adjacent vertebrae could also fracture. Sometimes the cement squeezed through the cracks between the bones, inflaming soft tissue, or the cement was accidentally injected into the disc or a vein, with grave consequences.

To eliminate these shortcomings, researchers hunted for a better cement formula. Norian, a Cupertino, California, biotech company, had a product that not only filled cracks but, once in place, acted like living, growing bone tissue. In 1999, six years after Jensen and Dion did their initial vertebroplasty procedure, Synthes, a Swiss medical device company, bought Norian. Shortly thereafter, the FDA approved the product for use in bones in the arm and the skull, but not for use in the spine.

Synthes wanted that labeling expanded to include treatment of vertebral fractures. But when the company's researchers injected the novel cement into pigs' spines, the bone cement caused blood clots to form in the pigs' lungs. In alarm, the FDA reinforced its earlier stance, adding a warning to Norian's label that said it was never to be used to treat vertebral fractures in humans.

In an ill-advised move, Synthes attempted an end run around the FDA, observed *Fortune* and CNN reporter Mina Kimes. In conjunction with his management team, Synthes's chief executive officer, Hansjörg Wyss, a Swiss billionaire, put Norian in fifty physicians' hands. They'd use the product in their vertebroplasty procedures, report their findings in peer-reviewed medical journals, and thereby convince physicians to give it a try.

Because it involved unsanctioned human experimentation, this plan was as unethical as it was illegal. At least one of Synthes's regulatory staffers voiced his objections, sending cautionary e-mails to the company's top executives. In February 2001, the first of Synthes's physician-consultants to inject the cement reported that two patients suffered associated rapid declines in blood pressure. Ultimately, four frail and elderly patients would die on the table.

That should have shut the project down. But instead, in the spring of 2003, Synthes issued a sales plan for Norian, predicting revenue of at least $20 million by 2005, with after-tax profit margins of 50 percent. At hosted physicians' dinner meetings and golf outings, the Norian sales team described how to use Norian in vertebroplasty. After one doctor injected the cement into the spine of an eighty-three-year-old Northern California physicist, whose heart stopped in the OR, the company sent letters to its physician-consultants observing that "deaths have been reported."

To clarify the procedure, Synthes published a technique guide, which included an image of the spine of a woman who had died during an operation performed in Texas. Belatedly, the FDA caught on and sent an investigator who interviewed executives at Synthes's headquarters and issued a condemnatory 114-page report.

Still, it would take five years before Pennsylvania's assistant U.S. attorney brought allegations of off-label marketing and illegal human experimentation, as well as false and materially misleading statements made to FDA investigators. The government prosecutors employed the "responsible corporate officer doctrine," a statute that permits the government to levy criminal charges against highly placed executives if they fail to prevent or to immediately correct corporate violations in regard to food and drug laws. That statute had never before been used to prosecute a health care industry executive. Significantly, it meant that even without adequate proof that the officer in question had direct knowledge of corporate malfeasance, he or she could still be prosecuted.

In November 2011 in a federal courthouse in Philadelphia, after two years of heated argument, four of Synthes's top executives were sentenced to prison terms ranging from five to nine months. The news shook corporate officers throughout the back pain industry, some of whom—as we will see—were culpable of similar or worse offenses. They'd understood that their companies might pay fines, but they had never dreamed that they would end up behind bars.

In a bit of courtroom drama, according to *Fortune*, one defense attorney refused to let his client, a Synthes executive, take the bullet for CEO Hansjörg Wyss, who was not indicted, but had already collected about $10 billion when he sold Synthes to Johnson & Johnson for $23 billion.

After suggesting, before the judge, that Wyss, rather than his client, might be culpable, the defense attorney suffered a dizzy spell, whacked his head on the side of a courtroom table, and lay bleeding and unconscious on the floor. The bailiff led the chief operating officer away in handcuffs, but two other executives were permitted to attend to personal business before paying their $100,000 fines to the federal government and serving their terms. (The hearing of the fourth executive was postponed until his lawyer recovered from his courtroom fall.) Synthes, with $3.4 billion in sales in 2009, paid just $23 million in fines—a drop in the bucket. And the doctors who performed the Norian procedures—including those who failed to report deaths to the FDA—suffered no legal action.

AT ROUGHLY THE same time that Synthes launched its unauthorized Norian experiments, neuroradiologist David F. Kallmes was in medical practice with Mary Jensen, the physician who had brought vertebroplasty, first performed in France, to the United States and who made developing the technique a major focus of her career. Kallmes ran a tiny pilot study that compared patients who received vertebroplasty with those who underwent a sham procedure, in which only anesthetic was injected. Kallmes made sure the two groups of patients were "blinded" to their designated procedure, meaning they would not know which one they would receive. In both cases, he opened a container of polymethylmethacrylate, which has a scent like nail polish, and banged on a bowl so that, to the patient, who couldn't see what he was doing, it sounded as though he was mixing cement. In both groups, Kallmes pressed heavily on the patients' backs to simulate the feeling of the cement injection. When outcomes were evaluated, it was evident that the sham procedure—where no cement was injected—was just as effective as actual vertebroplasty. Both groups experienced immediate and similar improvement in pain and disability. For Mary Jensen, who had trained more than one hundred thousand U.S. physicians in the vertebroplasty protocol, and who believed that the procedure was safe and that it offered significant benefits to elderly patients because it got them back on their feet as soon as possible, this was not good news.

Kallmes left Jensen's practice and moved to the Mayo Clinic, where he had a very hard time finding the funds and participants he needed to perform a larger study of vertebroplasty. On the shaky premise that such a trial would unfairly deny relief to the group allocated to the sham intervention, hospitals and doctors declined to participate.

Three years after Kallmes suggested that it might be a costly and un-necessary procedure, doctors were performing almost thirty thou-sand vertebroplasty procedures annually, at about $30,000 per case. It was not a business they were keen to give up.

Finally, in 2009, Kallmes published his second study's outcomes in the *New England Journal of Medicine*. In a larger trial of 131 patients, many of whom were recruited from abroad, there was no difference in pain relief, function, or quality of life, whether they'd undergone vertebroplasty or a sham procedure. "We aren't saying that verte-broplasty doesn't work—because somehow it does," Kallmes said. "But both sets of patients experienced significant improvements in pain and function a month following the procedure, whether they received cement injections or not." Those benefits, Kallmes added, could emerge from any number of variables, among them local anes-thesia, sedation, and the patients' own expectations.

Soon after Kallmes's *New England Journal of Medicine* publication, the American Academy of Orthopaedic Surgeons retracted its recom-mendation for vertebroplasty in patients who presented with osteopo-rotic spinal compression fractures, leaving physicians who performed the procedure in a quandary. Thus began the hunt for a new way to augment crushed vertebrae.

That new method was called "kyphoplasty." Instead of squeezing the cement between crumbling fragments of vertebrae, the physician inserted a needle that contained a tiny balloon. Once the needle was in place, the physician inflated the balloon and injected the cement. Because it was encased in the balloon, as the cement hardened, it did not stray. Minneapolis-based Medtronic, one of the largest med-ical device manufacturers in the world, produced the device in a kit, which it trademarked as "Kyphon Balloon Kyphoplasty."

The procedure, Medtronic's marketing team explained, could be performed by orthopedic surgeons, in hospitals, on an inpatient ba-sis. Those hospital stays could be billed to Medicare. That was good for business, and it meant that sales of Kyphon Balloon Kyphoplasty quickly outpaced vertebroplasty.

When federal prosecutors caught on, Medtronic was accused of health care fraud, under the provisions of the U.S. False Claims Act. The device manufacturer, no stranger to such lawsuits, settled with the U.S. government for $75 million. Subsequently, in repayment for incorrectly billing for overnight stays, 130 U.S. hospitals returned $105 million to Medicare.

Given the lack of evidence for either procedure, health policy experts anticipated that Medicare would shut down payments for both kyphoplasty and vertebroplasty. Additional clinical trials made it apparent that, typically, vertebral fractures did not require care beyond mild analgesics and a brief reduction of daily activities; in short, in most cases they healed by themselves in a matter of weeks. Although the government continued to pay for kyphoplasty, and interventional pain physicians continued to do it, the less profitable technique of vertebroplasty was mostly shelved.

Curious about how Mary Jensen had felt when vertebroplasty hit the skids, and what she thought of the procedure now, I gave her a call. It was still a great procedure for the right patients, she said. In fact, she explained, in a recent randomized, placebo-controlled, double-blind trial out of Australia, using a sham procedure as a comparison, vertebroplasty for osteoporotic fractures resulted in "early stand up" (getting patients mobile again), and "less narcotics use." In these ways, the technique worked better than both the sham procedure and standard nonoperative care. It was essential, said Jensen, to select the right patient; one with a fracture that was not more than six weeks old, who had not responded to standard medical care, and who was in truly debilitating pain.

The problem—and it was hardly a new or original one—was that many of the doctors she trained, especially those who were not radiologists, "vastly overutilized the procedure," choosing the wrong patients, for the wrong reasons. She said some of them were very cavalier about patient selection. "They saw that radiologists did vertebroplasty, so they figured it was a very easy procedure to do, and you could bill for it, and make money. So there was lots of self-referral, and often there were patients who, from years of experience, I would not have considered appropriate candidates. To be honest, it disturbed me greatly." In subsequent years, Jensen has served as an expert witness in legal cases where vertebroplasty has gone wrong. "I've been very much appalled at some of the things I've seen," she said. "The procedure has been poorly performed, on patients for whom it is not indicated."

When I told my friend, who was definitely on the mend, that she really didn't need the kyphoplasty that her doctor had recommended, she thanked me, said she would think it over—and then scheduled the procedure. She had to stay on her pain management doctor's good side, she said. And after all, Medicare—the government program funded by all U.S. taxpayers—would bear the expense. Two weeks later, just as her doctor had promised, she was as good as new—just as she would have been if she'd declined to undergo the procedure.

5

The Gold Standard

WHY LUMBAR SPINAL FUSION IS NEVER YOUR ONLY REMAINING OPTION

S PINE SURGEONS, WHO are typically trained as orthopedic surgeons or neurosurgeons, do essential things. They repair traumatic injuries; they excise spinal tumors; they fix congenital abnormalities. But except for top-tier physicians, who usually work at academic medical centers, such procedures are not their mainstay. About 60 percent of patients who walk into a spine surgeon's clinic have back pain that will be diagnosed as "ordinary," "axial," "mechanical," "degenerative," "functional," or "nonspecific." Those terms describe flattened discs, black discs, bulging discs, herniated discs (described as "prolapsed discs" in the United Kingdom), and the bony outgrowths known as osteophytes. Too often, surgeons point to these commonplace artifacts on an MRI and diagnose "degenerative disc disease," recommending lumbar spinal fusion surgery as the best option.

But there's a problem with this very common procedure, in which the intervertebral disc is excised and adjacent vertebrae are connected with cages, screws, plates, rods, and other medical devices. Studies show that lumbar fusion succeeds in barely 40 percent of patients. And in this context, the word "success" does not mean much. In one study, two years after spinal fusion, in "successful" procedures, pain had barely been reduced by half and most patients continued to use painkillers. In another study, two years after surgery, about one-third of the patients reported that their pain was as bad as it had been before they'd had the operation, and 14 percent believed that after spinal fusion they were in worse shape than before it.

Here's what surgeons told me: Eighty to 85 percent of the time, although they can visualize an anomaly on the X-ray or MRI, they cannot, with any certainty, determine the source of the pain. That's why ten spine surgeons will propose ten different solutions; one may recommend fusing the spine at three levels, while another sees no indication for any type of procedure. The ambiguity inherent in diagnosing back pain makes it possible for surgeons to do practically anything they want.

But what they do not want is to go under the knife themselves. At an American Academy of Orthopaedic Surgeons conference in the summer of 2010, a hundred surgeons were polled as to whether they'd personally have lumbar spinal fusion surgery for unspecific low back pain. The answer—from all but one—was "absolutely not." The risk-reward ratio just wasn't good enough.

Under such circumstances, why do surgeons continue to pursue this type of operation? They "have their own inherent conflict," explained prominent orthopedic surgeon and Cedars-Sinai Medical Center researcher Hyun Bae. "It's not only a financial conflict. It's an emotional conflict. We get paid to do the work. We want to make the patient better. So we concentrate on the good results and we dismiss the bad results." Nor can the surgeons be held entirely responsible, because they are under constant pressure, said Bae, from patients who beg them to "do something." Under the circumstances, it's hard not to want to be a hero.

But too often, even if the procedure goes well, recovery stalls within weeks. The *American Journal of Medicine* observed that, in the United States alone, about eighty thousand spine surgeries fail annually. Patients who have not done well are referred to as "failed backs," and they often return to the OR repeatedly, losing ground after each procedure.

About one in five patients who undergo spinal surgery for a degenerative disorder returns for a revision procedure—a second operation. Even when the fusion is deemed to be "radiologically

perfect"—meaning that on an X-ray the vertebrae have grown together and the hardware is positioned correctly—the fusion itself
imposes increased stress at other vertebral segments, which often
results in "adjacent segment deterioration," a condition where the
vertebral level above or below degrades, causing more pain. A second back surgery has a 30 percent chance of success. That prognosis
drops to 15 percent for a third back surgery, and 5 percent for a
fourth.

Oregon Health and Science University spine medicine researcher
Roger Chou believes that surgeons should be required to reveal the
odds to their patients before going forward. "If [the surgeon] said, 'Yes,
we can do this $70,000 surgery, but you know, there's still more than a
50 percent chance that you're going to have a lot of pain, and you still
won't be able to work, and you're going to need pain medicine, and
you'll have complications related to the surgery'—and all this is well
documented—then most people would say, 'I don't want it.'"

In an article in a medical trade journal, orthopedic surgeon Terry
Amaral made note of some of the things that can go wrong—things
that are rarely mentioned to surgical candidates. "The spinal cord is
right next to where we are putting the screws in; we are working
near where the nerve roots exit," he observed. "If you perforate that
area, the patient will experience weakness or even paralysis. Then in
the front of the spine, there are other things to be concerned about,
like the aorta, the vena cava, the lungs." There are other risks that
go unspecified: The spinal screws are misplaced in 5 to 10 percent
of all fusion procedures. After spinal fusion, infection is common.
Nerves may be jostled and inflamed, resulting in dull, diffuse, aching, or sharp stinging pain in the legs that may or may not ever go
away. Supportive spinal ligaments and muscles, disturbed during the
surgery, rarely work with the same efficiency, and that incompetence
may result in more back pain.

But in spite of risks and mediocre outcomes, the number of spinal fusions performed in the United States grew from 61,000 in 1993
to more than 465,000 in 2011—more than a 600 percent increase,
accounting for more than 60 percent of the spinal fusion surgery

performed worldwide. It's the most expensive form of elective surgery in the United States, costing about $40 billion annually.

For twenty years, the *Dartmouth Atlas of Health Care* has documented variations in how medical resources are allocated in the United States. In 2011, the university's Institute for Health Policy and Clinical Practice, which produces the atlas, reported a puzzling finding: The prevalence of spine surgery in Casper, Wyoming, was nearly six times higher than it was in the Bronx, New York. Even more baffling, the rate in St. Cloud, Minnesota, was twice that of Rochester, Minnesota, the home of the Mayo Clinic, only 150 miles away. Evidently, the decision to have spinal fusion surgery was based more on geography than actual medical need.

Although there are exceptions, most European and UK surgeons avoid the procedure. "I end up sending most of my patients with chronic pain to rehabilitation programs, and therefore end up fusing a tiny number of highly motivated patients," said Oxford University Hospital's orthopedic surgeon Jeremy Fairbank. "The busy guy argument—the one you get from the patient who somehow has time to have a major back operation but can't manage a rehab program—does not stack up. If you have a spinal fusion operation, you are off work for four to eight weeks, and sometimes longer. A rehab program takes one to three weeks."

Lumbar spinal fusion is an operation with a bad reputation. But as we will see, in Asia-Pacific countries, especially China and Japan, such procedures are expected to nearly triple in number between 2014 and 2020, and almost double in revenues, with more than a little encouragement from U.S. spinal device manufacturers.

VERY EARLY IN my research, I talked my way into a professional meeting of the North American Spine Society, held at a beach resort in Maui. It was there that I met orthopedic surgeon Alexander Ghanayem, chief of the division of spine surgery at Loyola University Medical Center in Maywood, Illinois. Although at the time I had no idea why they were avoiding me, most of the surgeons I asked for interviews politely declined, citing other urgent business. But Ghanayem was game and boldly suggested that we have our conversation in clear view of his colleagues and the device manufacturers' reps who had sponsored the meeting.

If he didn't take me under his wing, Ghanayem said, I risked being brainwashed by elitist surgeons from academic medical centers. At his clinic in Mayfield, at Loyola University Medical Center, he saw working-class folk, assembly line and machine shop workers—people whose bad backs threatened far more than their ability to play golf. I should come visit, he said, and join him for a morning in the OR. I could hang out with him as he saw patients. I jumped at the chance.

Four months later, I was in a cab at dawn, in the frosty Chicago exurbs, rolling past rows of identical houses that were lavishly decorated for Halloween. After he collected me in the parking lot, Ghanayem's surgical fellow described the day's first case. The patient was in his mid-forties, a machine operator who had injured his back on the job. Joe* was scheduled for an anterior lumbar spinal fusion at L4–5, the vertebral joint at approximately navel height.

After I dressed in surgical scrubs, a blue bouffant cap, and disposable shoe covers, Ghanayem asked whether I fainted at the sight of blood. I assured him that I'd be fine, but really, I had no idea how I would respond when I first peered inside a human being's abdominal cavity.

With seven on the surgical team and a reporter underfoot, the small OR was jammed. Except for a glowing orange square of flesh on his abdomen, the result of a Betadine antiseptic scrub, the patient was covered in sterile blue drapes. Ghanayem, a big man, pulled on a twenty-five-pound leopard-patterned lead apron and neck gaiter, meant to protect him from the radiation from the fluoroscopy machine, and passed me a drab model to wear. At the computer monitor, he clicked through a series of Joe's scans, starting with the disc herniation as it had appeared several months earlier. I could see a delicate protrusion of disc tissue, nestling up to a tender spinal nerve root. "It's gone now," he said, pointing to the same spot on a more recent scan. "But he's got mechanical symptoms. And the disc is a little black."

The surgical indication, as noted on Joe's chart, was "degenerative disc disease."

Ghanayem explained that he based his decision to operate not only on the imaging and Joe's symptoms but also on the results of commonly used provocative discography, a test meant to evaluate the function and integrity of a painful disc. On the plane to Chicago, the day before, I'd read what Eugene Carragee, then the chief of the Stanford University School of Medicine's spinal surgery department, had recently written about discography's diagnostic validity.

In provocative discography, the disc is punctured with a needle and injected with contrast medium, which elevates the pressure inside the tough annular shell. Typically, that increase in pressure causes pain, and that pain is considered evidence that the integrity of the disc has failed. But Carragee, a crackerjack researcher and spine surgeon with a penchant for questioning long-accepted procedures, found that a disc didn't have to be damaged to cause a patient to yelp in pain; on the contrary, an individual with a healthy disc exhibited the same painful response when the medium was injected. Furthermore, Carragee's research demonstrated that puncturing a disc with a needle, especially one large enough in diameter to allow contrast medium to flow through it, could cause that disc to fail in various ways.

When Carragee announced his findings at the annual conference of the International Society for the Study of the Lumbar Spine, attendees were aghast. A favored diagnostic tool, which health insurance providers had long accepted as an indicator of the need for lumbar spinal fusion, had just been outed as a charade. That year, physicians had ordered about two hundred thousand provocative lumbar discography procedures, at roughly $1,750 each. Spanish spine expert Francisco Kovacs, never one to mince words, declared: "Before Gene's study, discography was just useless," he said. "Now we know it's both useless and dangerous. Surgeons tell patients to have discography so they can sell the patient and the insurance provider the operation. The test is positioned as a diagnostic tool, to help make a decision, but that test will be positive, since it's positive in everybody."

In 2015, in spite of its lack of diagnostic or prognostic value and its evident risks, discography was still being performed about seventy thousand times a year—and health insurance providers continue to pay for it.

IN THE CHILLY OR, there was an acrid odor; I realized that, even naked under his drapes, Joe reeked of cigarette smoke. Because in heavy smokers the spinal vertebrae often fail to fuse properly after lumbar spinal fusion, it's common for surgeons to require patients to clear their bodies of stored nicotine prior to the operation. But Joe had been smoking more than ever. Having gained fifty pounds in under a year, he was also obese and dependent on painkillers. With a pending workers' compensation claim, the deck was stacked against him.

After some discussion, the surgical team chose Bob Marley and Fleetwood Mac as the sound track for Joe's procedure. As the general surgeon made the first incision and retracted layers of muscles, the rhythm of the first song matched the *beep . . . beep . . . beep* of the heart monitor. Up to his elbows inside Joe's abdominal cavity, the general surgeon moved aside the intestines, kidneys, and blood vessels. Then, as his nurse laid out long black strands of suturing material on Joe's draped legs, Ghanayem stepped onto a low metal stool, the narrow beam from his headlamp functioning as the only light source in an otherwise darkened room.

I stood in the corner, as motionless as if I'd been planted there, my view obscured. Carefully, I crept forward. I'd been warned that if I casually brushed anything draped in blue—for instance, the table of surgical instruments or a box of metal plates and screws, each in its own little cubbyhole—the surgical team would have to re-drape everything, a process that could take an hour.

A chunk of the intervertebral disc that Ghanayem had just removed whizzed past my ear, landing with a clang in a stainless steel receptacle. Yellow and striated, it had the texture of canned crabmeat. Ghanayem showed me the tough outer layer of the disc—the annulus fibrosus—and the squishy inner core of the nucleus pulposus. Up close and personal, the latter, which I'd heard described as being like the "jelly in a jelly doughnut," more closely resembled heavy phlegm. Although the annulus is commonly characterized as the disc's protective shell, in fact, there was no demarcation between the obliquely oriented layers of collagen fibers in the annulus and the gel-like material of the nucleus pulposus. The bands of collagen grew thicker as they moved from interior to exterior, anchoring the disc to the bony top of one vertebra and the bottom of the adjacent one. At that moment, Ghanayem explained, he was struggling to remove the anchor.

I'd assumed that with no notice, a disc could slide out from between the vertebral bones, like a hamburger escaping from a bun. But that was a fiction. As I watched Alex Ghanayem tugging and twisting, I realized that there was no such thing as a "slipped disc": Removing one was vicious work, like extracting a healthy tooth.

Once the disc space was picked clean, Ghanayem invited me to stand on my own metal footstool just behind his right shoulder, where I could see into the deep canyon of Joe's belly. Retractors pulled apart the abdominal walls, revealing six inches of gelatinous red fat. At the bottom of this gorge lay a queue of snowy white bones: the spinal column.

"Okay, here comes the delicate part," Ghanayem said, winking, before he took up a mallet to pound a section of milled cadaver bone into the gap between Joe's fourth and fifth vertebrae. The nurse wiped the sweat from the surgeon's brow. From the box of spinal hardware, he selected a plain metal plate and four screws, and set them in place.

After the surgery, Joe would spend a couple of days in the hospital and then begin walking a mile or so every day. If all went well, after a month he'd ride a stationary bike. After two months, if the X-ray looked good, he could start an exercise-based rehab program. I should understand, Ghanayem added, that this surgery was the best chance Joe had; otherwise, the big gut and the painkiller addiction ensured an early demise.

Alexander Ghanayem was optimistic. But the odds were not good. It remained to be seen whether Joe would become a statistic or get back to work; as a work comp claimant, he'd be the exception.

Typically, such patients continue to require painkillers after the operation, and that can spell disaster: Among middle-aged male workers' comp claimants, overdosing on pain meds after spinal fusion surgery for degenerative disc disease is the most common cause of death. Typically, such patients accidentally overdose on opioids and suffer respiratory failure. This accounts for about 20 percent of all deaths occurring within the first three months after surgery.

As the surgical fellow methodically stitched up the long incision in Joe's abdomen, Stevie Nicks sang an especially appropriate lyric of her song, "Over My Head:" "Sometimes I can't help but feel that I'm wasting all of my time." I couldn't help but wonder whether Ghanayem had just done the same.

WHEN MIXTER AND Barr excised that first intervertebral disc in 1934, they didn't know they'd done the easy part; encouraging the untethered vertebral bodies to grow back together would be the real challenge. In pursuit of a solution, surgeons tried contraptions made of celluloid bars and silk threads. They fiddled with wire and hooks, hoping to build a construct of spinal hardware that would stand up to harsh treatment.

One orthopedist of that era, frustrated with yet another failed effort, wrote that the random and scattered bits of metal revealed in his patient's spinal X-ray brought to mind the contents of the junk drawer in his kitchen. Patients were initially immobilized for a while with sandbags piled around them. Later, they wore neck-to-hip braces. And still the bones did not fuse, leaving patients in great pain, and sometimes relegated to wheelchairs or bedridden for the rest of their lives.

As a result, lumbar spinal fusion remained a procedure of last resort until 1982, when Arthur Steffee, an Ohio orthopedist and surgical hardware inventor, designed a headless screw that slipped into a slot in a stainless steel plate. With the plate screwed into position, anchoring adjacent vertebral bodies, bone could grow, filling the gap and providing a sturdy union.

With production already under way at Steffee's AcroMed factory, the surgeon rushed his invention through the FDA's newly established and still amorphous device approval process. The green light allowed Steffee to market the screws and plates for setting long bone fractures— but didn't permit AcroMed to market the product for use in the spine. But setting a precedent that many device manufacturers would follow, AcroMed took FDA regulations casually. Within a year, Arthur Steffee had trained hundreds of physicians to use his invention in lumbar spinal fusion.

Over the next twelve months, the number of lumbar spinal fusions performed in the United States, nearly all of them using Steffee implants, grew from a thousand procedures to three times that many. Other companies saw the opportunity to profit, and brought their own medical devices to market. In seven years, sales of spinal instrumentation increased from $225 million to well over $2 billion.

In the winter of 1993, around one hundred million people watched *20/20*, the *ABC News* show hosted by Barbara Walters and Hugh Downs. The anchors interviewed nine unhappy spine surgery patients, all of whom had received Steffee screws and plates. Painfully, they described how the devices had dislodged, broken, or both—and ruined their lives.

When Walters demanded that the FDA explain its failure to stop AcroMed from engaging in off-label marketing (promoting Steffee plates to surgeons for spinal fusion), the federal agency's chief declared that AcroMed had engaged in illegal off-label marketing. AcroMed's management team rejoined that there had been a misunderstanding; they thought they'd had the FDA's approval. For three years after the *20/20* spine surgery episode aired, personal injury lawyers urged TV viewers who had undergone back surgery to get in touch via a toll-free number so that they might sue AcroMed. Eventually, without admitting any wrongdoing, AcroMed agreed to pay $112 million to thirty-two hundred patients who claimed injury from the Steffee devices, a settlement that emptied the company's coffers and closed its doors.

But even in the wake of that controversy, dozens of new spinal devices were poised to enter the market. Fearing another fiasco, the FDA fought for more regulatory control. Instead, after device manufacturers and their lobbyists convinced members of Congress that the FDA's regulatory proposals were paternalistic, costly, and time-consuming, the agency's oversight was further constrained. In a policy paper, the Cato Institute, Charles Koch's libertarian think tank, cattily described the FDA as "a full-service government bureaucracy. . . . It is promulgator, police, judge, jury and executioner, all rolled into one." In the political climate of the moment, more regulation would not fly.

Thus vilified, the FDA took the easier tack and became industry's pal, moving products through the approval process as fast as possible. "It was part of the culture of 'Let's get this done, let's get things out fast, and don't ask too many questions.' There was no sense that we had to get the science right," said Larry Kessler, who was director of the FDA's Office of Surveillance and Biometrics at the Center for Devices and Radiological Health.

In the mid-1990s, the "interbody fusion cage," a hollow, perforated titanium cylinder, made its way into the market. After scraping the intervertebral disc from between the bones, the surgeon filled the cage with pulverized bone, and implanted the device in the resultant gap. In theory, the bone graft would encourage the growth of bone through and around the cage, resulting in a solid fusion. It was meant to make spinal fusion so simple that even a chimpanzee could do it, said its inventor, orthopedic surgeon and mechanical engineer Gary Michelson.

But in reality, in the heat of the moment, many surgeons had trouble selecting the proper size cage. Too often, as documented in X-rays I found online, the unsecured titanium cylinders drifted out of the disc space, coming to rest under a facet joint or in the shadow of a delicate nerve root. Surgeons concluded that the interbody fusion cage, which Michelson had designed to eliminate the need for screws, plates, and rods, would not reliably stay in place without the support of other devices. Helpfully, device manufacturers sent sales reps into the OR to aid surgeons in selecting additional screws, rods, securing nuts, and transconnectors. Each of those devices bolstered the bottom line, making spine surgery more profitable for all stakeholders.

AcroMed's scuffle with the FDA over off-label marketing clarified the risks manufacturers faced if they brazenly touted their own products for expanded uses. Over the next few years, industry players worked out a system of perks and payments for surgeon-consultants who could spread the word to other physicians without attracting the FDA's scrutiny—or so it seemed.

IN THE MID-1990S, as they competed for surgeons' business, device manufacturers began sponsoring training weekends in warm places like Maui, with rounds of golf interspersed with a few hours of "continuing medical education" (CME) presentations each day. Because the federal antikickback statute, on the books since 1972, made it illegal for medical device manufacturers or pharmaceutical companies to court doctors or to provide favors or cash in return for physicians' business, these were billed as "no strings attached" events—but it was no coincidence that surgeons began to use their hosts' products in the OR, to the exclusion of those from other companies.

Most device manufacturers wooed physicians with perks, but Medtronic was the first to get caught. The U.S. Department of Justice unveiled a spreadsheet listing the names of more than two hundred doctors who had attended a 2003 Medtronic meeting at a beach resort in Southern California. The document recorded each surgeon's annual spending on spinal devices. It identified which doctors were "100 percent compliant" Medtronic customers—meaning that they bought only from Medtronic—and which required "special attention" from sales reps, because they were not completely loyal. Despite the fact that the company had been caught red-handed, the feds went easy on Medtronic: In a year when the spine division's revenues were greater than $2.3 billion, the Justice Department limited the device manufacturer's settlement to only $40 million.

After that, Medtronic adopted a different approach, seeking to attract prominent surgeons who could serve as "key opinion leaders," or "KOLs." Patients were often aware of their doctors' influential status, but rarely grasped that a big-name surgeon might have a major financial conflict of interest.

In return for their help, referred to as "consultancy," such high-profile surgeons would receive patents and royalties that could be worth a great deal of money. Some physicians engaged in product development in significant ways. But others served essentially as cheerleaders, paid to persuade their colleagues to do business with Medtronic. The KOLs' real role would be to ensure a successful product launch and life cycle: Not only did KOLs develop new products; they took these products through FDA trials, published peer-reviewed papers about them, trained surgeons to use them, and later worked to expand their labeling. For a while, this airtight process allowed device manufacturers to skirt both the prohibitions of the False Claims Act and those of the antikickback statute.

Once inside the inner circle of KOLs, if a surgeon had reservations about the safety of a product, or believed that further clinical trials were required, or just wanted out of the deal, he risked being ostracized by his gung-ho colleagues.

BY THE LATE 1990s, many spine surgeons regarded the interbody fusion cage as a professional humiliation. Studies showed that no matter how many costly screws, rods, and plates were added to the original construct, the outcome of lumbar spinal fusion was not much improved. Still, giving up on the highly profitable procedure was out of the question.

In search of a better technique, a team of investigators led by orthopedic surgeon Scott Boden found a way to use recombinant DNA technology to create a type of hyperactive, genetically engineered bone cell. A decade earlier, researchers at the Wyeth-Genetics Institute in Cambridge, Massachusetts, had developed several methods of synthesizing the necessary proteins, which could then be purified, deposited into sterile vials, and freeze-dried. The resulting substance could be mixed with water, collected in an absorbent collagen sponge, and tucked inside the interbody fusion cage. Thus equipped, the interbody fusion cage was reborn as a delivery system for recombinant human bone morphogenetic protein-2, commonly referred to as BMP-2.

It would take years for BMP-2 to emerge as a profitable commercial application. For more than half a century, pulverized bone drilled from the patient's hip had been packed into the fusion site, to encourage bone growth. But "autograft," as the patient's own bone was called, could be extracted only in relatively small quantities, limiting the number of vertebral levels that could be fused during a single surgery. Post-op, some patients suffered hip pain from the drilling. BMP-2 was going to change all of that.

In 2002, Medtronic released a package containing a vial of BMP-2, a sponge, and Medtronic's patented Infuse Bone Graft/LT-Cage. BMP-2 had complex pharmaceutical properties, and there was no substantially equivalent product in use in spine medicine. According to many experts, that meant that BMP-2 should have passed through the FDA's most rigorous pharmaceutical approval channels instead of being studied as a device. But Medtronic, rushing to get a BMP-2 product on the market, did not send Infuse through the pharmaceutical approval process. Instead, the product was treated as an add-on to the already approved interbody fusion cage. Because the Medical Device User Fee and Modernization Act had recently switched the burden of paying for the approval process from the federal government to the device manufacturer, it's possible that the FDA, anxious to please one of its most important customers, rushed the new product through the pipeline.

This sidestepping of regulatory red tape turned the FDA's preapproval advisory meetings on Infuse into tense affairs. The FDA brought in industry experts. Medtronic's top brass and some of the company's KOLs were present, as were other interested outsiders. In the meetings, several people observed that the Infuse clinical trials were poorly designed—too brief, and with too few participants—to give a good reading on what would happen once the product arrived in the surgical suite.

Patsy Trisler, a regulatory consultant, who in the past had served at the FDA as a scientific reviewer and special assistant to the director of the Office of Device Evaluation, noted that, of the doctors who performed the premarket trials, nine were "key opinion leaders" who were engaged in financial relationships with Medtronic. "After this prototype is out in the marketplace," Trisler said, "if it is misused or misapplied, the potential for harm is great." What would happen, she asked, if BMP-2 turned out to be a cancer-promoting compound? What if the product, used off-label, spurred uncontrolled growth of bone in the spine or pelvis? A chorus of Medtronic's supporters dismissed Trisler's concerns as unfounded, bristling at the implication that the promise of a big payday could sway the judgment of a group of eminent surgeons.

At the advisory meeting, Oklahoma spine surgeon David Malone's cautionary letter was read into the record. Malone had served as one of Medtronic's clinical investigators in an early trial of BMP-2 in posterior lumbar fusion, but that trial ended prematurely, when more than 70 percent of those participating developed superfluous bone growth in the spine, with chronic radiating pain in their arms and legs. The excessive growth was so evident, wrote Malone, that "the secretaries in our clinic could look at X-rays and tell who got the BMP-2 and who did not." In response, the FDA explicitly restricted BMP's use to anterior spinal fusion (involving an abdominal incision) in future clinical trials. But Malone worried that if the FDA green-lighted the product, surgeons would use the product as they saw fit. In doing so, they could inadvertently endanger patients' health.

Despite such misgivings, the FDA approved Infuse Bone Graft, recommending that it should be used only in clinical situations where a fusion with pulverized bone was likely to fail. But in the months to come, key opinion leaders would publish papers in peer-reviewed medical journals, charting off-label uses well beyond the FDA's recommendations, and describing good outcomes, with remarkably few adverse events. Relying on the accuracy of what they read, surgeons in the United States, and in most other well-developed countries, embraced Infuse as a standard part of the fusion procedure.

Infuse hit the market in 2002. Within months, surgeons who might have performed a standard, inexpensive, and relatively safe decompression procedure on a patient with spinal stenosis, instead were opting to fuse four vertebral levels. With autograft from the patient's hip, it would have been difficult to extract enough bone, but Infuse arrived in handy packets and could be prepared as needed, in any quantity. Between 2002 and 2008, the number of complex operations for spinal stenosis increased fifteenfold. The product could boost the cost of a two-level spinal fusion by $17,000, without increasing other costs. The message to surgeons was clear: They were to fuse more levels because more levels meant more money.

Private health insurance providers, Medicare, and workers' compensation carriers were helpfully liberal in their reimbursement policies for BMP-2—at least until July 2008, when the FDA received thirty-eight reports of life-threatening complications, including documentation of life-threatening swelling of the neck and throat associated with the off-label use of Infuse in cervical spine operations.

While the FDA tried to alert physicians to the problem, authorities in the Justice Department and the U.S. Attorney's Office considered whether, yet again, Medtronic's use of off-label marketing had crossed the line. In its investigation, the Justice Department ordered Medtronic to hand over more than five thousand documents that described the company's payments to physicians over the prior fifteen years.

While U.S. federal prosecutors evaluated records, Tomislav Smoljanović, a young orthopedic surgeon at the University of Zagreb in Croatia, studied the data on Infuse. He noticed that some male spinal fusion patients whose procedures had included BMP-2 had developed a condition called "retrograde ejaculation," which leads to temporary or permanent sterility. (It occurs when sperm and semen go the wrong way, entering the bladder as opposed to the urethra. In patients who had undergone the standard bone graft procedure, this condition was rare.)

According to John Fauber, an award-winning investigative reporter at the *Milwaukee Journal Sentinel*, when Smoljanović asked Thomas Zdeblick, the editor of the *Journal of Spinal Disorders and Techniques* and professor and chairman of orthopedic surgery at the University of Wisconsin School of Medicine and Public Health, why his journal articles about Infuse failed to discuss this connection, Smoljanović got no response. So he wrote to other journals, until finally the letter was published in the *Journal of Bone and Joint Surgery*. Zdeblick published a response that denied a relationship "between the use of BMP-2 in stand-alone interbody fusion cages and the postoperative development of retrograde ejaculation."

Eugene Carragee, the Stanford surgeon, who was also editor in chief of the *Spine Journal*, had published papers reporting similarly excellent outcomes for Infuse. Smoljanović's letter attracted his attention, because his own surgical colleagues had also started to describe issues with retrograde ejaculation among their spinal fusion patients. Carragee set out to compare the outcomes of Stanford patients who had undergone spinal fusion with BMP-2 and the outcomes of those who had bone taken from their hips.

What he found shocked him: The patients who received BMP-2 had suffered adverse events that key opinion leader authors' papers had not even mentioned. When Carragee checked Medtronic's clinical trial data on Infuse, he concluded that a host of complications had been intentionally concealed. Disgusted that the articles he'd published might have caused the *Spine Journal*'s surgeon readership to practice bad medicine, Carragee set out to correct the record.

It helped that Carragee was one tough soldier, who had been awarded a Purple Heart and a Bronze Star after serving two deployments in Iraq. As a lieutenant colonel in the U.S. Army Reserve, he'd been injured when an IED exploded. To survive the vitriol that was to come his way after he blew the lid off Infuse, he'd need at least as much courage.

In an offensive that secured Carragee's position in the annals of medical history, the June 2011 issue of the *Spine Journal* laid bare the inaccuracies in thirteen peer-reviewed articles about BMP-2. "We were falsely reassured that there were independent people looking at the data," Carragee told *Milwaukee Journal Sentinel* reporter John Fauber, who would cover the story brilliantly. Carragee described what had happened as "a violation of the fundamental trust of peer-review." In the *Spine Journal*, Carragee explored BMP-2's ties to retrograde ejaculation as well as the incidence of inflamed nerves and the inflammation of other soft tissues, tumor prevalence, and the problem of extraneous bone growth. "There was evidence of a wide range of complications and adverse events in the early trials," Carragee told the *Back Letter*, the discerning and frequently critical monthly guide to back pain industry news.

The *Spine Journal*'s takedown sent shock waves throughout the back pain industry. In response, Medtronic's spin machine issued statements meant to bolster shareholders' confidence. In an interview with the *New York Times*, Medtronic's CEO and chairman, Omar Ishrak, asserted that "integrity and patients' safety" were his highest priority. He assured a *Times* reporter that "independent physician-scientist researchers," rather than staffers in Medtronic's marketing department, had written and edited the journal articles.

From the podium at the North American Spine Society's annual meeting in 2012, Eugene Carragee observed that surgeons were finding "tumors all over the place"—lung cancer, pancreatic cancer, prostate cancer, stomach cancer, ovarian and breast cancer—in patients whose spinal fusion procedures had included BMP-2. Carragee thought that rather than actually causing tumors, BMP-2 had "a cancer-promotion effect." It was possible, he said, that BMP-2 impaired the body's ability to eliminate cancer cells in their earliest stages of development. Carragee told thousands of uneasy spine surgeons that "a lot of injuries—and even deaths—could have been prevented" had the product been properly studied.

"If someone tells you that they have a really powerful bone growth factor," he told the audience, "and gave it to eight hundred study subjects without a single adverse reaction ascribed to it, I think your mother could tell you what to conclude there. This would be an incredible result for people taking an aspirin, never mind a powerful growth factor."

In response, Medtronic and its lobbyists assailed Carragee's credibility. When an orthopedic industry trade journal implied that Carragee's less-than-stellar surgical outcomes were the result of spending too much time away from the OR, on the edge of the Iraqi conflict, his colleagues were furious that such an unpatriotic premise was even advanced.

While that battle raged, the Justice Department's investigators found that Medtronic had paid more than $210 million over fifteen years to thirteen doctors (and their associated corporations) who had been authors of articles about Infuse for medical journals. Specifically, the device manufacturer had written checks for more than $34 million to Thomas Zdeblick, the University of Wisconsin surgeon and journal editor who had declined to publish the Croatian researcher's letter about retrograde ejaculation. The *Wall Street Journal* reported that, despite CEO Ishrak's denial to the *Times*, e-mail correspondence between physician-consultants and Medtronic marketing executives showed that the staff had pushed doctors to make questionable claims. Medtronic's marketing department, the *Wall Street Journal* contended, was "heavily involved in drafting, editing and shaping" of medical journal articles before they went to press.

In August 2011, Medtronic commissioned a panel of outside experts to analyze the complete patient data set from the Infuse Bone Graft clinical trials. No health care company had previously allowed proprietary data to be examined this way. Cardiologist Harlan M. Krumholz, director of the Yale New Haven Hospital Center for Outcomes Research and Evaluation, was in charge. Krumholz also led YODA: the Yale University Open Data Access Project. After Medtronic wrote a check for $2.5 million, Oregon Health and Science University's Pacific Northwest Evidence-Based Practice Center and the Centre for Reviews and Dissemination at the University of York (England) would run separate investigations under YODA's direction.

"Science has the power to be self-correcting," Krumholz observed, "but only if data are available. Imagine how much more careful [researchers] would be if they knew their results could be checked by any master's degree student."

With the trial data in YODA's hands, the Justice Department and the U.S. Attorney's Office closed the federal investigation, explaining rather feebly that, in terms of allegations of off-label marketing, there was "insufficient evidence" to allow the government to pursue federal, civil, or criminal charges.

In June 2013, YODA released independent reports on Medtronic's clinical data. Christine Laine, editor in chief of the *Annals of Internal*

Medicine, published these findings, making it clear that as far back as the days in the Wyeth lab, researchers knew about BMP-2's potential for causing retrograde ejaculation and superfluous bone growth. Beyond that, more than forty of the trials that YODA reviewed demonstrated that there was a risk of cancer.

Worse, it became evident that BMP-2, a product associated with multiple adverse events, offered no clinically significant benefit over the pulverized bone that had been used in fusion procedures for decades. BMP-2 did have one indisputable advantage, however. It increased the profit margin on spine surgery.

At its peak, in 2010, Infuse had sales of $809 million. By 2014, in light of the Carragee controversy, those sales had declined to $409 million. The *Back Letter* observed that "the chairman of the department of orthopedics at a large urban university hospital in the Eastern United States" had reported that BMP-2 was "dead in the water" in his region. "No one is using it at our hospital because of concerns about litigation." Lawsuits were mounting quickly, but Medtronic did not acknowledge any wrongdoing in regard to Infuse, which, by that time, had been implanted in a million patients' spines. Instead, the company reaffirmed its commitment, promising to "vigorously defend the product and company actions in the remaining cases."

By late 2014, as a result of litigation, Medtronic was on the hook for $22 million. The eventual severity of the device manufacturer's financial exposure would depend on how courts around the nation interpreted the statute known as "immunity by federal preemption." The term refers to the invalidation of a U.S. state law that conflicts with federal law; in this way, federal laws supersede state consumer-protection laws. Because the FDA, a federal agency, had already approved the medical device in question, it was possible that state courts would not agree to hear cases against Medtronic, making it impossible for personal injury lawyers to win them or collect their fees. Some legal experts believed that the application of immunity by federal preemption would not hold up in cases when FDA policy had been blatantly derailed in clinical trials, and Medtronic would have to pay up. In early 2016, patient Patricia Caplinger, whose surgeon used an unapproved posterior approach to spinal fusion, leading to "exuberant bone growth in her lumbar spine," (and whose case had already been dismissed by an Oklahoma state court), asked the U.S. Supreme court to "reconsider whether Medtronic could be sued under state laws for promoting Infuse for uses that the FDA never judged safe and effective." At the time, she was one of more than six thousand patients who were suing Medtronic for injuries related to Infuse. Abiding by its traditional stance on immunity by federal pre-emption, the Supreme Court declined Caplinger's petition for a hearing, without further comment, and in an increasingly pro-business political climate, it was anticipated that lower courts would follow suit.

THE INFUSE CONTROVERSY made it clear that spine surgeons were as vulnerable to financial conflicts of interest as stockbrokers or politicians.

Charles Rosen, the orthopedic surgeon who founded the spine center at the University of California–Irvine hospital, felt that the problem arose not only from the large paychecks that device manufacturers issued to surgeons, but also as a result of the lack of financial transparency surrounding these transactions. To establish standards for conflict of interest disclosure for drug and device manufacturers and physicians and associated hospitals and research facilities, he and medical marketing pro Gemma Cunningham built the Association for Medical Ethics, designing a searchable database that would allow anyone who was interested to scrutinize device company payments.

In Washington, D.C., Rosen implored Congress to make this reporting a federal requirement. The regulatory mechanism he endorsed was the Physician Payments Sunshine Act (PPSA), which would require drug and device companies to track and report every financial transaction involving doctors and hospitals that collect Medicare and Medicaid payments.

Health insurance providers might have continued to issue blanket approvals for spinal fusion if the Infuse travesty had never occurred—or if Eugene Carragee had not had the courage to expose it.

But the news about Infuse snapped their pocketbooks shut. (Throughout this ruckus, and despite robust data that should have raised questions, the Centers for Medicare and Medicaid Services kept paying.
Several years earlier, CMS had hired a Duke University research team
to examine the advantages and risks of spinal fusion surgery in an
older population. When the Duke investigators found no conclusive
evidence of short- or long-term benefits, CMS didn't change a thing.)

But private insurers began to look more closely at outcomes, and
more frequently declined reimbursement for lumbar fusion when the
indication was degenerative disc disease. Increasingly, before health
care plans would agree to pay for lumbar spinal fusion, surgeons
had to document that the patient had received extensive conservative care. If those requirements weren't satisfied, insurance providers
could "claw back" reimbursements for the surgical procedure, as well
as unnecessary diagnostics such as MRI and discography.

First, Blue Cross and Blue Shield of North Carolina said no. Then
BCBS of Illinois announced that it would not pay for spinal fusion if
the sole indication was disc herniation, degenerative disc disease, or
facet syndrome. This digging-in of heels, with the potential to slash
revenues, so panicked spine surgeons that nine medical societies
drafted a letter they titled their "Call to Rationality," fairly begging
insurers to come to their senses. The San Diego medical device and
imaging guidance company NuVasive, one of Wall Street's favorites,
with revenues growing at more than 10 percent a year, kicked in
$100,000 to help with advocacy efforts.

Surgeons' compensation is based, in part, on the number of "revenue hours" they spend in the OR. A full-time neurosurgeon makes an
average of $1.7 million per year for his hospital, while an orthopedic
surgeon pulls in about $2.7 million. A significant part of that revenue
is generated by spine surgery, and hospitals depend on the proceeds to
help out departments that are not nearly as flush. As insurers balked
on reimbursement, both surgeons and hospitals felt the pinch.

Spine surgeon Paul Slosar bemoaned the difficulty he'd had in getting BCBS to preapprove spinal fusion surgery. "Frankly, it made me
acutely depressed and angry . . . when I heard about and then read the

BCBS policy statement, it just hit me," he wrote in an e-mail to his colleagues, quoted in *Orthopedics This Week*. Slosar told reporter Robin Young, "I can't do the job I've trained my whole life to do. It sucked the wind right out of me."

Because bills coded for "degenerative disc disease" did not generate private health insurance providers' prompt approval, spine surgeons looked for another way to get patients into the OR. As a diagnosis, "spinal instability" was vague enough to be promising. No defined metrics existed for what degree of instability, or "slip," qualified a patient for surgery. Thus, even though they suspected that the procedures would not be effective, surgeons sometimes ordered multiple-level disc decompression procedures, where bits of stabilizing bone and disc material were excised. Post-op, when such patients' vertebrae slid perilously over one another, those physicians could cite spinal instability as their new diagnosis, and get approval for spinal fusion. In short, the disc decompression cases of today often became the lumbar spinal fusion patients of tomorrow.

At its peak, the U.S. spinal device industry earned $5 billion a year and luxuriated in two decades of double-digit growth, making stock market investors very happy. Between 2012 and 2013, as insurance providers cracked down on spinal fusion, those gains declined to about 2 percent a year. To keep shareholders engaged, manufacturers pursued international markets, where they found developing health care infrastructures, favorable reimbursement policies, and large middle-aged and elderly populations.

India, South Korea, Japan, Brazil, South Africa, Russia, and Eastern Europe were all promising markets for spinal device manufacturers, but with a population of 1.35 billion and a rapidly increasing proportion of old people, China was the main target. The number of spinal fusion procedures in that nation was slated to triple by 2020. Between 2014 and 2018, the medical device market was expected to grow by 75 percent. To gain access to Chinese doctors and patients, Medtronic spent more than $800 million to buy a hospital corporation, and also made extensive investments in other parts of Asia.

As the promise of the spinal fusion market in the United States dimmed, the Texas Back Institute, a dedicated spine surgery clinic and hospital with multiple facilities, began to establish a network of freestanding orthopedic surgery hospitals in China. Every six weeks it shipped its own "key opinion leader" surgeons from the United States to Asia, where insurance coverage was not an issue and there were plenty of patients who were prepared to pay for their spinal fusion procedures in hard cash.

IT'S HARD TO say whether the high-profile surgeons who touted Infuse knew of its shortcomings from the start, or discovered them when they were already in too deep. But when spine surgeons bought shares in physician-owned medical device distributorships, referred to as "PODs," they should have known that they would run afoul of federal law.

Legally and ethically, physicians are required to maintain arm's-length relationships with medical device manufacturers, as the federal antikickback statute requires. Before he operates, the surgeon tells the hospital purchasing department what surgical instrumentation he needs for the procedure, and the purchasing department orders it from the distributor. Although the device manufacturer, the distributor, and the hospital all profit from this transaction, it is understood that the physician does not.

At least that was the way it worked until 2003, when a handful of spine surgeons bought ownership stakes in physician-owned distributorships. The plan was to cut out the big-name manufacturers by pushing business to a generic device maker that would sell cut-rate products to the POD. In turn, the POD would sell the devices to hospitals. Explaining that this approach would cut costs and increase profits, surgeons who owned shares in PODs convinced their hospitals to buy exclusively from their distributorships. By 2011, physician-owned spinal device distributorships had put down roots in twenty states. In California, forty PODs were registered.

Because the profit distributions were tied to the number of devices each surgeon used, the more operations a POD-owning surgeon scheduled, the more money he made. With a POD generating cash, a surgeon who did two or three fusion procedures weekly could bring in an extra half million dollars in a year.

Surely, some surgeons who owned shares in PODs behaved sensibly, ordering the same number of devices as they had in the past. But, on average, when a hospital switched to buying from a POD, the spinal fusion rate at that hospital increased by more than 20 percent. Although POD-owning surgeons promised hospitals that they would save money, purchasing departments sometimes paid seven times as much as if they'd bought from a big-name supplier, producing inflated bills that went straight to insurers. The scam took about a decade to register, but finally the U.S. Senate Committee on Finance, which oversees Medicare and Medicaid, took notice.

In 2010, within weeks of his purchase of a five-thousand-dollar stake in Apex Medical Technologies (one of roughly a dozen physician-owned distributorships belonging to spinal hardware manufacturer Reliance Medical Systems), neurosurgeon Aria O. Sabit began implanting dozens of extra devices in patients.

Before he bought his Apex share, Sabit had performed sixty-four instrumented spinal fusions over eight months at Community Memorial Hospital in Ventura, California. But after he inked the deal, Sabit's numbers more than doubled. Haste made waste: In just eighteen months, the surgeon generated nearly thirty malpractice suits. The Community Memorial Hospital whistleblower physicians, stunned by his speed in the OR, turned him in to the FBI, noting in testimony that Sabit's procedures were "plagued with high infection rates, high return-to-surgery rates, violations of operating room protocols, failures in instrumentation, surgical mishaps, inappropriate case selection, high complication rates, poor medical record documentation and poor patient management."

Despite his record, Community Memorial Hospital allowed Sabit to keep working, possibly because he was a "rainmaker," bringing the facility $8.4 million in Medicare revenue in a year and a half. Sabit himself made almost $440,000 from his Apex dealings and received more than $800,000 in Medicare reimbursements.

Finally, Sabit's hospital fired him, and the California state medical board revoked his license. But before he lost his right to practice in California, Sabit moved to Birmingham, Michigan, where a new medical license awaited him. There, he opened a spine surgery clinic, received OR privileges at three hospitals, and continued to schedule back-to-back spinal fusion procedures. In many cases, as subsequent scans of his miserable patients' spines would reveal, Sabit implanted no hardware, but had instead billed insurers for ghost devices.

In November of 2014, federal agents arrested Sabit in Michigan. Because he was considered a flight risk to his native Afghanistan, he was denied bail and put behind bars. In a tricky move, the California and Michigan legal cases were combined under the jurisdiction of Judge Paul Borman, a federal judge on the U.S. District Court for the Eastern District of Michigan. Half a year later, still cooling his heels in jail and hoping for a shorter sentence, Sabit agreed to help the Justice Department go after Apex and Reliance. He pleaded guilty to four counts of health care fraud, one count of conspiracy to commit health care fraud, and one count of unlawful distribution of controlled substances. By that time, he had cheated Medicare, Medicaid, and private insurers out of $11 million.

Shortly before he was due to hand down the reduced prison term that Sabit's legal team had negotiated with Michigan prosecutors, Judge Borman received heart-rending testimony from patients whose lives the surgeon had ruined. In response, the judge tossed out Sabit's guilty plea. In January 2017, after more than a year of legal wrangling, Sabit was sentenced to nearly twenty years in prison. Upon release, he will be under lifetime supervision.

What at the time appeared to be an insignificant change in state law had opened the door to this mayhem, allowing PODs to catch on. In California, in 2002, the state legislature passed a bill including a statute called the "spinal pass-through law." Under that statute, in workers' compensation cases, a spine surgeon was free to select hardware from any vendor he preferred and to direct his hospital's purchasing department to buy it for him. This policy was intended to make sure that the hospital did not railroad the surgeon into using bargain hardware. For its role in managing the transaction, the hospital netted $250.

That worked passably, until the administrators of two small Southern California hospitals saw their chance for a tremendous payday, at the expense of workers' compensation carriers. In time, an incestuous relationship began with PODs that would earn a total of more than a half-billion dollars for Tri-City Regional Medical Center in Hawaiian Gardens and Pacific Hospital in Long Beach.

With ownership in several companies in the distribution chain, these hospitals' administrators could siphon off profits each step of the way, adding to the cost of each device. The more spine surgeries that were scheduled, the more the scam was worth. Court documents claim that the administrators evolved a "capping, running, and steering" arrangement. Allegedly, they paid $15,000 per patient to doctors and chiropractors who agreed to send spinal fusion cases to their surgeons, who were apparently also in on the deal.

Between 2001 and 2010, surgeons at Pacific Hospital performed well over five thousand spinal fusion surgeries, billing $533 million for them—three times as much, in the same time frame, as any other hospital in California, including major medical centers. The *Wall Street Journal* reported that Tri-City Regional Hospital showed a similarly stratospheric increase in revenue: In 2007, the hospital collected just $3 million from insurers. Three years later, the bill for spinal fusion rose to $65 million.

The patients were typically Latino workers, many of them pulled from the agricultural fields, who spoke little English and were drawn into a system that promised to provide very expensive health care, at no cost to them, in addition to substantial paid time off to recover. Often, at their doctors' behest, they traveled hundreds of miles to have surgery far from home. To close the loop, hospital administrators provided translators and transportation, chauffeuring patients to surgical evaluations and to MRI facilities they also controlled.

For a while, these hospitals ordered their hardware from obscure vendors and then doubled or tripled the price on hospital invoices, before submitting them to workers' compensation. But then they figured out a way to make even more money.

Prosecutors allege that the hospital administrators made a deal with an elderly tool-and-machine shop owner to manufacture what legal documents refer to as "false, fraudulent, fake, counterfeit, and non-FDA-approved 'knock-off' medical devices" that were designed "to give the appearance of being authentic, FDA-approved spinal fixation devices." The fake instrumentation might have been similar in appearance, but FDA-approved hardware is milled from medical-grade titanium on calibrated machines. The local tool-and-die maker's equipment made ordinary industrial machine parts.

Not surprisingly, compared with medical hardware, the local products were cheap. While a set of pedicle screws used in spinal instrumentation can sell for many hundreds of dollars, the tool-and-die maker sold a single screw for $65. By the time that screw was transferred from one sham distributorship to the next—and marked up each time—the bill to the hospital was more than $12,000. Prosecutors found that by the time the invoice reached the hospital, various partners in the scam had marked up the cost of devices for sixteen surgeries from $326,000 to $1.1 million.

So that devices can be identified if they fail or must be recalled, post-op surgical notes always record the serial numbers from implanted hardware. But to elude detection, when surgeons used the tool-and-die maker's hardware, this step was skipped. Therefore, when patients in excruciating pain began to come forward in February 2014, with broken hardware in their spines, there was no way to identify what type of instrumentation they had received.

IN 2014, *CBS News* reporter Ben Eisler published a list of the highest-billing spine surgeons in the United States. Certainly, on Eisler's list were superstar surgeons who corrected congenital deformities at the top medical facilities in the United States, and who shored up spines shattered by trauma or cancer. But only a few were high-profile specialists. In an extraordinary feat of data journalism, Eisler ferreted out community spine surgeons who, between 2011 and 2012, had operated on ten times the average number of patients. Some had already been suspended from their hospitals. Others were settling multiple medical malpractice lawsuits. But they had this in common: They were all churning back pain patients who had arrived in their clinics expecting ethical treatment.

Near the top of the list was forty-four-year-old spine surgeon Abubakar Atiq Durrani, whose Center for Advanced Spine Technologies had clinics in Kentucky and Ohio. Durrani's alleged MO was to inform patients with normal spines that they needed immediate surgical intervention. To convince them, he said that without intervention, they could suffer paralysis, or that "the head would fall off," noted the U.S. Attorney's Office "because there was almost nothing attaching the head to the patient's body." The complaint described, in horrifying detail, injuries to at least three hundred patients who opted to go to the OR. Why, under the circumstances, Durrani's hospital allowed him to continue to operate is unclear, but from a financial perspective, he was an MVP: He'd brought in $7 million in Medicare reimbursements in a thirty-six-month period.

In 2013, the state of Ohio brought charges against Durrani for performing unnecessary spinal surgeries and then billing private and public health insurance companies for millions of dollars in fraudulent claims. Medical boards in both Kentucky and Ohio suspended his medical licenses. Facing a thirty-six-count federal indictment and 285 pending lawsuits, the surgeon fled to his native country, Pakistan, leaving his wife and three children behind. One lawsuit charged that he had never actually attended medical school. It was "highly doubtful" that he would return to the United States, his attorney said. In 2015, one of several hospitals in which Durrani had OR privileges agreed to reimburse the U.S. government for more than $4.1 million. The personal injury lawsuits remain unsettled, and Durrani is still a fugitive. According to *Orthopedics This Week*, by 2015 he had established his own spine surgery clinic in Lahore, Pakistan.

In Florida, between 2000 and 2012, in part owing to the active surgical practice of Daytona Beach neurosurgeon Federico C. Vinas, the number of spinal fusions rose fivefold. Nearly half of those surgeries were performed on patients diagnosed with "degenerative disc disease." In a whistle-blower case in 2009, Halifax Health's compliance officer sued the hospital, asserting that kickbacks, illegal physician contracts, and unnecessary back surgeries had occurred. The *Washington Post* reported that Vinas performed three or four spinal fusion surgeries every day at Halifax Health Medical Center, roughly three times the customary number, sometimes operating four or five times on the same patient. When external hospital auditors inspected the records, they found that 90 percent of the surgeries he performed were not considered medically necessary.

When the feds got involved, they alleged that Vinas, and other doctors, had been compensated based on the number of patients they referred to the hospital. Under the Stark Law, such contracts compromised patient safety because they offered doctors a financial motive. (Vinas disputed the findings, and Halifax Health has said that subsequent reviews validated the surgeries.)

The hospital insisted that all its contractual agreements with physicians were in accord with federal requirements. The facility declined to pursue Vinas, and also left two other high-roller neurosurgeons untouched. The *Washington Post* reported that the three doctors each generated more than $2 million in hospital profits, which considerably enhanced their personal bonuses.

Ultimately, Halifax Health agreed to pay $90 million to settle the case, avoiding any admission of wrongdoing. Halifax Health also maintains it never delivered inappropriate care.

Despite his troubles, at the time of writing, Federico C. Vinas's physician profile still appeared on Halifax Health's website. Yet, when I called the hospital to check on his status, the person I spoke to said that she had no record of him. His office phone number had been disconnected. But his Healthgrades web profile, probably the first mention that a prospective patient would find in a Google search, listed no sanctions, no malpractice claims, and no board actions against him.

6

Google Your Spine Surgery

THE TRUTH ABOUT "CUTTING-EDGE"
PROCEDURES, AS ADVERTISED
ONLINE AND ON TV

IN THE SPRING of 2008, when I began looking for a solution, I knew
nothing of the mayhem I have just described. I was still convinced
that surgery was the way to go, and I was determined to find the best
surgeon in the business, even if it meant traveling to another city.
My husband, a big sports fan, did some research and discovered that,
down in Marina del Rey, near Los Angeles, eminent orthopod Robert
Watkins III was "the spine guy" for Joe Montana, Peyton Manning,
Wayne Gretzky, and Dwight Howard. With some of the highest-
earning athletes in the world as his patients, he could not afford to
make mistakes.

To my surprise, it took just a few weeks to get an appointment
with Watkins. In June, on the short flight south, I carried my yellow
envelope of scans and a stack of completed medical forms that had
been sent from his office. One of those forms included a coloring book
outline, front and back, of a human figure. As directed, I'd drawn
dashes to identify areas of numbness, circles for pins and needles,
crosshatches for burning sensations, slash marks for stabbing pain,
and plus signs for aching. Accordingly, the lower right quadrant of
my low back was tattooed black with crosshatches. Slashes tumbled
down the right buttock, hip, and thigh and then trickled to speckles
from the knee down to the foot.

Within moments of my arrival at the Marina Spine Center, Robert Watkins III, white-haired and gently self-assured, joined me in the exam room. I told him about my rounds of physical therapy and why in the past I'd avoided spinal injections. When he asked what prescription drugs I was taking, I said I took Aleve, and stayed away from painkillers because I could not afford to have a fuzzy mind.

After he performed a hands-on exam, checking my range of motion, gait, reflexes, and motor strength, Watkins sent me over to the hospital for a CT scan of my facet joints to see if inflammation there might be causing the pain. He said that his office would be in touch with the results and handed me a note to give to the security detail at the airport, where the radioactive dye that remained in my body after the scan would be likely to set off alarms. In a few weeks, he said, I should plan to return to Marina del Rey for more tests, including discography and electromyography (EMG). I left with the feeling that I was in exceptionally good hands.

Regrettably, that call never came. Every couple of days, I telephoned the office, only to be shuttled to a voice mail recording that answered the call by chirping "prescription drug line." In mid-July, Watkins said that his assistant would schedule my diagnostic procedures in Los Angeles, immediately. A few days later, as I headed for the airport, anxious to get the show on the road, that assistant let me know that the electromyography machine was broken and my appointment had been canceled. I rescheduled, only to learn, less than twenty-four hours before I was supposed to arrive, that Watkins had "canceled the day," evidently because one of his athletes was in duress. Beyond that, because two months had slipped away since my initial visit, my health plan's preapproval for the diagnostic procedures had expired, and Watkins's office would have to obtain these again. Exasperated, I told the receptionist that I'd be in touch when I returned from a two-week, multicity speaking gig. I should have been eager, but frankly, it was hard to think of anything beyond the thudding pain in my back and hip, and how much worse it was going to get when I was on the road.

ROBERT WATKINS IS a leader in his field, a highly respected "conventional" spine surgeon, which means that he sticks with well-accepted protocols and avoids faddish procedures. But, as I was about to discover, there were other options.

As my plane took off for Philly, an ad featuring a bikini-clad woman on a beach, a Band-Aid stuck to the small of her back, grabbed my attention. The copy read: "Just two weeks ago I had back surgery. Thank you, Laser Spine Institute." Reading further down the page, I learned that 97 percent of patients recommended this safe, fast, and apparently bloodless minimally invasive procedure, which took less than an hour. Apparently, you could expect to "get your life back" immediately.

As soon as I was on the ground, I found a wireless connection and went directly to the Laser Spine Institute's website. Happy patients at LSI's facility in Tampa, Florida, waxed euphoric, including their full names and hometowns in their endorsements. Patients had to be incredibly impressed to be willing to do that, I reasoned, feeling my journalist's customary skepticism ebb away.

Laser Spine Institute described itself as "the premier health care provider in spinal surgery." Physicians there employed "a wide variety of laser-assisted techniques," performed while the patient was "under local anesthetic." The Band-Aid on the woman on the beach covered "only one three-millimeter incision at the surface." Naively, I reasoned that an incision that small meant that the disruption of the bones and soft tissue beneath the skin was also minimal. Desperate for a solution, and just as LSI's direct-to-consumer marketers hoped that I would, I picked up the phone.

BEFORE WE MOVE on, a quick explanation. There is a type of minimally invasive spine surgery that's so sophisticated that only a short list of spine surgeons who were fellowship-trained in this super-specialty ever perform it. They do their work at university hospitals, accomplishing remarkable things through many small incisions.

They straighten the spines of patients with scoliosis, and repair those of patients who have suffered devastating disease. These procedures are minimally invasive only in comparison to open procedures that involve ten-inch-long incisions.

But those advanced procedures do not involve lasers. They are not sold through consumer marketing channels. For the most part, the advertisements that pop up in your Internet browser sell two approaches. In a "percutaneous procedure," the physician makes a tiny incision, just long enough to slip a narrow tube containing a probe and a laser beneath the skin. The probe breaches the disc's tough shell, entering the nucleus, where a laser vaporizes a bit of tissue, thereby reducing pressure on the nerve root.

In the other type of procedure, referred to as "endoscopic," the physician inserts one or more tubular retractors, which hold crochet-hook-sized surgical instruments, as well as a fiber-optically equipped video camera that sends images to a computer monitor. Although endoscopic procedures are described as "minimally invasive," in many cases, they require several inch-long incisions, as well as cutting through muscles and ligaments and grinding away at bone. Therefore, an endoscopic disc decompression is not necessarily "less invasive" than a conventional microdiscectomy.

The laser spine surgery craze took hold in the mid-1990s, but it took more than a decade for a well-designed Cochrane Collaboration review to show that the minimally invasive procedure, which resulted in higher levels of nerve root injury, dural tears, and reoperation rates, was not safer than a conventional microdiscectomy. The minimally invasive group had a 38 percent revision rate, more than double that of the group that underwent the standard procedure. Patients who had conventional microdiscectomy recovered faster than those in the laser surgery group, and they required fewer than half as many return trips to the operating suite.

Despite conventional microdiscectomy's superior performance, when compared with a minimally invasive approach, it should not be assumed that the procedure is always successful. As I mentioned earlier, both Golden State Warriors head coach Steve Kerr and golf legend Tiger Woods would tell you that plenty can go wrong. Kerr's conventional microdiscectomy in the summer of 2015, to relieve sciatic pain, culminated in a dural tear and a cerebrospinal fluid leak, leaving him to suffer excruciating headaches and fatigue. Even after a second surgery, to fix the leak, Kerr was stuck at home for more than half the Warriors' season.

Tiger Woods, the winner of more than one hundred pro-golf events worldwide, had a conventional microdiscectomy in 2014 and yet another in 2015. Both failed, leading to a third procedure in October 2015. Eight months later, at a press conference, Woods was downcast. He did not know when or if he would be able to play again. "I have no answer for that. Neither does my surgeon or my physio," he said. "There is no timetable. There's really nothing I can look forward to, nothing I can build toward."

Despite such unpredictable outcomes, patients remain drawn to the mystique of the quick and bloodless minimally invasive procedure. The Cedars-Sinai spine surgeon Hyun Bae explained that the high incidence of "failed backs" had put patients off conventional procedures. Stepping into that vacuum, direct-to-consumer marketers had made minimally invasive spine surgery look much better than it actually was. "It's not because the procedure is good," he said, "It's because of errors that spine surgeons have made over the last quarter century. We've done it to ourselves."

WITHIN FORTY-FIVE MINUTES of my first call to LSI, I heard back from the bubbly patient coordinator, who invited me to FedEx my MRI for a free assessment. In the course of a long discussion about what I might expect at LSI, I explained that I was a journalist and thought I might write about my experience in Tampa. In less than forty-eight hours, the coordinator called back, to say she had great news for me. LSI's physicians had already reviewed my scans and determined that I was a candidate for surgery. Two weeks hence, LSI could do my procedure in Tampa.

The bad news was that my health plan, Anthem Blue Cross, was not part of LSI's provider network. The cost for LSI's standard five-day stay, to be paid in advance, was $30,000 out of pocket, a tariff that did not include airfare, accommodations, or meals. When I called Anthem, I learned that if I used any of the company's in-network surgeons, my out-of-pocket costs would top out at $8,000. Accordingly, I told the LSI patient coordinator that $30,000 was way out of my budget.

A few weeks later, a direct-mail solicitation from LSI arrived. If I was willing to schedule my surgery "off-season," just prior to Thanksgiving or Christmas, the fee for the five days would be $8,000, exactly what I'd have to pay if I used one of Anthem's in-network surgeons. The $8,000 could go on my credit card once I arrived in Tampa. As so many of us do, I reasoned that I'd given conservative treatment and conventional spine medicine my best shot—and gotten nowhere. Intent upon wearing my own post-op Band-Aid to the beach, I called LSI to book my dates.

I'd arrive on a Thursday, have my evaluation and tests on Friday and Monday, and undergo the procedure on Tuesday. Wednesday I'd recover, and Thursday evening I'd be on a plane to New York, where I planned to celebrate a pain-free Thanksgiving with my parents, spouse, and children and the rest of my extended family.

Working from the full names and locations that were posted on LSI's website, I contacted several recent LSI alums, identifying myself on the phone as a prospective patient. The few people I reached told me it had been a great experience. The LSI team was fabulous. When I asked how their backs were, some said they felt great. Others were not so sure; only time would tell. I figured that the half dozen or so who didn't return my calls were out playing eighteen holes, or strolling down the beach, or just didn't feel like talking about medical things with a complete stranger.

With my departure for Tampa just a few days away, I hustled to obtain the pre-op testing that LSI had ordered. On Thursday evening, limping after the cross-country flight, I made my way to my room at an extended-stay Marriott, equipped with a kitchenette. On Friday morning, LSI sent its van, the Shuttlefly, to collect me. A half-dozen patients, staying at other local hotels, were already on board, as ebullient as if they were tourists off to view the Taj Mahal. The shuttle driver told us about LSI patients who had come from places as distant as Canada, Japan, Europe, South America, Russia, and Lithuania. Conspiratorially, he revealed that the president of Cameroon, accompanied by his entourage, had been treated at the Tampa facility. As we made our way into LSI's showy marble-clad lobby, we congratulated one another. Clearly, we'd made the right decision.

Standing in line to drop off my scans, I chatted with a handsome, older Mobile, Alabama, couple, and a Moravian family from Indiana. The Moravian women wore ankle-length dresses, caps, and aprons, while the men were dressed in overalls, their beards brushing their collarbones. A college student whose bad back had benched him, and who was at LSI hoping to avoid the loss of his athletic scholarship, sat with his dad. A tattooed young man in a sleeveless undershirt tried to get comfortable lying on the floor, at the feet of his pregnant wife, who occupied a chair. No matter where, or under what circumstances, we'd started our journeys, we were now boats in the same hurricane, seeking safe harbor.

As I listened to people's stories, I recognized that nearly everyone had discovered LSI online. Often the researcher was a worried relative or spouse, who searched for help on the company's website. For many, coming to Tampa meant major financial sacrifices. Patients' out-of-pocket costs could amount to tens of thousands of dollars. To pay the fees, people had mortgaged or remortgaged their homes, emptied their retirement accounts, and procured high-interest loans. Boats, cars, and trucks had been hocked. One Canadian woman, in her seventies, explained her thinking: "What good is money if you're in pain? If you can't enjoy every living, breathing moment?"

Between appointments, several dozen patients and their support teams hung out in a dozen or so zero-gravity recliners, lined up along the walls of the large, sunny dayroom, referred to as "the café." At the buffet, we helped ourselves to hot dishes and got lattes and cappuccinos from the high-tech coffee machine. In that room, there was a powerful feeling of camaraderie.

By midday, the patients who had undergone procedures that morning began to return to the café, with stretchy flesh-colored lumbar braces wrapped around their abdomens. Their eyes were glazed and they walked gingerly, but their smiles were exultant.

As I chatted with people in the café, I asked what had brought them there. Because she saw this operation as his last hope, Sheryl Weber, a vital woman in her late sixties, had driven her husband from Palm Beach all the way across the peninsula. In his mid-seventies, John had Parkinson's disease. He'd already had eight spine surgeries, and for years, he'd relied on painkillers to get through his days.

Rob and Ginger Stage had also seen the LSI ad in an airline magazine. A retired US Airways employee from Pittsburgh, Rob observed that not so long ago, he had prided himself on his ability to lift anything—including a filled water bed. These days, he said morosely, he could hardly manage a bag of groceries.

Lauren,* who after many conversations would request that I use a pseudonym, was pale in the aftermath of a long car ride from her home in Nashville, Tennessee, with her husband. Until three years earlier, she'd been an executive recruiter for technology companies. She'd herniated a disc while carrying a large, soil-filled flowerpot from one side of her patio to the other, she explained. Her doctor prescribed increasing doses of Vicodin, and eventually sent her to pain management, where she was prescribed extended-release opioids, which left her weak, nauseated, and so exhausted she couldn't get out of bed—and still in terrible pain. Her teenage daughter, who felt that she deserved a more attentive mother, wasn't talking to her. This trip to LSI was a birthday present from her loving husband, who really wanted his wife back.

ALTHOUGH MINIMALLY INVASIVE spine surgery didn't become a big deal until Internet marketers started selling it, the approach began to develop in the early 1980s. That's when physicians tested a method of injecting chymopapain, an enzyme derived from the latex of the papaya tree, into the disc's gelatinous interior. The enzyme dissolved proteins inside the disc, which softened and shrank in size, thereby reducing pressure on the spinal nerve root. When the FDA approved chymopapain in 1983, for use in chemonucleolysis, the American Academy of Orthopaedic Surgeons endorsed it. Because this procedure was expected to eliminate half of conventional microdiscectomies, (and thereby cut deeply into revenues), over the next few years seven thousand doctors showed up for one-day training sessions, and treated tens of thousands of patients. In a relatively small number of patients, instead of finding its way into the disc, chymopapain was accidentally injected into the patient's spinal canal, injuring soft tissues and nerves, and causing pain and paralysis. Even when chemonucleolysis was performed correctly, some patients experienced allergic reactions, including anaphylactic shock, which could be fatal.

Almost ten years after chymopapain was introduced, a study showed that chemonucleolysis, perhaps because it had been poorly administered, was not what it had been cracked up to be. In reality, it was hardly more effective than a placebo injection of inactive saline solution. In 2003, the only company that had continued to produce chymopapain finally took it off the market.

At that point the procedure was shelved. With chemonucleolysis out of the picture, two physiatrist brothers, Jeffrey and Joel Saal, invented a procedure called "intradiscal electrothermal treatment," or IDET. This "percutaneous" procedure, which required a minuscule incision, employed a flexible catheter attached to a wire probe that, once inserted into the disc, could be heated to 190°F. The Saal brothers designed their own clinical trials, publishing glowing outcomes in peer-reviewed medical journals. They offered various theories about how IDET worked. Possibly the extreme heat destroyed threadlike nerve endings that infiltrated the annulus of the unhealthy disc and caused pain. Maybe the high internal temperatures broke the collagen bonds in the nucleus pulposus, allowing the fibers to contract and reducing the pressure on adjacent spinal nerve roots. At least in public, the Saal brothers did not acknowledge the possibility that the procedure did nothing at all.

Lured by the prospect of a cheaper, faster procedure, in 1998, private health insurance providers and Medicare agreed to reimburse physicians. Over three years, in a pattern that was already familiar, twenty-five hundred doctors, many of them interventional pain physicians, performed more than seventy-five thousand IDET procedures at roughly $6,000 each.

But in 2005, independent clinical researchers compared IDET with a sham procedure where no electrical current was administered—the patient was merely poked with a needle—and learned that the $6,000 procedure produced outcomes that were no better than those of the sham intervention. Medicare and private insurers stopped paying for IDET, leaving interventional pain physicians in the lurch.

BACK AT THE Laser Spine Institute, Friday and Monday were frenetic days for me. I signed medical releases and credit card receipts, had yet another MRI scan, and met with physicians' assistants and nurse-practitioners. When that was accomplished, the Shuttlefly transported a dozen of us to the pharmacy at CVS, where we stood in line to collect our prescription painkillers, which we'd need after our procedures. I left with a big vial full of hydrocodone tablets.

On Monday night, with pre-op jitters, I set my clock and also ordered a wake-up call for six a.m. Although fifteen to twenty procedures would take place that morning in LSI's very busy ambulatory surgery center, we were all treated as if we were revered guests. With a warm blanket over my legs, I settled into my recliner, and eavesdropped on the conversations beyond the privacy curtains on either side. The women in those chairs, I gleaned from their conversations with nurses and technicians, were both yoga teachers with enduring low back problems.

Soon, four masked and robed physicians conferred in front of a nearby light box to peer at my scans. The plan was to give me a diagnostic injection—a spinal nerve block. This would help them decide whether they should operate on L4–5 or L5-S1. The injection hurt like the dickens, but the usual pain did not abate. They'd do their magic on L4–5, they said. Later, one physician said casually, I might need another procedure at L5-S1. That made me nervous, but gowned and ready to go to the OR, I tried to ignore the possibility that I would not "get my life back," as LSI's advertising had promised.

I'd been told I'd have "twilight anesthesia," but the intravenous sedation I received left me on the distant shoals of consciousness. More than once during the procedure, the surgical team had to rouse me so that I could respond to questions about the location and severity of my pain.

Facedown, on my stomach, my head braced and cushioned, I could see nothing except the anesthesiologist's shoes on the linoleum floor. But if I'd been a fly on the wall, I'd have watched the surgeon insert a laser, burning at 7,500 degrees F, inside a wire probe through the skin alongside my spine, just above the facet joint, sending spidery nerves up in a puff of blue smoke. Then, in a procedure reminiscent of the failed IDET, a heated probe was inserted into the disc, elevating the temperature inside the nucleus pulposus.

Those preliminaries accomplished, the surgeon prepared for the endoscopic part of the procedure. Working ambidextrously, guided only by the procedure's mirror image on the computer monitor, the surgeon held the probe with the camera in his right hand and the suction device in his left. He passed dental-sized cutting and scraping tools back and forth, to make more room for the nerve roots at L4–5. When the laminotomy-foraminotomy procedure was complete, he inserted a large-gauge needle through the skin at the tip of my tailbone, delivering a hefty dose of anti-inflammatory medication, painkillers, and anesthetic, in a "caudal" injection.

ACCORDING TO INFORMATION on LSI's website, most patients' treatments are limited to "puff of blue smoke" nerve ablation and the heated probe procedure. Because those are very minor, it's not surprising that such patients hop merrily off the gurney, prepared to take the famous LSI post-op victory stroll. (Those spidery nerves regenerate within months, unfortunately, and the heated probe has never been shown to work better than a sham intervention.)

But personally, in the hours after the far more invasive laminotomy-foraminotomy, I was so sedated on Demerol, Flexeril, and Percocet that walking anywhere was out of the question. After an hour in post-op, when a nurse tried to help me to my feet, I became shaky and nauseated, broke into a cold sweat, and nearly sank to the floor. It was five p.m., many hours after I'd left the OR, before a sweetheart of a nurse drove me back to the Marriott, where my overnight caregiver, a home health aide, took over. As I staggered from the car and into a wheelchair, it occurred to me that this was nuts: In my condition, I didn't belong in a hotel suite. I belonged in a hospital bed, under medical supervision.

Dutifully, I took my hydrocodone tablets and settled into some lively dreams. In the morning, after breakfast and more drugs, I felt okay as I climbed the two steps onto the Shuttlefly van. Two physical therapy appointments were included in the LSI package. The PT was a straight shooter from South Africa. It was good I had shown up for my appointment, she said, because many LSI patients didn't bother: they had the surgery and left it at that. When she asked me to show her how I rose from a chair, I staggered to my feet without bending any part of my spine, and nearly toppled over backward. That wouldn't do at all, she said, showing me how to wiggle to the edge of the seat and use my arms to push off.

She told me to avoid lifting or carrying anything over five pounds for at least several weeks, and to abstain from hauling heavy items or lifting them over my head in the future. Numbly, I tried to imagine how that would work. What about the dreaded overhead compartment? What about the stacks of documents that went with me everywhere? What about the boxes of groceries from Costco? That *was* my life. Wasn't I supposed to be getting it back?

On Day Two, as the payload from the caudal injection washed over the soft tissues, calming inflamed nerve roots, I felt better than I had in years. In fact, I called an old friend to tell him I was cured, and was dancing around the hotel parking lot. When he asked me what I was on, I thought he was trying to be funny.

I WAS CLEARED to leave Tampa on Thursday afternoon. The morning before my scheduled departure, the nurse who had returned me to the hotel room knelt beside me in the café, and asked if I would like to provide a testimonial. I felt amazingly great, I told her; of course I would. I still had not recognized that my pain-free euphoria had more to do with the opioids in my bloodstream than with a sustainable improvement—or that the same situation prevailed for many of the patients in the room. Instead, I took up the clipboard I'd seen in others' hands, to write a glowing, if narcotics-addled, account of my experience. Glassy-eyed and deadly pale, I smiled for the camera, so that my picture might also hang in the gallery of satisfied customers.

Flying to New York three days after surgery was not the best idea, especially while I was stoned on painkillers. But for several days that followed, I strolled the city streets, feeling as if I owned Manhattan. On Thanksgiving Day, defying the PT's orders, I pulled a large casserole of baked yams and marshmallows out of my sister's lower oven and humped it across the kitchen, as if I were once again invincible.

Ten days later, back at home in California, and exactly twelve hours after taking my last hydrocodone tablet, I was sure I'd come down with the flu. The vial was empty, and I was sweaty, shaky, and sick to my stomach. My back ached, but so did every other joint in my body. I wouldn't realize for many months that it wasn't a virus. After two weeks on the drugs, I was going through opioid withdrawal.

When a staffer from LSI called me to check on my progress, I said that although my leg pain was improved, the pain that gnawed at me as I sat at my desk was unchanged. After years of dealing with a right foot that was numb, I was glad to reacquaint myself with my toes, but my feet were either ice cold or far too hot, prickling with "pins and needles." The LSI physician who phoned back said that the pressure on the spinal nerve had been released, and my foot had come back to life. The paresthesia would last for a while; my central nervous system was just confused. To deal with the pain from sitting, he advised, I might consider undergoing a series of epidural steroid injections. Or, if I wanted to return to Tampa for a second procedure at L5-S1, he could offer $500 off the standard $30,000 fee. The $8,000 I'd paid for the last go-round was definitely a onetime thing.

I hung up, with a lump in my throat, a familiar pain in my right buttock, and a bad case of buyer's remorse.

OVER THE NEXT twelve months, I checked in regularly with the friends I'd made at LSI. Sheryl Weber related that before she and her husband, John, left LSI for good, they'd spent $37,000 on several unsuccessful procedures. Later, at the Mayo Clinic, Sheryl was distressed to see doctors grimace and raise their eyebrows when they heard that the couple had been to LSI. John was taking such high doses of opioids, Sheryl said, that at any time he could suffer a fatal overdose.

"I never stop trying, because the person I love is in such pain," Sheryl said. "They should not have accepted him as a patient at LSI. They should have been able to identify that he was not a candidate because he'd had so many failed surgeries before and he was obviously in poor condition."

Nor did Rob Stage's wife, Ginger, have good news. The couple had returned to LSI three times, for four procedures. After the first operation, there was a tiny bit of improvement—enough to make him want to try again, and again. "It's like he went to Las Vegas and got slot madness," Ginger said. By the summer of 2010, after the fourth surgery, Rob couldn't stand unsupported for more than five minutes. He'd undergone lumbar spinal fusion, which did not help. "He still has pain, every day, and although I've tried to encourage it, he's done almost no rehab," his wife said sadly. Her husband was worn out, and frankly, so was she. And she'd just about used up her considerable storehouse of empathy.

Lauren, whose birthday present from her husband was surgery at LSI, said she'd left Tampa in great pain. She had also lost all sensation in her left leg. Back in Nashville, she had two disc decompression procedures. Although her goal, prior to surgery, had been to taper her dose of painkillers, instead she needed more: 180 milligrams of morphine a day, supplemented with Percocet for breakthrough pain. Her husband was working in another city, coming home only for weekends.

When her pain management doctor refused to write any more prescriptions, she found a new doctor, who helped her taper her morphine dose by half. She felt the depression lift slightly, and reignited an old passion, becoming a singer in a rock band. When some pictures from that gig turned up on my Facebook page, I offered my congratulations. Maybe things were looking up? "That's Facebook life," she lamented. "That's not real life.

"I want to be positive, to believe that the Lord can heal me," she said. "But there's really no cure. I think about death all the time." I worried about Lauren; I had the feeling that one day, I would find my e-mail message returned to sender, and I would know she had not survived. But just before this book went to the printer, I saw a picture of her on Facebook, in a hospital bed, oxygen tubes in her nostrils, with her fingers raised in a hopeful "V" for victory. After a decade of pain, she'd just had a lumbar spinal fusion. The message accompanying her photo read, "Hi, Facebook family. I have not been on here for a while because of waiting on this. . . . Doc told us it could not have gone any better." I asked her to let me know how she was doing as soon as she was able. I heard nothing, and that image of her in the hospital bed stayed at the top of her Facebook feed.

ALTHOUGH MY CONFIDANTES were not among the success stories, there were LSI patients who were very happy with their outcomes. Laser Spine Institute's CEO, Bill Horne, introduced to me several, among them, a Texas investor in slick cowboy boots and khaki slacks named Carl Karnes.

He told me that before his stint at LSI, he was "sucking down ten Percocet tablets each day." Just in his early fifties, he walked only with a cane. For eighteen months, his high-flying Dallas spine surgeon had ordered imaging and physical therapy. He sent Karnes for epidural steroid injections and wrote prescriptions for painkillers. When that conservative treatment failed, the surgeon recommended a two-level lumbar spinal fusion. "He said I'd spend three to four weeks in the hospital," Karnes recalled, "and it would be six months before we knew if the surgery was going to be any good. There was a 50 percent chance I would be worse. And I had several friends who were living proof of how badly fusions can fail."

Soon after he'd started taking Percocet, "I just sort of stopped showing up at work one day," he said. After his divorce, although he was granted partial custody of his preteen son, he couldn't "reliably get up in the morning and take a shower, never mind get the boy breakfast and off to school three days a week. It was the drugs, and I knew it was the drugs, but they make you so lazy, so bored with everything, that you can hardly find the energy to make a phone call. You just lie there in your sheets and you don't care."

The day before his pre-op consultation with the surgeon, Karnes joined his girlfriend at a corporate Christmas party. "I was sort of crumpled on a bar stool," he said, "when the guy sitting next to me picked up on the fact that I was in agony." The man was James St. Louis, the anesthesiologist who was preparing to launch LSI. "He told me exactly what he did—how he'd invented this method where instead of cutting through massive amounts of muscle, he inserted tiny metal straws, working them down toward the spine," Karnes explained. "He said that his patients went for a long walk that same afternoon."

The next morning, in preparation for his pre-op appointment, Karnes printed out everything he could find on the Internet about laser and endoscopic surgery, which at that time amounted to barely two pages. "When I handed those over, the surgeon looked at me like I was the devil himself," said Karnes. "And then he told me that what LSI was doing was 'witch doctoring,' and if I ever went to see them, he would release me from care and never write me another prescription for painkillers."

Unhappy with what he perceived as a threat, Karnes canceled his surgical date and pushed to be LSI's first patient. From what he remembers, the entire procedure, which in his case was limited to facet joint ablation—the puff of blue smoke—took about fifteen minutes. Within a month, Karnes reported, he was in the gym three or four times a week. He weaned himself off Percocet, started eating right, and swore never to go near another opioid.

Karnes was so pleased with his outcomes that I wondered if I'd somehow fallen in with a misbegotten crowd in Tampa. In order to perform a more rigorous evaluation, I tracked down the phone numbers of sixty people who had undergone procedures at LSI in 2009. About twenty-five of them answered their phones or returned my calls. When I explained that I was a journalist, and not an LSI marketer, barely a quarter reported satisfactory—but not brilliant— results. Most felt they'd been misled into thinking that they could "get their lives back." More than half planned to return to LSI for additional surgery. Notably, thirty-five people out of the sixty did not respond to my repeated attempts to call. This time, instead of assuming that they were out on the golf course, I wondered whether they had nothing good to say and therefore preferred to say nothing at all.

But the fact that so many were planning to make return trips for more surgery concerned me the most. In a macabre way, the tried-and-true "get the return customer" approach was paying off. David Armstrong, reporting for *Bloomberg Businessweek*, estimated that between 2006 and 2009, LSI's business model consistently generated nearly a 35 percent profit margin, which, wrote Armstrong, made LSI "more profitable than Google." In 2009, Goldman Sachs valued the company at $428 million as part of its proposal for an initial public offering, although ultimately that deal did not go forward. Barely adolescent, it was already a big business—and it was just reaching its growth spurt.

BEHIND THE LASER Spine Institute's ascendancy, there was a soap opera's worth of drama. The cast included Alfred Bonati, the owner of the Bonati Spine Institute; Sam Bailey, an Arkansas preacher/entrepreneur; James St. Louis, the founder and medical director of the Laser Spine Institute, whom Carl Karnes had met at the bar; Lawrence B. Rothstein, an anesthesiologist turned inventor; and Chris Lloyd, a certified public accountant.

Many would say that Alfred Bonati started it all. Long before the Internet offered a broad net in which to catch back pain patients, he developed surgical instruments and techniques for minimally invasive spine surgery and put them to the test on such patients in his clinic in Hudson, Florida. Sam Bailey, the Arkansas preacher, met Bonati in 1996, when he brought his wife Annette to the physician for treatment. He was pleased with her outcome, and the two men talked about Bonati's marketing strategy. Bailey agreed to run seminars at his church, back in his hometown. According to Chris Lloyd, who would eventually go into business with Bailey, after the first seminar, Bonati got fourteen new patients. Ultimately, Bailey ran about 150 "educational seminars," generating hundreds of prospects for Bonati.

In 2002, anesthesiologist James St. Louis, the physician who would eventually lead LSI, joined Bonati's thriving practice in Hudson. For a while, Bailey, Bonati, and St. Louis were a team. But understandably, after the Florida Board of Medicine sanctioned Bonati for performing unnecessary, inappropriate, and harmful procedures, and he settled the first of several pending malpractice cases for $3.1 million, St. Louis and Bailey decided that Bonati was not a great bet. With the backing of several investors, the men prepared to launch Laser Spine Institute. At the eleventh hour, when the financiers announced that they wanted a bigger piece of the pie, the one to sacrifice his share was Bailey, the Arkansas preacher, which made him so furious that later he would pursue LSI for reparations amounting to hundreds of millions of dollars.

Having been involved in developing the business plan, Sam Bailey recognized that LSI had a problem in the OR. One of the local anesthetics used in the procedure rapidly reached a neurotoxic dose. It meant that Laser Spine Institute doctors had to get in and out fast, and therefore were restricted to operating on a single vertebral level in one session.

Bailey was starting over, and this time, he went hunting for bells-and-whistles technology that would eliminate the one-level-only restriction. When he met Dayton, Ohio, anesthesiologist Lawrence Rothstein, who had recently developed a surgical instrument he called the AccuraScope, he called his business associate Chris Lloyd to evaluate the technology's financial prospects.

Specifically, Rothstein had connected a conventional steerable catheter equipped with a video camera to a 2.5 mm laser. The steerable catheter could be threaded through the skin and into the tiny opening in the sacrum, at the base of the spine. From there, as the video-guided camera/catheter/laser combo traveled upward, in the space between the bony walls of the vertebrae and tough covering of the dural sac, the laser burned away the disc material that impinged on spinal nerves. Using light as an energy source, the laser carved away soft tissue with bursts of heat, but did not whittle through bone. To patients, as Bonati had discovered, "laser surgery" sounded state-of-the-art. But in truth, in the presence of delicate nerves, lasers were hard to manage, and in the spine this made it remarkably easy for something to go wrong.

Chris Lloyd and Sam Bailey were so impressed with the Accura-Scope that they overlooked Lawrence Rothstein's many pending malpractice lawsuits, as well as the temporary 2001 suspension of his Ohio medical license after his arrest for felony cocaine possession. The three formed North American Spine, a Texas-based LLC. According to court documents, Rothstein's deal, as chief medical officer, involved a salary of $700,000 a year, plus a $5,000 bonus for each surgery. Three months after Rothstein joined North American Spine, the courts awarded a $1.3 million judgment for an epidural steroid injection that resulted in permanent nerve damage to a patient who had been injured prior to the company's formation. Seven months later, in another malpractice claim, a patient who suffered brain damage in Rothstein's clinic, from a post-op overdose of pain medication, was awarded $5 million.

I asked Chris Lloyd why he'd gone into business with Rothstein. "I knew exactly who I was getting in bed with," he replied. "I read him spot-on from the get-go. He had a horrible bedside manner. He tended to overpromise relative to what he had a statistical chance of delivering, and he was rather cavalier about building really high expectations in patients." Still, Lloyd and Bailey felt that Rothstein could be "handled" and that the AccuraScope procedure was promising enough to make up for its inventor's foibles.

By 2010, faced with more than forty pending malpractice suits, Rothstein filed for bankruptcy. The courts dismissed most of the lawsuits, leaving many injured patients with no recourse. Anxious to cut their ties with him, Bailey and Lloyd agreed to pay Rothstein $3.5 million over five years for the right to market the AccuraScope and quickly shifted the company's operations from Dayton to Dallas.

In April 2013, the State Medical Board of Ohio permanently revoked Lawrence Rothstein's medical license. The surrender document, as lurid as any I have read, recorded his "inappropriately utilized laser endoscopic technique" and noted that he performed procedures "that were clinically contraindicated," for which he "failed to provide appropriate follow-up care." It included a list of twelve patients who had been hurt, and specifically detailed their grisly injuries.

With ample evidence of how wrong things could go, Chris Lloyd and Sam Bailey sought to bulletproof the company against future medical malpractice lawsuits. On its website and in TV commercials and infomercials, North American Spine seemed to be a medical facility. But if you read the very fine print, you'd see that the company did not provide medical services. Instead, it sold marketing and office services to "partner physicians," primarily pain management doctors looking to add another tool to their kit. Under Bailey and Lloyd, North American Spine would be folded into a larger company that also owned ambulatory surgery centers.

Health plans might not pay for the AccuraScope procedure. But often they'd reimburse generously for the use of an ambulatory surgical center, making up for the loss of other fees. North American Spine's bills could get very high indeed. After her procedure, one woman reported a total bill of $94,514, according to the *Dallas Morning News*, with charges that included "$25,000 for the operating room and $9,000 for anesthesia supplies, for a procedure that took only about 45 minutes." The "recovery room" fee was $6,000.

Even without Rothstein in the OR, outcomes were not always great. Since North American Spine did not actually employ physicians, the company was not liable for medical malpractice suits resulting from the surgeons' use of the AccuraScope. The *Dallas Morning News* reported that Myrda Sue Ford sustained a severe neurological injury during the procedure, according to the expert witness in her case. When it was settled, she received $199,000, a third of which went into the pockets of her lawyer and her insurance company.

When I contacted some North American Spine patients who had posted negative comments on Facebook and elsewhere, I heard back from several, including Ken Miller, a sixty-four-year-old cop at the Tulsa, Oklahoma, airport, who suffered from painful spinal stenosis. He told me that prior to his procedure at North American Spine in Dallas in 2012, a spine surgeon had recommended a two-level spinal fusion, which Miller felt would end his career as a beat cop. Because he didn't want to spend his days sitting in a windowless office, he sent his MRI to North American Spine. According to Miller, the representative who phoned the next day cited an 87 percent success rate. She assured him that doctors could "get him squared away in Texas" and that most patients were "running around within two weeks."

His health insurance provider would have paid for conventional spine surgery, but it identified the AccuraScope procedure as experimental, and turned it down. Miller got a loan on his truck in order to pay $18,500 in cash.

"After it was done and I went home," Miller told me, "I didn't feel better at all. I was in severe pain, day and night." He saw an orthopedic surgeon who compared his MRI from before his AccuraScope treatment with a brand-new one and pointed out that the two were identical. In 2013, Miller went elsewhere to have a procedure to treat his spinal stenosis, but the operation left him with a severe infection and considerable spinal instability. It seemed certain that, despite his effort to avoid it, a multiple-level lumbar spinal fusion was in his future. While he was still in the hospital recuperating, he got a call from a doctor at North American Spine who advised him that if he agreed to hold the company harmless from further lawsuits, he'd get a check in the mail to reimburse him for $18,500.

FOR THE FRUSTRATED patient, direct-to-consumer medicine, such as exists at LSI, North American Spine, and countless other entities crawling the Web, appears to be the best way to skirt the relentless red tape of the medical-industrial complex. But it's essential to realize that health care companies that market their services this way on the Internet exist in a regulatory netherworld. The institutions that patients expect to safeguard them—among others, the FDA, the American Medical Association, and the Joint Commission on Accreditation of Healthcare Organizations (JCAHO, or the Joint Commission, for short)—exercise little or no authority over how such entities conduct their businesses. Although ads that drugmakers pay for typically carry disclaimers, there are far fewer such requirements for outfits that sell surgical procedures, so they can tout convenience, speed, and the size of the incision without ever discussing risks.

To stay afloat—especially when outcomes are at best mediocre—direct-to-consumer marketing organizations must consistently expand their sales territory. More than 80 percent of LSI's patients come from outside the state of Florida. To grow, and to compete in what would become a fierce war for customers, North American Spine had to go after and capture LSI's territory—with Google serving as the battleground.

That meant that North American Spine would have to spend at least as much as LSI on Google advertising to ensure that when a person typed in a relevant search term, the company's name would be at the top of the list of what are known as "organic" search engine results, rather than paid advertising. In 2010, LSI spent more than $200,000 a month to secure the company's premier position. The company also spent money on television commercials that ran on daytime cable TV and during the six o'clock news, featuring putative LSI alums as they went out jogging with the dog, hoisted grandkids, and worked in the garden. By 2013, with North American Spine nipping at its heels, LSI's marketing budget approached $10 million. Still, North American Spine would strategize so cunningly that by 2014, that company appeared to have edged out LSI in Google search results for "laser spine" or "minimally invasive spine surgery," in ads that consistently popped up in my browser.

To keep a steady stream of patients coming in, LSI needed a brand extension. The company introduced "minimally invasive stabilization" or "MIS," extolling it as an alternative to conventional spinal fusion surgery. But there were more similarities than differences. Like spinal fusion, MIS was performed under general anesthesia and also involved surgical implantation of hardware. But while lumbar spinal fusion patients typically spent at least a couple of days under scrutiny as hospital inpatients, LSI's "minimally invasive stabilization" patients departed the ambulatory surgery center for their hotel rooms within hours of the operation. The prospect of a fast turnaround surely attracted some patients, but it meant that no medical staff or rescue equipment was at hand.

LSI's other new product, called RegenaDISC, was meant to capitalize on the public's increasing interest in regenerative medicine. After they extracted mesenchymal stem cells from a patient's bone marrow, LSI's physicians introduced these "endogenous" cells (meaning they were extracted from the patient's body) into damaged intervertebral discs, using a laser to stimulate their growth. If things went according to plan, the cells would differentiate into cartilage cells, and continue to divide and reproduce, strengthening a disc's tough annulus and bulking up the nucleus pulposus.

This procedure was fast and easy and left no scar. On the surface, it made sense. But sadly, it didn't square with what scientists like now-retired Oxford University professor Jill Urban had learned about cartilage and intervertebral disc biology. Urban, whose career was devoted to studying cartilage metabolism in the intervertebral disc, recognized that stem cells require blood and oxygen to survive. In knee, hip, and shoulder joints, such nutrients are plentiful. But a healthy intervertebral disc is as hydraulic as a jellyfish, absorbing fluids at night and expelling them during the day. A degenerated disc could barely manage to feed itself, never mind find a way to nurture tender implanted stem cells, which were likely to shrivel and die. Because the FDA had not approved any kind of stem cell protocol for routine clinical use, insurers regarded these protocols as experimental. A patient who wanted this procedure could pay as much as $25,000 out of pocket for the RegenaDISC treatment.

Many scientists have expressed concerns about endogenous stem cell implantation. In an article in *Nature*, Harvard stem cell biologist George Daley said he would be very wary about infusing these cells into patients, and "certainly concerned if practitioners are charging patients for medical procedures that haven't been proven to work and could in fact be harmful."

While patient coordinators at LSI were explaining MIS and stem cell implantation to prospective patients, management was dealing with a flurry of lawsuits. "It's a litigious world out there," sighed Dotty Bollinger, who at the time was LSI's COO. "There are so many sharks in the water that I don't sleep at night." Bollinger was such a bright and congenial woman that I felt sorry for her. The Bailey lawsuit was still pending in appeals court. A new lawsuit had been filed by Alfred Bonati, who contended that LSI had sent spies into his Hudson, Florida, facility. Beyond those legal hurdles, professional wrestler Hulk Hogan (real name: Terry Bollea) had filed a medical malpractice lawsuit for $50 million.

By any measure, Hogan was in tough shape, after more than thirty years of being slammed to the mat with enormous force. He suffered from a number of health conditions, including degenerative scoliosis, spondylolisthesis, and severe spinal stenosis.

Hogan's lawyers asserted that LSI's direct-to-consumer marketing team had sold the wrestler a set of inappropriate procedures over nineteen months. They claimed damages of $50 million in "past and potential future income" because the minimally invasive procedures at LSI left their client physically incapacitated. It had not helped that, after the procedures failed, Hogan discovered that a headshot he'd autographed for the personal use of an LSI employee was hanging on the wall of patient testimonials and had also made its way onto the company's website.

At the end of 2010, Hogan underwent a three-level 360-degree lumbar spinal fusion with doctors from the University of South Florida's neurosurgery team. As of July 2016, his lawsuit with LSI remained unresolved. (Hogan had, however, won a jury award of $115 million from Gawker Media, which had published on its website an excerpt of a tape that featured the wrestler having sex with a friend's wife.)

By that time, LSI had expanded to seven ambulatory surgery centers strung across the United States and professed to perform five thousand spine operations annually. Having outgrown the building where I'd had my surgery, the company was developing a large dedicated "campus" in Tampa. The website still bristled with testimonials, in many cases obtained from patients who were only a few hours post-surgery, but the last names had disappeared. Dotty Bollinger told me in an e-mail that too many patients had been bothered when prospective customers ignored the list of spokespeople that LSI provided, instead tracking them down and peppering them with questions.

IN 2008, WHEN I started searching for it, the term "minimally invasive spine surgery" brought up half a page of entries on Google. Seven years later, that same search term produced about three-quarters of a million hits, including dozens of pages containing references to the Laser Spine Institute, the Bonati Spine Institute, and North American Spine. At times, the search engine was tone-deaf: I'd find a paid ad for a particular doctor or clinic beside a link to a news article that reported malfeasance at the very same clinic. Major hospitals, desperate not to lose patients to direct-to-consumer medical facilities, began advertising their commitment to minimally invasive spine surgery approaches, not because it was safer or more effective but because it was a sexy buzzword and the only way to compete for patients with sophisticated direct-to-consumer marketers.

Scattered through the search results, there were countless links to small ambulatory surgery centers, helmed by "board certified" physicians who were typically pain management doctors and not certified by the American Board of Medical Specialties in orthopedic surgery or neurosurgery. New Jersey anesthesiologist Richard Kaul ran one of those clinics. In early 2014, the trade journal *Orthopedics This Week*, a publication that is generally unswervingly supportive of the back pain industry, made an exception and posted an article titled, "What's Next for Spine's Most Notorious Rogue?" He was the founder and medical director of New Jersey Spine and Rehabilitation, about an hour northwest of New York City. Born in India and raised and educated in Britain, where he received his medical degree in 1988, Kaul completed his training in the United States, including a three-year fellowship in anesthesia at Albert Einstein College of Medicine. In turn, he received a medical license from the state of New Jersey. But when he learned he'd need another year and a half of training to qualify for hospital privileges, he returned to the United Kingdom. He and his brother invested in a dental clinic in East London, where he administered anesthesia.

In 1999, a patient who was heavily anesthetized for a tooth extraction went into cardiac arrest and died six days later. A British jury found Kaul guilty of negligent manslaughter and gave him a six-month suspended prison sentence, ultimately removing his license from the national physician registry.

Permanently out of business in the United Kingdom, he returned to the United States. The state of New Jersey graciously renewed his medical license and did not discover his negligent manslaughter conviction until a year or so hence, at which time his license was suspended for six months. While he waited out his suspension, Kaul began attending CME courses in minimally invasive spine surgery, including a two-week course in South Korea.

Preparing to set up a minimally invasive spine surgery practice, Kaul put up a website, where he described himself as a "certified Minimally Invasive Spine Specialist, with expertise diagnosing and treating spinal conditions using Non-Surgical Interventional Pain Techniques." Since there are no established standards for training in minimally invasive spine surgery, he was within his rights. But then he blundered: According to court documents, he began performing very complex spine surgeries, on an outpatient basis, in a one-room ambulatory surgical suite. Physicians who operate in one-room suites in New Jersey are required to have hospital privileges or board permission, but Richard Kaul had neither.

Many of Kaul's patients found him on Google or were referred by doctors, chiropractors, or personal injury lawyers after car accidents. The Bergen County *Record* reported that the auto insurance company Geico filed a lawsuit against Kaul, claiming that he bilked it out of $1 million by paying kickbacks to doctors and chiropractors "to get patient referrals and that most of the treatment he provided to accident victims was unnecessary and billed at inflated rates."

Over several years, he performed about eight hundred procedures, mostly on people whose insurance plans included out-of-network coverage, among them members of unions and people who had personal injury claims. After multiple patient complaints, New Jersey's attorney general demanded that the board of medicine intervene. In March 2014, after twenty-three days of deliberation, the New Jersey medical board took away Richard Kaul's license and fined him $300,000, ordering him to pay the state's litigation expenses of $174,000. The court order states that given the lack of any formal surgical training, Kaul "repeatedly subjected multiple patients to significant complex spinal surgery in a one-room surgery center with no hospital privileges or access to manage life-threatening complications that might occur."

The sworn testimony from eleven patients was unnerving: The Bergen County *Record* reported that "one man . . . testified that he went in expecting an injection for pain and ended up with hours of surgery to remove a disc and fuse two bones in his spine. Others showed long scars from surgery they'd been told would be minimally invasive. They described crippling injuries, intractable pain and the betrayal they felt at the hands of a doctor whose credentials and skills they trusted."

Kaul carried the minimum insurance that the state required of an anesthesiologist, but not the higher level of coverage required to perform spine surgery. When the lawsuits rolled in, the physician's financial resources were quickly exhausted, and he declared bankruptcy. Since he had no hospital affiliation or OR privileges, there was no one else for lawyers to sue, and patients who were harmed would receive minimal compensation.

Instead of slipping away with his tail between his legs, Kaul stepped up his Internet presence. He set up a Facebook page, promoting his philanthropic work at an African clinic, and touted his status as a "humanitarian physician." He posted videos of patients who vouched for him; they said that he was the victim of a smear campaign by jealous orthopedic spine surgeons who wanted to put him out of business. He pointed out that owing to years of course attendance, his background in minimally invasive spine surgery was far more extensive than that of most community spine surgeons. He said he was a victim in a battle for patients, between New Jersey orthopedic spine surgeons and interventional pain physicians, in what he described as a "scope of practice controversy." Ultimately, he sued New Jersey governor Chris Christie, and several New Jersey neurosurgeons, including the state's primary witness against him.

The real question was a tough one. Should interventional pain physicians be allowed to perform spine surgery? Where should the line be drawn? In most states, as long as they did their work in ambulatory surgery centers, there were no restrictions on how far interventional pain physicians could go. For years, they had nibbled away at board-certified spine surgeons' territory. In light of the poor evidence regarding epidural steroid injections, discography, and a slew of other catheter-based spine procedures, there was no reason to think they would stop adding invasive and profitable procedures to their armamentarium. And as a result, many patients who assumed that the guy standing over them in the OR had actually been trained in spine surgery, would discover their error when it was already too late.

Given how discouraged I was when I failed to get help at my community spine clinic and then at the Marina Spine Center, I might have easily become Richard Kaul's misbegotten patient—or one of Alfred Bonati's or Lawrence Rothstein's. I could have joined the club of LSI patients who pursued additional procedures until their bank accounts ran dry. In spite of the fact that I'd agreed to have an operation that left an $8,000 hole in my bank account, and permanently rearranged my spinal anatomy, I was fortunate: Nothing life-destroying happened to me at LSI. Although ultimately, the relief I got from my procedures was minimal, it was the kick in the pants I needed to get started on what would become my real mission: my own physical rehabilitation. That story begins in chapter 10. But first, we must contemplate a couple of other pitfalls.

7

Replacement Parts

WHY A BIONIC LUMBAR SPINE
IS NOT IN THE CARDS

MONTHS AFTER I left LSI, sitting for more than ten minutes was still very difficult. In an airplane or a theater, anywhere you are expected to sit quietly, my squirming bothered the people seated around me. Several of my friends had already had new hips or knees. Once again, they were out riding bicycles, playing tennis, and climbing mountains. If hips and knees could be so readily replaced with artificial joints, why couldn't I get the same deal on a couple of vertebral segments?

I wasn't the first to think of this. For decades, spine surgeons have hunted for a way to preserve motion. The goal was to eliminate the adjacent segment deterioration that is so often a consequence of lumbar spinal fusion.

Alf Nachemson, the innovative Swedish surgeon and researcher, was the first to attempt to engineer a flexible joint in the spine. In the mid-1950s, he stashed a salt water–filled testicular implant between two metal vertebral plates and anchored the hybrid in the disc space. The testicular implants, not designed to bear loads, exploded and collapsed, which quickly ended that experiment.

Ten years later, another Swedish surgeon, Ulf Fernstrom, implanted industrial ball bearings from a local factory in the spines of more than one hundred patients. (President John F. Kennedy, whose back pain was legendary, was rumored to be one of his patients, but that's unconfirmed.) The ball bearings quickly migrated out of the disc space and into the adjacent soft tissues, wreaking havoc with nerves—and yet another effort was scrapped.

Over the next two decades, European surgeons and engineers tested dozens of other designs. In 1982, a promising East German model called the Charité, made with a hard plastic dome sandwiched between two metal plates, finally reached the European market. The Charité wasn't very good: Papers published in European journals noted that the device failed to relieve pain, broke, or worked its way out of the disc space. The vertebral bones sometimes grew together around the device, immobilizing the joint, just as a lumbar spinal fusion would have done. And there was another drawback: After the replacement disc was implanted, scar tissue grew, engulfing the vascular system in the region of the fifth lumbar vertebra. That made removing a failed disc dangerous or impossible.

Despite these drawbacks, the prospect of being the first to bring disc replacement to the U.S. market attracted American device manufacturers. And spine surgeons—aware that interventional pain physicians, using chemonucleolysis and then IDET, were chipping away at their market share—were attracted to a procedure so technically demanding that only they themselves could do it. In 2000, a group of spine surgeons formed the Spine Arthroplasty Society, a professional society intended exclusively for surgeons who wanted to pursue disc replacement.

The Charité, designed in Berlin, was the first artificial disc replacement to enter the FDA regulatory process, in 2004. The proposed labeling would permit the device to be used only in patients no older than sixty, on the premise that younger people would heal faster and better than older people. Two members of the FDA's Charité approval panel, wary of the iffy outcomes of the device's clinical trials, asked the agency to delay a decision until more data could be collected. At the same meeting, André van Ooij, a Dutch surgeon who had performed nearly fifty disc replacements and tracked the performance of hundreds of others, said that after the disc was implanted, many patients suffered from unrelenting leg and back pain. He showed slides revealing broken disc replacement devices with flattened polyethylene cores.

Dallas spine surgeon John Peloza questioned whether the Charité's proposed labeling, for those sixty and younger, was appropriate. What would happen to a thirty-year-old when the disc stopped functioning? Peloza reminded panel members that revision surgery ought to be considered "potentially life-threatening in every case."

FDA administrators decide who will speak at approval panel meetings. That offer was not extended to Berlin-based surgeon Michael Putzier, who was engaged in a retrospective clinical and radiological study of fifty-three Charité implant recipients, about seventeen years after they underwent disc replacement. Sixteen months after the approval panel meeting, when Putzier published his findings, it would be clear that in half those patients, the disc prosthesis had not done its job: The intervertebral joint had fused. For the few patients in whom motion had been preserved, the news was even worse. They were the least satisfied with their outcomes, and the most likely to have undergone dangerous revision surgery. Possibly because they did not have the benefit of Putzier's commentary, the FDA's approval panel voted unanimously to permit the SB Charité III disc, manufactured by DePuy Synthes Spine, a division of Johnson & Johnson, to enter the U.S. market. Beyond excluding patients older than sixty, the approval's labeling barred patients with degenerative disc disease at more than one level.

That was puzzling, because in most instances, disc degeneration—those very common flattened, black, or otherwise damaged discs—occurred at more than one level. Barring patients with degeneration at multiple levels was like saying that the surgery was appropriate only for redheads who didn't have red hair. Still, a JPMorgan medical device analyst forecast that six years after approval, the disc replacement business would be worth $1.7 billion. To substantiate that projection, the Charité would have to find its way into the spines of tens of thousands of patients.

Soon after the FDA's approval, Johnson & Johnson began to train the three thousand American spine surgeons who signed up for sequential three-day hands-on sessions at the company's teaching facility. *Wall Street Journal* reporters described what happened in the classroom, where pairs of surgeons set to work on calf spines, while observing the instructor on a television monitor. "At one operating table," they observed, "Dr. Toselli, the J&J spine-research chief, cut through ligaments covering the front of the spine to reveal the calf's glistening, whitish disk. He removed it methodically with long-handled surgical gouges. After determining the proper size and angle for the implant, Dr. Toselli pried the spine bones apart with a pair of forceps and drove the implant into place with a steel hammer."

During those weekend training sessions, instructors allotted time to explain how to sidestep the greatest stumbling block of all: the prospect that Medicare and private health plans would refuse to reimburse for the procedure. By fall of 2005, surgeons thus trained had implanted more than three thousand devices.

IN THE UNITED States, the "dawn of the motion revolution" got a lot of press, in unlikely places. In *Boston* magazine, a local orthopedist hailed the disc prosthesis as "the most exciting thing in spine surgery in the last 50 years." Anticipating continuing double-digit increases in spinal device sales, Wall Street was enraptured.

Enthusiastic patients asked their surgeons about disc replacement. One of those surgeons was Charles Rosen, the University of California–Irvine spine surgeon who later would help facilitate the passing of the 2010 Physician Payments Sunshine Act.

Rosen's interest in the disc replacement procedure began soon after the FDA approved the Charité disc. "Patients were coming in to see me, clutching folders of printouts they'd found about artificial disc replacement on the Internet," he said. "I was curious, as I am about all new surgical gadgets. I thought I might want to do the procedure. I wanted to see if it made sense.

"There is [among patients] a personality that wants to be the first to do something medical," he added. "They are early adopters. They say, 'I read about this, and it's the newest thing, and I want to try it.' To get it done, they'll mortgage their homes. They'll pay in cash.

They are certain that with *Star Trek* medicine, there is a way to make them better."

But when Rosen studied the three-hundred-page transcript from the Charité's approval meeting, he noted imperfections in the devices' open-jaw design. "Real discs," he explained, referring to ones we are born with, "are squishy and compress easily. They absorb shock. But the Charité was made out of solid metal and plastic. And when you put a big plastic and metal thing into the disc space, you can't compress it or flex it sufficiently, so the force—which a normal disc would absorb—is directed into the back of the spine, crushing the facet joints."

Beyond that, he learned that seventeen of the surgeons who had been involved in the FDA clinical trial had undisclosed financial relationships with the manufacturer. Also, in its clinical trial, the Charité disc was compared with a device known for dismal outcomes—the failed BAK cage. And instead of measuring important benchmarks, such as pain relief, the clinical trials evaluated how well the surgeon had positioned the device, and other end points that Rosen thought were not entirely relevant to the patients' health. That there were no specific provisions in the approval for what to do when the disc wore out made Rosen especially wary.

When the surgeon learned that nearly every major spinal implant manufacturer in the United States planned to follow Charité with a similar product, he issued a formal request to the FDA recommending that Charité's parent company, Johnson & Johnson, should be compelled to withdraw the device from the market. That would prevent new but not significantly different iterations of the disc replacement from riding to FDA approval on Charité's tattered coattails.

When the FDA ignored his request, Charles Rosen teamed up with Gemma Cunningham. A public relations and medical marketing pro, she helped Rosen set up interviews with the *Wall Street Journal* and *The Street*, another investor-focused publication. (Later, Cunningham would become CEO of Truth MD, a company that describes its mission as providing consumers with unbiased information about doctors, drugs, devices, and hospitals.) The Charité's approval, Rosen told reporters, put "the American people potentially at great risk for receiving operations that could fail at a high rate and result in untreatable pain and disability."

But again, Rosen's warnings went unheeded, at least among FDA regulators. The agency moved steadily toward the approval of a next-generation disc prosthesis, the ProDisc-L Total Disc Replacement. The start-up capital to develop the device came, in part, from Viscogliosi Brothers, a private banking and venture capital firm specializing in the orthopedic industry. This time, among the investors were high-profile spine surgeons who would receive an ownership stake, in return for their help in getting the product through the FDA's regulatory process. Just as they had with Charité, the surgeons set the benchmarks for a successful outcome, choosing a 360-degree spinal fusion with instrumentation as the comparison surgery. If ProDisc outcomes measured up, the FDA would allow the disc replacement to enter the market, and the investors *cum* clinical investigators would receive shares in the business worth a total of $175 million.

RUDOLF BERTAGNOLI, A German orthopedist and mechanical engineer, whose ProSpine clinic is located in Bogen, Germany, would train more than three thousand surgeons in fifty-five nations to implant the ProDisc. His wizardry was legendary. Considered one of the most talented spine surgeons in the world, he took on challenging cases that other surgeons would not consider.

In October 2010, Bertagnoli and I (and several thousand others) attended the European Spine Conference, that year held in Warsaw, Poland. After a long morning in a frigid auditorium, listening as papers were presented, we convened as scheduled at his hotel. There was a tempting Viennese café just off the lobby, but Bertagnoli preferred to talk in the privacy of his suite, where his colleagues would not be privy to our conversation. "You know," he said as soon as the elevator doors slid closed, "with fusion, we are just doing a brutal thing to the spine. It's almost medieval to fuse everything and eliminate the function, and take the muscles away from their insertion points, so that the spine can no longer work properly."

He'd found a better way, he said; a miraculous fix. He tapped his laptop's touchpad, to bring up the image of a spinal MRI. But this was no ordinary spine; it was basically bionic. At each of five vertebral levels, there were two metal plates sandwiching a plastic dome. "We are the only clinic that has done five levels," Bertagnoli said proudly. "We usually do two or three." In Germany, the FDA's labeling did not apply: There were no restrictions on the number of levels or the age of the patient. "We do all ages," Bertagnoli said. The owner of the bionic spine on the screen in front of us, he said, was in his sixties, and after this surgery, he was doing wonderfully.

The FDA's determination that the disc should be implanted only in younger people made little sense, Bertagnoli said. He was worried about longevity. No one knew for sure how long the discs would last, and revision was very difficult. "It could be ten years," Bertagnoli said. "It could be twenty—but if you are young or middle-aged when you get that disc, this is not a final surgery." By the time the discs he had implanted wore out, he explained, he expected to have developed the technology and finesse to replace them.

In expert hands, the surgery was complex but still manageable, Bertagnoli said. But disc replacement manufacturers wanted the procedure to become part of every spine surgeon's tool kit. As a superstar surgeon and expert trainer, Bertagnoli would be expected to make this happen. But what he saw in the course of two- or three-day training programs left him with grave doubts.

"The manufacturers act as if this is a simple procedure," Bertagnoli said, "but it is not a matter of installing a replacement part, as we do with automobiles and TV sets. We are using this device in human bodies, and it is the surgeon's job to know what that individual's problems are and how to correct them."

After Bertagnoli introduced them to the procedure, many surgeons tried a few "training cases" and recognized that they didn't have the requisite skills. Others continued to perform disc replacements, but did not do them well. Both groups left a trail of damaged patients behind.

Several European surgeons, based in Germany, France, and the

Netherlands, advertised their clinics and disc replacement procedures on the Internet. In Europe, the procedure cost between $30,000 and $40,000, including hospitalization and rehab. In the United States, a disc cost about $11,000, but by the time associated costs were included, a patient was on the hook for tens of thousands more. Convinced that these European physicians knew something that U.S. doctors did not know, American patients who had struggled to find surgical solutions at home began to travel abroad for disc replacement procedures. Most paid out of pocket, but some had the kind of federal or municipal health insurance coverage that did not require preapproval, and would pick up the bill.

To ease the process, "international patient coordinators" who could be readily located on the Web, were prepared to set surgery dates, arrange transportation, and book hotels. On patient-oriented websites, designed to appear independent but often subsidized by surgeons, they described a stream of "advanced products" that were not yet available in the United States. After surgery, when the going got rough, many patients would discover that these helpful coordinators were no longer interested in advocating for them.

Back pain forums dedicated to artificial disc replacement were rife with stories of Americans who had traveled to Europe, certain that they'd found a cutting-edge approach, circumvented stodgy FDA regulations, and were going to get the best possible care. Brian Bohn, who worked as an engineer for the Federal Aviation Administration and therefore had excellent federal health insurance coverage, was one of those patients. A few weeks before he headed for Stenum Hospital in Bremen, he'd sent his MRI scan and X-rays to Germany. Quickly, he heard that he was a perfect candidate for a two-level disc replacement surgery and could be scheduled immediately. Bohn was one of a group of nine patients who arrived in Bremen. The others had paid in advance, out of pocket.

In his forties, Bohn had been in pain since he'd had a surfing accident in 1988. He "was eating Vicodins like bananas," he said, "and not sleeping for two or three days at a clip. I didn't care what they did. I was ready to swallow a bullet." Bohn's surgery went so far wrong that he built a website called "My Stenum Hospital Nightmare," greatly upsetting the hospital's administrators. (The site has since been removed from the Internet, and has been replaced with another web page, on which Stenum Hospital management rebuts what Bohn claims happened to him.) In even worse pain after his surgery, Bohn had another MRI back in the United States; it showed that the vertebrae had fused. He had elected to have disc replacement surgery so that motion would be preserved. "I went halfway round the world, to avoid fusion, and I'm fused anyway," he said glumly.

In 2002, another patient—an athletic Californian named Mark Mintzer—had undergone a two-level disc replacement procedure at yet another hospital in Germany. Initially, he was ecstatic: Six months after the procedure, Mintzer felt so well that he was "roller-blading backward with two Golden Retrievers on leashes." To convey what he'd learned, he launched an online forum called iSpine, where patients could share information about disc replacement and related issues. Interest in artificial disc replacement was so strong that many patients asked him for guidance and personal introductions to experienced European surgeons. In 2004, still feeling terrific, and sensing a business opportunity that would help people, he started Global Patient Network. Patients paid him to shepherd them through the entire process.

By the time I met Mintzer in 2010, he'd arranged for dozens of patients to have disc replacement procedures in Europe. That put him in a difficult position, because in the interim, his own pain had returned. He required extended-release opioid therapy to make it through his days, which made him wonder how well the operation had served him or those he had taken to Europe. Disc replacement, Mintzer realized, was not a miraculous antidote to back pain. A good outcome did not mean that you could hop onto your bike or play tennis or waterski. "Now, if I meet someone who is basically able to go to work and live life," he told me, "but who is in enough pain to be considering the procedure, I say, 'You have to understand that where you are right now would be considered a success after this operation.'"

There were a lot of failed artificial disc patients in the United

States, he said, because it could take fifty or sixty trial procedures for a surgeon to get it right. "The device manufacturers can set the bar for training," he added, "but it doesn't serve them to make that bar too high, or to say that only certain surgeons can learn to use the product." The worst problems occurred when patients fell into the hands of what he described as "second- or third-tier surgeons," whether American or European. "Some of them just have their heads up their asses," Mintzer observed sadly. "As a patient, if you're not a success, you're a nightmare."

In 2009, a Virginia law firm filed a medical malpractice lawsuit for an American patient, alleging that after spending $60,000 there, she left Stenum Hospital partially paralyzed below the neck. The press release associated with the lawsuit decried that a "foreign hospital like Stenum is actively soliciting patients in the United States through unlicensed sales agents, performing risky surgeries with implants not approved in the United States and without the proper medical equipment and preparation," and that the hospital "refuses to take any responsibility for medical malpractice, once the U.S. patients have paid for surgery and are back home." Even before it was filed, the legal community recognized that the lawsuit was unenforceable. It was impossible, personal injury lawyers knew, for an American patient to succeed in a suit against a doctor or hospital on European soil.

Just to test the waters, I sent a request to Stenum Hospital, to "international patient mediator" Malte Petersen, who asked me to send my MRI, my X-rays, and a completed data sheet for a "no-charge evaluation." A few days later, I had a response: I was definitely a candidate. Karsten Ritter-Lang would implant the Spinal Kinetics M6, which Petersen assured me would "provide shock absorption" and "graded variable resistance to motion." This disc, Petersen said, would not be available in the United States "for years." In his two-page letter, he promised a success rate of ">90%."

If I wished, I could arrive in Bremen on any Tuesday in May and have surgery on the following Friday. The whole package—which included seven days in the hospital and seven in a hotel—would cost under $30,000. At the end of the letter was all the banking information I'd need to issue a wire transfer that would reserve my space immediately.

IN THE WAKE of Rosen's interview with the *Wall Street Journal*, he and Cunningham had launched the Association for Medical Ethics, their watchdog organization. As a result, Rosen had come under heavy fire at his UC Irvine hospital. "Every time my superior returned from a medical meeting," Rosen said, "he'd tell me that people were demanding that he get rid of me. And those people, it seemed, were always enmeshed in consulting arrangements with the device industry." According to an article in the *Orange County Register*, Rosen's department chairman threatened to dismiss him. But there was an eleventh-hour dustup: Instead of firing Rosen, the department chairman himself lost his position. His replacement not only determined that Rosen would stay on board but also encouraged him in his quest to clean up the spine business. "[Rosen] was ahead of his time," Rajan Gupta told the *Register*. "He was met with a lot of resistance. People were not thrilled."

Among his colleagues, Rosen still felt like a pariah. But he could not escape his conviction that what was going down in the back pain industry was a violation of patients' human rights.

After we'd gotten to know each other pretty well, Rosen entrusted me with a stack of letters from patients with identifying information redacted. Most were in their thirties and forties. They'd opted for the device specifically because they'd been told that a disc replacement would preserve motion and function better in the long term than spinal fusion.

Those letters broke my heart, as they had broken Rosen's. The words "unbearable" and "desperate" appeared repeatedly. Patients wrote that they planned to kill themselves unless Rosen could intervene. They described themselves as "completely disabled," with maddening neurological symptoms—burning feet, numb toes, and electrical shocks that shot through their limbs. Some could not find comfort even while lying in bed; for them, sleep was a thing of the past. In their correspondence, they noted that they had lost jobs, spouses, and homes as a result of their failed procedures.

When they returned to their surgeons, in desperate need of help, they were told that their disc replacements were perfectly positioned in the X-ray, which meant that the surgeon had done his job. With no options remaining, they were sent to pain management, where they required increasing doses of extended-release opioids and faced a lifetime of disability.

One letter sent to Rosen stood out. It came from a forty-five-year-old disabled Medicaid patient. In 2005, he'd received a Charité disc, implanted by a Kentucky surgeon who was an investigator in that device's clinical trial. The patient wrote: "I dont know what to do, I was hopeing may you could PLEASE give me some kind of info that could help." He explained that he was on high-dose opioids, but "there helpfulness is fading fast. Im afraid to ask for anything more because I get treated like a pill head or a junky. . . . Im sorry this letter hops around but in trobbing & burning from the tops of my hips down & my head is spinning, and Im tring to keep my composier & not cry in front of my daughter. I hope you understand."

Charles Rosen understood. He'd predicted exactly this kind of disaster. Under the pressure of the implant, the frail butterfly-shaped facet joints in this patient's spine were cracking, just as Rosen anticipated.

With two colleagues at UC Irvine, Rosen launched an investigation of twenty-nine patients with implanted artificial disc replacements and facet joint fractures. In ten patients, with a posterior surgical approach, Rosen was able to remove the broken facet joints and fuse the replacement discs in place. At best, he recognized, this was salvage surgery: Six or seven of those patients got some relief, while the remainder experienced no change.

The other nineteen patients, whose spines had problems that Rosen didn't believe would respond to removing broken facet joints and fusing the replacement discs, posed a far worse situation. Other surgeons had opened up patients' abdomens to remove the discs and found that "everything was scarred over," Rosen said. When they tried to move the iliac vein out of the way to reach the surgical site, either it didn't move or it moved and tore, resulting in dangerous, and possibly fatal, blood loss. For those patients, Rosen could do nothing, and when he was concerned about such an outcome, he did not operate. The decision weighed on him. They were young, and they would live in torment for decades. The worst part was that "most of these patients did not fit the criteria for any operation whatsoever," he said. "It's not like they should have had a fusion instead. They should have had nothing."

Some patients regarded their pain as penance for choosing the wrong surgery. Walking my dog one spring afternoon, I got into a conversation about back pain with a woman who asked me to contact her dear friend on Long Island, Gary Silverman. His disc replacement surgery, she said, had ruined his life.

Silverman, who had worked for years as a fund manager in financial services, agreed with his friend's assessment. A year prior to receiving two Charité discs, he had been one of the individuals featured in a Fox News segment on various means of avoiding spine surgery. He had undergone physical therapy and acupuncture—but he was still in pain. His physiatrist, who had been his friend since childhood, referred him to the head of spine surgery at a major New York hospital.

Silverman had several ongoing health issues, including severe asthma. As a young man, he'd been badly burned. During his recovery, he'd taken high-dose steroids, which had left him with osteoporotic bones. He did not meet the FDA's criteria for even a single device, but his surgeon explained that he would implant two Charité discs, off-label.

"He said he liked the challenge of a unique case," Silverman recalled. "But after that surgery, what had been a basically great life changed instantly, and forever." While he was still in the hospital, one of the replacement discs broke, shattering his vertebrae. In an emergency surgery that left him in the hospital for weeks, that disc was removed.

Many evenings, Silverman said, the surgeon stopped by his bedside to check up on him. "He said it was the first time he'd had a disc replacement surgery fail," Silverman recalled. "He was very upset over what was happening."

The once-successful fund manager required high doses of opioids. His pain was still terrible. His keen mind turned so foggy that he could not work and had to apply for Social Security Disability Insurance. He hired a lawyer, who had already begun to file suits against DePuy Synthes Spine and Johnson & Johnson in a Massachusetts court, alleging that the Charité was defective and that the victims, including Silverman, were due millions in compensation. But once again the federal preemption doctrine came into play, this time with teeth: In 2008 the U.S. Supreme Court had upheld the doctrine of preemption as it concerned FDA approval. Instead of paying out millions to injured Charité patients, J&J issued a settlement, which Silverman described as a "pittance," to four hundred claimants. His lawyer had told him from the start that he wouldn't sue the surgeons involved because most were the biggest orthopedists in the spine business, and it would have been impossible to find colleagues of similar stature who were willing to testify against them.

IN 2006, WITH ProDisc slated to enter the U.S. market, Rosen, representing some three hundred AME members, wrote a strongly worded letter to Republican senator Charles Grassley. Once again, Rosen explained that the approval and monitoring of disc replacements had "occurred under suspicious and secretive circumstances that suggest that this is the work of undue influence by industry." He requested that the feds take a closer look.

In response, Senator Grassley's staffers did begin to study the problematic financial conflicts of interest between the surgeon-investigators who ran ProDisc's FDA clinical trials and the manufacturer, DePuy Synthes Spine. (In the wake of the Norian controversy, Johnson & Johnson had absorbed Synthes, rolling it into its DePuy subsidiary.)

By that time, DePuy Synthes Spine was also under scrutiny in New Jersey, Pennsylvania, and New York, where subpoenas had been issued, seeking information about the investment backing that had funded ProDisc's development. New Jersey's attorney general, Anne Milgram, launched an investigation of New Jersey surgeons who had invested in ProDisc with Viscogliosi Brothers and participated in the clinical studies that moved the product through the FDA. Upon Pro-Disc's FDA approval, as previously arranged, they'd received their $175 million in ownership.

In a remarkably plainspoken letter, Milgram upbraided the FDA for not insisting that DePuy Synthes Spine disclose the surgeons' financial conflicts of interest. Milgram alleged that the FDA had ignored some very obvious omissions, while approving DePuy Synthes Spine's applications for premarket approval "without any delay or further inquiry into this issue." Such transgressions prevailed throughout the health care industry, Milgram explained, and it was time for them to stop.

In response to Milgram's salvo, DePuy Synthes Spine agreed to limit corporate payments to high-profile surgeons to about $600 an hour. It also agreed to collect information on physicians' conflicts of interest, to be made public on the company's website and, in a token punishment, to pay $236,000 as reimbursement for fees and costs related to the investigation. That year, DePuy Synthes Spine's revenues were about $3 billion. With ProDisc integrated into J&J's product line, the company finally took the SB Charité III off the market.

AS NEWS OF poor outcomes for disc replacement procedures surfaced in the literature, insurance providers increasingly kicked back requests for reimbursement. Medicare had never paid for the discs, because the FDA's labeling was for patients aged sixty and younger. But even without insurance reimbursement, there was still a market for disc replacement in affluent older patients who were willing to pay out of pocket.

Rick Delamarter, the director of the Spine Institute in Santa Mon-

ica, California, attracted such self-payers to his practice. Considered
a master of the most complex aspects of the implantation procedure,
Delamarter had been one of the investigators in the ProDisc's FDA
trial. He was also an author of several papers describing how Pro-
Disc could be used to treat patients who fell outside the "under sixty,
degeneration at one level only" limitation. During our interview in
2010, he told me about several successful patients, including a twenty-
seven-year old female LAPD police sergeant, who received a ProDisc.
Four months later, she'd returned to work. When I spoke to the officer, Hayley Smith, she couldn't have been happier. "From the second
I woke up from the anesthesia, it was amazing. Four months later,
I was back in a police car in my uniform, which meant thirty-five
pounds of extra weight—a leather belt, two pairs of handcuffs, two
bullet magazines, radios, batons, keys, spray, bulletproof vest, boots,
and a gun." She stopped using painkillers about a month out of surgery. Five years after her surgery, she won the LAPD's Medal of Valor,
after she entered a burning apartment complex and pulled out five
families. "The heat was so intense," she told me, that "the cars were
exploding in the carport. But my back lasted through all that."

When Rick Delamarter and I met, the ProDisc's future still looked
rosy. I asked him whether he thought it could work for me, at the age
of fifty-three. Without reviewing my chart and my films, and getting
more imaging and diagnostics, he couldn't say. But he could tell me
that despite the FDA's labeling for patients sixty and younger, age was
not the defining factor. "This is Southern California," he said, "and
we have affluent sixty-eight-year-olds running marathons and eating
tofu. They plan to stay active. They think they're forty."

In subsequent weeks, Delamarter would arrange an introduction
to Lou Gram, one of his star patients, who was in his late sixties. I
sat with Gram in a restaurant in Los Angeles. His feet, shod in glove
leather driving moccasins, were in perpetual motion. He wiggled and
tapped them, he explained, to relieve his ongoing pain. He'd forgot-
ten to bring his X-rays, but he had "four little beauties lined up in
there," he said.

Years earlier, Gram had gone to see Marina del Rey orthopedic surgeon Robert Watkins III, who had been much more attentive to him than he was to me. "He was a very ethical guy," Gram said. "He did the MRIs, diagnosed degenerative disc disease, and said right off that he couldn't see anything surgical that could be done." He had many epidural steroid injections, but they never helped for more than three weeks. "The walls in the office were decorated with portraits of famous athletes, who wrote, 'Thank you Dr. Watkins for the miraculous results,'" Gram recalled. "But he had no answer for me."

After Watkins sent him to pain management, Gram became dependent on opioids. "I was taking more and more drugs and playing less and less golf," he said. The drugs didn't help much: By the time he was in his mid-fifties, he couldn't walk for more than one hundred yards without stopping to sit down. Golf—his enduring passion—was out of the question. He couldn't bear to swing a club, and the opioids made his brain too fuzzy to strategize on the course. His father had been similarly afflicted. "God rest his soul," Gram said. "He lay around the house in his later years, taking Percocet."

On one of his visits to Watkins, he laid it on the line. "I said, 'Bob, we can't go on like this. There has to be something.'" The surgeon told him about Rudolf Bertagnoli, whom he described, said Gram, as a surgeon who could do things that others would not even consider. Watkins said he'd send Gram's charts to Germany.

After he studied the material on Rudolf Bertagnoli's ProSpine website and talked with several of his prior patients, Gram and his wife made the trip to Bogen. "After a very cursory examination—he didn't even ask me to bend over—Rudy told me that he could definitely help me, with a five-level disc replacement. He said I had come to the right place: He was the only surgeon in the world who could do that operation," Gram said.

The southern Californian was not thrilled with the logistics: After the surgery, he would have to remain in Germany for at least a month for rehab. "I don't speak German, and although the town of Bogen was quaint and pretty, the thought of spending a month convalescing in Germany did not knock my knickers off," he said. When he returned to L.A., he discovered that he might not have to go to

Germany after all: Rick Delamarter's clinic was just twenty minutes away from Gram's Bel Air home.

"I wanted to be the only American with replacements at five levels," said Gram. But Delamarter would consider doing only four, with a lumbar fusion at L5-S1, the lowest lumbar vertebral joint. Delamarter could not predict how his patient's body would react, but he wanted Gram—who was in poor physical condition, to get in shape before the operation. Dutifully, Gram—whose pain had limited his activity for a long time—swam regularly, dieted, participated in gentle yoga classes, and did strength training. He quit smoking.

Realizing that I was treading on thin ice, I asked Gram how he—a man who was in too much pain to walk around the block—adopted such a demanding exercise program. "You do what you gotta do," Gram shrugged. "It was the only way I was getting that operation."

The surgery occurred in January 2007. Gram, who was heavily sedated for weeks afterward, does not recall much from the immediate post-op period. But what came later, he will never forget. After the surgery, he was two inches taller because the ProDiscs expanded the spaces between his vertebrae. That meant that all his soft tissues— nerves, muscles, and ligaments—had to stretch to accommodate the change in disc height. "I experienced the most extreme pain I'd ever had in my life," he said.

"We are talking about incessant and unending burning pain up and down my legs and feet, no matter how many drugs I took," Gram said. "At the height of it, my legs felt like I had third-degree burns. Even satin sheets felt like sandpaper. I'd wake up at night and start to weep because my legs felt so bad."

He relied on painkillers, muscle relaxants, and drugs to treat neuropathic pain. Seven months after surgery, still completely miserable, he watched everyone else playing golf at Pebble Beach and believed that he'd ruined the rest of his life. It was not until fifteen months after surgery, when he could finally begin to swing a golf club again, that he began to think that his grueling ordeal might have been worthwhile.

He did not blame Rick Delamarter. "He never promised me a life without pain," Gram said. "We were in uncharted waters. I took a shot at being better. None of us knew what the outcome would be, but it was a bitch of a procedure and a brute of a recovery."

By the time we met, Gram felt that he was over the hump; the procedure had been worthwhile. Two years after surgery, he and his wife walked across the Great Wall of China. He was back on the golf course, with a handicap of 17, only three points off his lifetime's best. He could play golf five or six days a week.

Among Gram's golfing buddies, Gram observed, there were several who had multilevel lumbar spinal fusion with top Los Angeles spine surgeons. They too were miserable for months. The main difference, Gram said, is that he could play golf every day with no pain, "and they were lucky if, with pain pills, they could get in one round every four days."

PRODISC-L, HAILED BY its manufacturer as superior to Charité in many ways, would appear less promising in 2011, when the *British Medical Journal* published results of an investigation comparing Pro-Disc patients' outcomes with those of a group of patients who had not had surgery, but instead had participated in a well-designed exercise and cognitive behavioral therapy (CBT) program.

The *BMJ* paper reported significant post-op complications in the disc replacement group. Notably, one ProDisc patient had a leg amputated after the polyethylene segment of the disc replacement dislodged and the revision attempt failed. More than three-quarters of the "successful" ProDisc patients remained dependent on opioids. Based on the data, and given the procedure's risks and its expense, it was impossible to claim that ProDisc offered any significant advantage over the much safer exercise and CBT protocol. By that time, more than thirty-five thousand ProDiscs had been implanted in patients.

By the time the Cochrane Collaboration reported in 2013 that, as a class, the artificial disc replacement was not yet ready for routine clinical use, the product had been on the market for a decade.

In May 2013, after eight years of sporadically covering a single-level ProDisc surgery, Anthem Blue Cross said that it was ending reimbursement for the FDA-approved indication of degenerative disc disease at a single level. A few months later, Aetna followed with a similar policy, denying coverage for all but a handful of patients. The market that had once looked so promising had evaporated.

The artificial disc business would never be worth $1.7 billion annually, as the financial analyst had once predicted. Sales would peak at an unimpressive $150 million in 2009, sinking to $35 million by 2013. Still, some very influential surgeons were convinced that given more time—and the money and perks required to recruit top talent to do the work—device manufacturers would eventually get it right.

By 2014, it was hard to find a current reference to lumbar disc replacement on the Internet, except in patient forums, where the mounting carnage was discussed in blood-soaked detail. Not everyone was unhappy. When I checked in with Gram, he responded to my e-mail right away. Eight years after his surgery, he was still out playing golf five or six times a week. The pain in his feet had never relented. "It's intense all the time, and unbearable some of the time," he said. "At certain times of day, my feet start to burn, and the skin on my legs is tender." He needed painkillers and other drugs to deal with that. "I guess it is something I will continue to suffer for the rest of my life," he said, "but I'm still a miracle."

Lou Gram did have one nonnegotiable demand. "I want to be sure I leave this earth before those discs wear out. I wouldn't want Delamarter to open me up and redo it for all the tea in China."

IN THE WAKE of Infuse and Charité and ProDisc, Charles Rosen and Gemma Cunningham fought to change the way that device manufacturers did business. In 2014, under the Physician Payments Sunshine Act (which was signed into law as part of the Affordable Care Act), the Centers for Medicare and Medicaid Services reported this information, in a database that was searchable and comprehensive, including the manufacturer's name; the physician's name, specialty, and address and the specific payment information; and the value of the payment. The initial database report listed 4.4 million payments made to more than half a million physicians, amounting to $3.5 billion. At Policy and Medicine, a website that addresses transparency and compliance issues in health care, Thomas Sullivan explained that the Sunshine Act, if implemented in full, would allow physicians and patients to make more informed choices.

Failure to comply with the posting requirement—thereby defrauding the federal government—would result in fines to the device manufacturer of between $1,000 and $10,000 for each instance, up to a maximum penalty of $150,000 a year. But medical ethicists argued that these fines weren't nearly injurious enough; as long as corporations and physician-scientists were financially entangled in any manner, scientific integrity and patients' welfare would remain at risk.

In the aftermath of the 2016 election, the future of the Affordable Care Act, and therefore the Physician Payments Sunshine Act, remained ambiguous. It seemed unlikely that President Donald Trump's avidly pro-business cabinet appointments at both the FDA and the Department of Health and Human Services would see fit to maintain a statute that existed to exert control over device manufacturers' and pharmaceutical companies' shenanigans, limiting their profitability.

8

The Opioid Wars

HOW CHRONIC OPIOID THERAPY
KEEPS YOU IN PAIN

IN MEDICINE, CHANGE comes very slowly—unless, of course, it happens overnight. When I began my research for this book, opioid therapy was the standard treatment for people who suffered from chronic pain. Along with most of the other patients at LSI in Tampa, I filled my prescription and swallowed my hydrocodone tablets, unaware of the implications. We understood the drugs to be perfectly safe if taken as directed.

Over the months and years to come, I would meet dozens of back pain patients whose opioid use had gotten the better of them. These were not street corner addicts, nor were they typically young and impressionable; on the contrary, they were often middle-aged people who reminded me of me. Pam, the woman who waited in Saint Peter's Basilica because she was in too much pain to tour Vatican City, had filled increasingly strong prescriptions for a decade. For Carl, who sought help at LSI, it was no different: Without resolving his pain, the drugs had drained him of the motivation to get out of bed. Two long-standing chronic pain sufferers—Bruce, fifty-five, from a town near Palo Alto, California; and Kim, a New Yorker, also in her mid-fifties—were taking towering doses of OxyContin, but they were still in terrible pain, out of work, and desperate. In time, I realized that such stories were not exceptional. For the back pain patient with a chronic condition, being dispatched to "pain management" was a standard part of care.

When I began my research, hardly anyone mentioned risks or side effects. The first time I encountered someone with doubts was when I sat down in 2010 with epidemiologist Michael Von Korff at the Group Health Research Institute in Seattle. He was one of the few scientists who questioned the efficacy of opioid treatment in non-cancer chronic pain patients. In his office, with a view of the Seattle Space Needle and Mount Olympus, I learned that the drugs were not as safe as people seemed to think. For a medical journal, Von Korff had written a highly controversial editorial, enumerating the risks of chronic extended-release, high-dose opioid therapy, including the potential for addiction and overdose; the possibility that the patient would develop "opioid-induced hyperalgesia," or increased pain; and the lack of evidence for pain control. On opioids, patients could become lethargic or depressed, or suffer from severe constipation, memory problems, weight gain, muscle wasting, fatigue, hormonal imbalances, mood swings, or insomnia. He pointed out that, short of suggesting a drug rehab clinic, or a 12-step program, neither of which were designed for chronic pain patients, doctors had few options when it came to tapering their patients off high doses of opioids. His little editorial had not gone over well with opioid manufacturers, pain management doctors, or pain foundations. In fact, Von Korff had been denounced for trying to prevent people in pain from seeking relief they deserved.

When I left Michael Von Korff's office, I was thoroughly disturbed. I had no idea that I'd spend the next four years tracking a story that had more twists, turns, and corrupt characters than a Le Carré spy novel.

THE HISTORY OF opium, a nectar milked from the pod of the poppy, is almost as old as the history of the human race. But it was not until 1803, when a pharmacist's assistant discovered a crystallizable isolate of opium he called "morphine," that it became the palliative used to treat almost every human woe. By the end of the nineteenth century, the anodyne's drawbacks were already obvious. Although a pharmacist's reference guide of the period observed that regular use led to "tremors, paralysis, stupidity and general emaciation," in 1898, the German pharmaceutical firm Friedrich Bayer & Co. offered a new product: a cough suppressant called "Heroin." Three times more powerful than morphine, the syrup induced such an alluring sense of well-being that it begot hundreds of thousands of opioid-dependent people on both sides of the Atlantic.

Sixteen years later, the cough suppressant had wrought such devastation in American cities that the U.S. Congress passed the Harrison Narcotics Tax Act, requiring physicians to register with the government if they wished to prescribe it. Physicians who ordered the drug, for patients who they recognized to be addicted, could wind up in jail.

Most doctors stopped prescribing painkillers, except for patients who were hospitalized. For those who suffered from arthritic conditions, at that time referred to as "rheumatism," they recommended good strong whiskey, or sticky, inflammatory capsicum plasters. These approaches dominated until the 1950s, when Arthur M. Sackler, a brilliant strategist and psychiatrist by training, invented the field of medical marketing, cunningly devising lists of brand-new ailments, like "anxiety" and "psychic tension." Under Sackler's tutelage, Americans learned that pain or distress, whether emotional or physiological, could and should be resolved pharmaceutically, with drugs like Librium and Valium. Sackler's drug company clients sponsored and funded "patient advocacy organizations," which dutifully advanced corporate agendas. Sackler also invented industry-sponsored "continuing medical education" for physicians, and then, to identify high-volume prescribers who could convince their colleagues to get on board, he developed methods of quantifying prescribing habits. He planted favorable articles in the mainstream press, published ostensibly scientific journals that made unfounded claims for clients' products, and developed the hybrid sales tool we know as the "infomercial."

In 1952, having lost interest in advising others on how to make money, he and his younger brothers bought Purdue Frederick, a small, privately held New York City pharmaceutical firm that produced Gray's Glycerine Tonic Compound, a sherry-based elixir. In 1987, after years of adding nothing more lucrative than laxatives and earwax remover to the inventory, Purdue Frederick received FDA approval for its first blockbuster. MS Contin was a morphine-based drug in tablet form. It allowed terminal cancer patients and others in great pain to escape the intravenous morphine drip.

Arthur Sackler died the year that MS Contin entered the market. His two brothers, aware that copycat products were about to emerge from the pipeline, were working on another new drug, with an extended-release formulation—one that offered twelve hours of pain relief. The plan was to expand the FDA's labeling to allow doctors to prescribe it liberally to "non-cancer" chronic pain patients. But that would not be easy. It was hard to imagine that physicians would risk prescribing highly addictive drugs to patients with low back pain and arthritis, when they knew they could go to prison under the provisions of the Harrison Act.

Over the next decade, employing the strategies they'd learned from their late brother, the remaining Sackler siblings set out to alter the way the medical community had viewed opioids for more than half a century. They were remarkably successful.

OxyContin arrived on the market in 1996. Six years later, the drug produced annual sales of $1.5 billion. Over the two decades that followed, OxyContin would rack up revenues of $35 billion, making the Sacklers the sixteenth-richest family in America.

Arthur Sackler had already demonstrated that the best way to capture physicians' hearts and minds was to have one of their own do the wooing. To that end, Purdue harnessed the supremely charismatic and handsome Russell Portenoy, a young anesthesiologist who had completed his medical residency in pain management. Under the supervision of superstar neurologist Kathleen M. Foley at Memorial Sloan Kettering, he was investigating better ways to assuage cancer patients' misery.

In 1986, Portenoy and Foley published a paper in *Pain*, the journal of the American Pain Society, establishing that thirty-eight patients who had been treated with low doses of morphine over a short period had *not become addicted to the drug*. The authors concluded that, under the correct circumstances, opioids could "be safely and effectively prescribed . . . with relatively little risk of producing the maladaptive behaviors that define opioid use." In support of these findings, Portenoy and Foley cited a five-sentence, hundred-word letter to the editor published in the *New England Journal of Medicine*, which noted that just 1 percent of hospital patients who were treated had become addicted. For the three decades that followed, that off-the-cuff letter to the editor, from authors Jane Porter and Hershel Jick, would serve as the pharmaceutical industry's basis for promoting prescription opioid use. By 2015, Porter and Jick's un-fact-checked letter, often described incorrectly as a "study," would have been cited 635 times.

Soon after the publication of Portenoy and Foley's paper in *Pain*, the former commenced what would be a meteoric rise to influence. When Portenoy became the director of analgesic studies at Memorial Sloan Kettering, Purdue Frederick helped fund his department's research. When, in his early forties, he left Sloan Kettering to become founder and chair of the department of pain medicine and palliative care at Beth Israel Hospital, he brought pharma money with him.

On archival television footage and in interviews with the media, he was Arthur Sackler's dream of a doctor-educator, self-assured and quotable. "There's a growing literature showing that these drugs can be used for a long time," Portenoy told the *New York Times*, "with few side effects and that addiction and abuse are not a problem." Doctors should not worry about "a ceiling dose" (a dose at which risks exceeded benefits), he explained. In fact, when the patient's pain was insufficiently relieved, it was both safe and prudent to escalate the dose, because this was evidence of normal "physical tolerance." When he became president of the American Pain Society, the media adopted Portenoy as the spokesman for all matters related to painkillers, and he continued to convey the message that for physicians engaged in treating chronic non-cancer pain, high-dose, extended-release opioids were the way to go.

IN THE FIRST five years that OxyContin was on the market, Purdue Frederick conducted over forty national pain management and speaker training conferences. Physicians who were willing to spread the word could expect to make up to $3,000 for telling their colleagues, often at lavish dinner meetings or continuing education medical seminars, why Oxy worked so well for them. The strategy could not have been more successful; in record time, ordinary musculoskeletal pain was recast as an enemy to be battled and subdued. Physicians who allowed patients to suffer needlessly were labeled as lacking in compassion. For general practitioners, who found themselves with agonized recipients of the Steffee Plates and other devices entrusted to their care, OxyContin appeared to be a gift: Instead of telling such patients they'd need to learn to live with their pain, they could write an Rx for opioids.

To help Purdue deliver its message to doctors, British-born physician Alan Spanos, who practiced in North Carolina but spoke with a pearly English accent that lent gravitas to his comments, was invited to address its largest physician groups. Purdue made a videotaped version of Spanos's presentation, titled *I Got My Life Back: Patients in Pain Tell Their Story*, for distribution among fifteen thousand doctors across the country. The video included interviews with six patients, including the robust, middle-aged Johnny Sullivan, who made his pitch from a construction site. Standing beside heavy machinery, which presumably he operated, Sullivan told viewers that he was thrilled to have found a drug that did not turn him into a zombie. Before OxyContin, "even a good day was hell," he said, but now, his future "looked just great." The five other patients of Spanos who were interviewed described similar levels of satisfaction.

In his narration, Spanos described his patients as "well-maintained on long-acting painkillers." With conviction, he cited Porter and Jick (the hundred-word letter), and of course Portenoy and Foley, contending that "the rate of addiction amongst pain patients who are treated by doctors is much less than 1 percent."

Two years after *I Got My Life Back* was released, Purdue, rosy with success, distributed another promotional video, *From One Pain Patient to Another: Advice from Patients Who Have Found Relief.* Copies of this video were distributed to physicians' waiting rooms; patients could watch them there, or check them out to view at home. At the end of the tape, the OxyContin label scrolled across the screen.

Purdue also produced a sequel to *I Got My Life Back*, in which Spanos assured viewers that in the two years that had elapsed, not one of his patients had become addicted, nor had it been necessary to increase their opioid dose. But the footage told a different story. On screen, Johnny Sullivan, whose future had looked so promising twenty-four months earlier, murmured semi-incoherently that he'd "done well with it, and it's wonderful . . . there's never a drowsy moment."

Purdue's marketing team may have believed that Spanos's informal, documentary-style videotapes were not advertising, and therefore could fly under the federal regulatory radar that requires pharmaceutical manufacturers to submit all promotional materials to the FDA upon their first use. But when Purdue distributed the videos without the FDA's okay, the company violated the Federal Food, Drug, and Cosmetic Act, a misstep that would have costly repercussions.

BY THE YEAR 2000, Purdue had doubled the size of its sales force, in an effort to accumulate a roster of seventy thousand "committed" physicians who would prescribe OxyContin for the treatment of chronic non-cancer pain. Reps were encouraged, legal records show, to tell doctors that extended-release opioids should be substituted for other analgesics, including short-acting ones like Vicodin and a subgroup of NSAIDs (nonsteroidal anti-inflammatory drugs) called COX-2 inhibitors. For Purdue's pharmaceutical sales reps, who were expected to make about thirty-five physician calls per week, it was a lucrative business: The average income for a Purdue rep, including bonus, exceeded $120,000 annually.

Purdue's collateral patient advocate website, positioned as an impartial and valuable patient resource, listed thirty-three thousand physicians who were ready and willing to prescribe opioids. These physicians, the website explained, would provide suitable patients with a starter coupon that they could take to the pharmacy for a free thirty-day supply. (Later, this freebie was reduced to a week's supply.) By July 2001, patients had redeemed roughly thirty-four thousand coupons, and the number of primary care visits that resulted in an opioid prescription had increased, in less than a decade, by 44 percent. Within two years, primary care doctors would write half the prescriptions for OxyContin.

Under pressure not only from the pharmaceutical business, but also from physicians who wanted to be sure they had the federal stamp of approval for this rampant prescribing, the Joint Commission declared pain to be "the fifth vital sign," adding it to measurements of pulse, blood pressure, core temperature, and respiration. This would turn out to be a grave error. The standard vital signs were readily quantified—either they were normal, or they were not—but only the patient could identify his pain level. Nevertheless, the Joint Commission directed all accredited U.S. hospitals and health care facilities to instruct personnel to monitor pain and to provide compassionate care. In the Joint Commission's monograph, published in 2001, the organization noted that "in general, patients in pain do not become addicted to opioids."

If Purdue hadn't been on hand to help make the transition, maybe doctors and nurses would have offered compassion, rather than narcotics. But the company sent out a specially trained team of sales reps to call on and further educate personnel in hospitals all over the United States. As part of the effort to help a patient identify his level of discomfort, so that he might be appropriately treated, Purdue provided nursing staff with paper copies of the "smiling-to-crying" pain scale. Soon, that scale would become a common evaluation tool in most doctors' offices, where any patient who circled an unsmiling face became a potential candidate for analgesia.

Many state medical boards responded to the Joint Commission's new standard by making it clear that not only was it safe for physicians to write opioid prescriptions for patients in chronic pain, but if they failed to do so, they could lose their licenses. As Oregon physician Jim Shames explained on a public radio broadcast, back in the days when he prescribed opioids to all comers, he felt that he was abiding by his state medical board's directive to become more compassionate about treating pain. "You walk in, we close the door, we spend fifteen minutes," he said. "You expect a pill, I expect to give you a pill, and out you go and everyone's happy." It would be years before he realized, to his regret, that pharmaceutical companies had fed him and his state medical board this view, ultimately resulting in many addicted patients.

Even the Drug Enforcement Administration (DEA) climbed on board, signing an agreement with twenty-one medical professional societies that allowed doctors to prescribe the drugs without fear of prosecution. If physicians had lingering doubts, and some did, these were dispelled in President Bill Clinton's last weeks in office, when he signed legislation declaring the upcoming decade, 2000 to 2010, to be the Decade of Pain Control and Research.

FOR A LONG while, it was understood that opioid addiction was the outcome of misuse or abuse, and was unrelated to doctors' prescribing habits. "The reality is that the vast majority of people who are given these medications by doctors will not become addicted," Russell Portenoy told those assembled for a media gathering at a D.C. press conference. Repeatedly, Purdue described a "bright line" between the state of addiction and that of physical dependence in the treatment of chronic pain. For patients who needed pain control, Purdue said, access to chronic opioid therapy was really no different from providing insulin to a diabetic.

Some regarded that comparison as outrageous. Andrew Kolodny, at the time an addiction psychiatrist at Maimonides Medical Center in New York City, had founded a group called Physicians for Responsible Opioid Prescribing (PROP). (Subsequently, he would be chief medical officer at Phoenix House, before accepting the position of co-director of opioid policy research at Brandeis University.) In 2011, in the first of many conversations I'd have with him, Kolodny explained that physicians who overprescribed to patients with non-cancer chronic pain were largely responsible for having created the epidemic of addiction, not only to prescribed opioids but also to heroin. "The reason we have a severe epidemic of opioid addiction," Kolodny said, "is that we have overexposed the U.S. population to opioid pain medicine. The people who are using heroin are out there using heroin because they were first addicted to opioid pain medicines." In 2010, enough painkiller prescriptions were written and filled to medicate every American adult around the clock for a month.

Kolodny was both persuasive and persistent. At a press conference, he told the assembled media: "When anyone starts to take opioids every day, or needs an extended-release round-the-clock drug, within a week, that person is dependent on opioids. If you use OxyContin for a week, when you quit, you will feel sick. There is positive reinforcement when you take it—you feel better—and negative consequences when you don't. When you stop, life can feel like one prolonged panic attack."

Michael Von Korff, who was a PROP member, had been right on target when he pointed out the risks, including opioid-induced hyperalgesia, endocrine disruption, insomnia, depression, and constipation, and faced his colleagues' derision. Even if physicians immediately stopped writing new opioid prescriptions—and they wouldn't stop, unless it became legally perilous to continue to do so—we were in it for the long haul. Kolodny explained that for the next sixty years or so, we'd be dealing with a "lost generation" of patients whose "moderate to severe opioid-use disorders" (this term had replaced "addiction" and "dependence," which suggested that patients had brought it on themselves) were doctor-driven, and their troubles would be epic. Many people, finding it hard to fill their long-standing prescriptions for high-dose opioids, would move on to heroin, Kolodny predicted, unleashing a scourge that would afflict Americans of all ages and socioeconomic levels.

In gratitude for Kolodny's help with his own disorder, a patient donated funds that the psychiatrist hoped to use in the production of a documentary about the risks of prescription painkillers. Kolodny had just commenced work on that project when he ran into Russell Portenoy at a medical meeting. To Kolodny's surprise, Portenoy agreed to be interviewed on the spot.

Earlier that year, Portenoy had appeared on *Good Morning America*, offering his usual thoughts to upwards of four million viewers about the impressive benefits of long-term opioid therapy for chronic pain. When pain was properly treated—in the absence of a major psychiatric disorder or a personal or family history of drug abuse—addiction was "distinctly uncommon," Portenoy said. But just months later, Portenoy offered Kolodny's video camera what appeared to be a genuine admission of personal error. Kolodny sent me the footage so I could see and hear it for myself. (Later, I'd speak with Portenoy on the phone to confirm that I had not misinterpreted a random sound bite.) "If I'd had an inkling of what I know now, *then*, I wouldn't have spoken in the way that I spoke," he said. "It was clearly the wrong thing to do. And to the extent that some of the adverse outcomes now are as bad as they have become in terms of endemic occurrences of addiction and unintentional overdose deaths, it's quite scary to think about how the growth in that prescribing—driven by people like me—led, in part, to that occurring."

ONCE ANDREW KOLODNY opened my eyes, I spotted trouble in every corner. A colleague introduced me to Olivier Laude, an effusive and talented photographer who had at one time made a fine income while working for ad agencies and magazines, at least until a life spent schlepping cases full of heavy camera equipment, spending too much time on airplanes and in rental cars, personally renovating his multi-story house, and simultaneously going through a hellish divorce had finally wrought havoc with his back.

Following the usual path, he tried a half-dozen sessions with a chiropractor, then epidural steroid injections, then physical therapy. Nothing helped.

Because his priority was to continue working—with kids to support, and his bank account evaporating fast—a prescription for painkillers held strong allure. "I won't lie—I really looked forward to that little hit of euphoria that accompanied the pain relief," Laude said. At first, two Vicodin tablets made the pain disappear, but the relief didn't last: Within a few weeks he was taking four Vicodin a day, and then six. When he tried to cut back, he felt nauseated and feverish, as if he'd come down with a terrible case of the flu. His primary care doctor, concerned about his escalating dose, sent him to pain management, where 10 milligrams of methadone, a drug which most people associate with the treatment of heroin addicts but is commonly used as a painkiller, was prescribed. "The experience was totally seamless, with no peaks or valleys," Laude said. "I thought that maybe I could stay on it for the rest of my life." As it turned out, that was wishful thinking; again, before the month was out, he needed more. He wouldn't learn, until much later, how quickly a methadone dose can climb into the danger zone—at one point, the drug was involved in a third of the prescription painkiller overdose fatalities in the United States—nor how hard it would be to kick the habit.

As so many of us do, in his search for answers, Laude consulted Google. That's where he found a discussion of sciatic nerve entrapment in "piriformis syndrome." Checking further, he learned that a surgical procedure existed that involved slicing through the thick gluteus maximus muscle, and freeing the nerve. Many orthopedists and neurosurgeons did not think it was a worthwhile or safe procedure; others doubted that "piriformis syndrome" even existed. But when he tracked down a maverick surgeon to do the operation, Laude didn't know about the naysayers. He thought it was his last hope.

Because methadone has a long half-life, it remains in the body well after its pain-relieving properties have elapsed. The surgeon explained that the combination of residual methadone and surgical anesthesia could be lethal. Before the operation could take place, Laude would have to taper his methadone dose, which could take months. Inadvisably, Laude decided to go cold turkey—to get off methadone over a long weekend. "It was hideous," he said. "It was like having every shit disease you ever heard of, all at once." As the methadone left his body, he skidded into the harshest kind of withdrawal, plagued with violent nausea, respiratory distress, chills, fever, and diarrhea, coupled with overwhelming anxiety and depression—the same brutal symptoms that torment a person trying to kick a heroin habit.

Briefly, he was clean—but as soon as the post-surgery drugs wore off, the pain returned, and it was worse. "It felt like my leg was being drowned in acid," Laude said. "The prospect of living like that for the next forty years made me want to throw myself out the window." Within days of his piriformis procedure, he was back on methadone.

Because Laude was born in Corsica, he had access to the French national health care system. Hoping for a better outcome, he underwent a minimally invasive laser disc procedure at a Parisian clinic, to no avail. The following summer, on an ever-increasing dose of methadone, he returned to France, this time to be evaluated by a top neurosurgeon. "After he did all the tests and imaging," Laude reported, "he said that it was criminal for anyone to have ever operated on me, because there was nothing on the scans that needed to be fixed." Not only had the chronic, high-dose opioids made Laude abnormally sensitive to pain, the neurosurgeon said; the side effects were probably the source of many of his other symptoms. He warned Laude that it was time for him to quit obsessing about his pain and leave the methadone behind for good. If he didn't take this advice seriously, the doctor warned him, he'd overdose and die.

Duly chastened, he began to taper his methadone dose slowly. Although it was extremely difficult—again, he felt ill for weeks—Laude found the motivation to begin to rebuild his body, signing up for Iyengar yoga classes, and weight-resistance training at a gym. He discovered that tight, overworked hip flexors—the plague of all who sit for a living—commonly caused low back and leg pain, just like his own.

The more he exercised, the stronger and better he felt. Six months after Laude and his romantic partner and new baby moved to Asia, I called him on Skype. His update was encouraging. He rarely thought about his back pain anymore, he said. He'd gone back to work. Several times a week, he practiced Muay Thai boxing, in which he was becoming a formidable opponent. He had escaped by the skin of his teeth, he acknowledged. Olivier Laude could have easily switched to heroin, and become a statistic. Andrew Kolodny observed that, according to a government study, four out of five current heroin users reported that their opioid use began with medically prescribed drugs. And exactly as he had forecast at our first meeting, the prevalence of addiction and fatal overdose continued to rise.

For several years, John Fauber, the *Milwaukee Journal Sentinel* investigative reporter, had covered the opioid crisis in depth. Aware of Purdue's promotional videos, he'd gone looking for Spanos's patients. Around the same time, Andrew Kolodny also checked in with Spanos, who informed him that of the six patients featured in the original film, two had "moved away" and thus were lost to follow-up. A third had "died in an auto collision," Spanos said, commenting that there was "no suspicion that intoxication was involved."

Both Fauber and Kolodny went searching for Johnny Sullivan, who had informed untold thousands of patients about how well Oxy-Contin worked for him. But it was Sullivan who, in 2008, had died in the auto collision. Specifically, he had fallen asleep at the wheel of his truck, and flipped it. His widow explained that she knew her husband was addicted to OxyContin. He fell asleep everywhere, she said, and he'd overdosed several times before he died. "I knew eventually it was going to kill him," she told Kolodny. "He might have said he got his life back, but it took his life in the end."

FOR YEARS, THE epidemiologists at the Centers for Disease Control and Prevention had left the question of how to handle opioids to the FDA and the DEA, agencies that have greater regulatory authority than that of the CDC. By 2009, it was clear that although the FDA had made feeble attempts to implement requirements for state-run prescription drug registries (which would make it harder for patients to doctor-shop), such registries were useless when patients crossed state lines, and started afresh, making their rounds of potential prescribing doctors.

To make physicians more aware of the challenges and risks involved in opioid prescription, the FDA also began to develop a Risk Evaluation and Mitigation Strategy, or REMS, which went through several iterations, only to be declawed repeatedly at the hands of pharmaceutical industry interests.

At the heart of the REMS was the Opioid Risk Tool (ORT), developed by Utah anesthesiologist and pain management doctor Lynn Webster, a man whose credentials were impressive. With many publications to his name, he was senior editor of the journal *Pain*, president of the American Academy of Pain Medicine, and the director of the Lifetree Pain Clinic. He'd developed the counterfactual, but nevertheless well-accepted construct of "pseudo-addiction," which held that some patients, who showed evidence of addiction, in fact just needed a higher dose of pain medicine. He also proposed that "breakthrough pain," long established as an issue for cancer patients, also afflicted chronic pain patients—and should be treated with more opioids, to support the opioids already on board. His five-question patient survey, the ORT, hailed as both convenient and cost-effective, could be administered in one minute. But it was easy for a patient to find the questions online and prepare answers in a way that would allow him to get the prescription he sought.

As the FDA prepared to make the ORT part of its risk management plan, the DEA raided Webster's Utah clinic. The doctor was arrested on charges of inappropriate prescribing, and the DEA carted off his documents and patient charts. Later, Webster would shift the blame for several patient deaths to his staff, suggesting that his nurse-practitioners or physicians' assistants, who generally took care of refills, had made errors. For a time, it looked as though the DEA was going to make an example of Lynn Webster, but ultimately, the feds were unable to gather enough evidence to convict him, or prove "criminal wrongdoing beyond a reasonable doubt," and he went free. Promptly, he resumed his mission of securing the right to dispense opioid prescriptions for patients suffering from chronic pain; he even wrote a book about his quest. But it was becoming clear that there was no tool—not Webster's ORT, or any other scale—that could discern the risk of addiction or the legitimacy of the pain complaint. Meanwhile, the FDA continued to approve new—and considerably stronger—opioid formulas.

Thomas Frieden, the director of the CDC, exercised admirable restraint. The FDA and the CDC are sister agencies, and they go out of their way to avoid arguments, but it was becoming increasingly obvious that the FDA did not have the resources, or perhaps the inclination, to clean up its own mess. That's when the theoretically objective Institute of Medicine (IOM), part of the National Academies of Sciences, Engineering, and Medicine, stepped into the fray. Federal decision-makers asked the IOM to provide a report that would analyze the prevalence of chronic pain in the United States. The result was a most embarrassing bungle.

The institute's report, called *Relieving Pain in America: A Blueprint for Transforming Prevention, Care, Education, and Research*, was 338 pages long. Among other things, it revealed that since the 1990s, the prevalence of chronic pain in the United States had grown by a factor of four, to encompass some 116 million adults. As a nation, we appeared to be on our last legs.

Ultimately it became clear that the IOM's panel had run into serious trouble—with threatened open warfare between competing factions—while trying to nail down a single, comprehensive definition of what constituted chronic pain. Those playing on the pharmaceutical industry's team—and nine of the nineteen experts on the institute's panel were engaged in financial relationships with opioid manufacturers—wanted to make sure that the definition would encompass any patient with an ache that lasted more than three days.

At first, the IOM issued an erratum statement, decreasing the number of patients in chronic pain to a hundred million. But it seemed that this new figure had been drawn from the published work of Michael Von Korff, the same Group Health Research Institute epidemiologist who had been accused of lacking compassion after he published an editorial questioning rampant opioid prescribing. Von Korff was not pleased that his work had been shanghaied for this purpose, and besides, the hundred million figure had been plucked out of context. "Nobody asked me before they used it," he said.

Reporter John Fauber got in touch with Philip A. Pizzo, the IOM committee chairman and a professor and former dean at the School of

Medicine at Stanford University, to ask him about the sudden change and whether there might have been an error. "I totally disagree that we are using numbers that are not credible," Pizzo declared. "That was our best estimate of the data."

By 2015, the IOM's tally of the number of people in pain had been downsized again—to about 19 percent of the population, or 39 million adults. In the year that followed, the number would be revised downward yet again, first to 25 million and then to between 9 million and 12 million, a long way from the 116 million the IOM report had initially described. Although media outlets around the world had given substantial ink and airtime to the original 116 million, the news cycle had moved on, and very few saw fit to revisit the topic.

WHILE THE FDA shepherded powerful new painkillers onto the market, scientific investigators continued to establish that for chronic pain patients, the drawbacks of the drugs—established side effects like opioid-induced hyperalgesia, lethargy, sexual dysfunction, and constipation—exceeded their benefits and could actually impede effective care. Expert groups like the Cochrane Collaboration stated that they could find no clinically significant benefit for opioids over NSAIDs like naproxen—the over-the-counter medicine commonly sold as Aleve. An investigation in the United Kingdom revealed that patients who were prescribed daily opioids for chronic pain were more disabled at the study's six-month follow-up than they were before they began taking the drugs. A Scandinavian study complemented those findings, showing that the odds of recovery from chronic pain were almost four times higher for patients who did not take painkillers, compared with those who used opioids. Medical professional societies got on board: The American Academy of Neurology (AAN) told its members that the risks of opioids in the treatment of non-cancer chronic pain patients far outweighed the benefits. If physicians stopped using the drugs to treat such conditions as fibromyalgia, back pain, and headache, the AAN observed, long-term exposure to opioids could decline by as much as 50 percent.

Several years earlier, the CDC's director, Tom Frieden, had made it clear that he'd wanted something done about the ninety-two thousand opioid poisoning visits to hospital emergency departments each year, at a national cost of about $1.4 billion, and the nearly nineteen thousand overdose deaths in the United States associated with prescription opioids. There had been no improvement—in fact, the chilling and well-publicized news, derived from a study by Princeton economists Anne Case and Angus Deaton, was that among white, middle-aged men with limited education, deaths caused by drug and alcohol poisoning had risen fourfold. Mortality among white women, especially those from rural areas, was not far behind; Case and Deaton found that twice as many working-age whites died in 2014 as in 1999. There was no question that the United States was in the grip of an epidemic, leaving Frieden with no alternative except to act.

In September 2015, after initiating a comprehensive evidence review, the CDC sent out a preliminary guideline on the best approaches to treating chronic non-cancer pain. As anticipated, there was a hue and cry from opioid manufacturers and their patient advocacy organizations. The Washington Legal Foundation, funded in part by grants from Purdue Pharma, asserted that the CDC's guideline had been developed "behind closed doors"; beyond that, said the legal foundation, by refusing to release the names of the members of its "Core Expert Group," the agency had violated federal law. Six months later, the agency issued a mostly unchanged guideline. In sharp contrast to the FDA's pharma-pleasing REM (Risk Evaluation and Mitigation Strategy), the CDC's recommendations were mostly non-pharmacologic, including exercise therapy, weight loss, psychological therapies such as cognitive behavioral therapy, and interventions to improve sleep. Non-opioid treatments, the CDC found, "could be better tolerated and were superior for improving physical function while conferring little or no risk of addiction and substantially lower risks of overdose and death."

Several important new issues were brought to the fore: Polypharmacy—the co-prescription of benzodiazepines (Ativan, Xanax, Valium)—was involved in many of incidents of overdose fatalities; in a North Carolina study, in which a remarkable 80 percent of patients received co-prescriptions, those who received benzos with their painkillers were ten times more likely to have died than those who did not. Beyond that, the CDC guideline pointed out that there was no such thing as a "safe" threshold for opioids; when they are combined with benzos, alcohol, or sedatives, as they often are, any dose could be fatal.

Chillingly—and conclusively—the new guideline included the following statement: "Overall, one out of every 550 patients started on opioid therapy died of opioid-related causes a median of 2.6 years after the first opioid prescription; the proportion was as high as 1 in 32 among patients receiving doses of 200 MME [morphine milligram equivalent] or higher. We know of no other medication routinely used for a non-fatal condition that kills patients so frequently."

AMERICAN ADULTS SPEND nearly $18 billion annually on drugs meant to treat non-cancer chronic pain. The CDC acknowledged that its recommendation to stop prescribing them would be difficult to achieve: Health insurance carriers and Medicare and Medicaid had never covered most of the proposed alternatives. In many parts of the country, cognitive psychologists trained to treat pain and opioid-use disorders were in short supply. Exercise specialists trained to deal with the vagaries of back pain were also scarce. It would take a while to ramp up, and it would happen only if practitioners could depend on reimbursement. This would require the cooperation of several federal agencies—the CDC, the FDA, and the Centers for Medicare and Medicaid Services, as well as the American Psychological Association and the American Medical Association. There were the usual questions about who would shoulder the additional costs of care; if you didn't take into account the considerable downstream costs of addiction, cognitive behavioral therapy and exercise were more expensive than painkillers.

Just as the CDC released its guideline, the Comprehensive Addiction and Recovery Act (CARA), a bill that the Senate had fiddled with for at least a year, passed almost unanimously and began its trek through the House. CARA was designed to throw cash at the national epidemic of opioid abuse, primarily by improving options for treatment and recovery. In 2013, the National Survey on Drug Use and Health had revealed that in the United States, about one-tenth of the people who needed treatment for a substance use disorder actually got it.

There are about eleven thousand short-term substance disorder treatment programs in business in the United States, but very few of them are oriented toward treating people with opioid use disorders and chronic pain. Long-standing, multi-week programs at the Cleveland Clinic, Silver Hill, Mayo Clinic, and the now combined Hazelden Betty Ford Foundation have generally employed the 12-step model, focusing on detox and abstinence. But years of poor outcomes, coupled with the new science on how opioids affect brain chemistry over the long term, suggest that for many—or most—detox and abstinence are not an option.

The alternative to the conventional, 12-step-oriented residential treatment model is medication-assisted treatment (MAT), usually accomplished with a drug called buprenorphine, or "bupe." Buprenorphine is a partial opioid agonist, which means that it plugs into opioid receptors in the brain, thereby reducing or eliminating the drug craving without delivering the euphoric hit of other opioids. It is used to help heroin- or painkiller-addicted patients withdraw from these substances. It is delivered in various ways, but most commonly in a film that dissolves under the tongue.

The premise behind the care protocol is that individuals who have been dependent on high-dose opioids or heroin can never actually leave those drugs behind. Their brain chemistry has been permanently altered and the drug cravings—along with the dangers of relapse and fatal overdose—will forever be present. Today, addiction researchers and many public health experts regard buprenorphine as an immensely valuable tool, the best hope for patients with opioid-use disorders. From a philosophical standpoint, especially for chronic pain patients, it has its drawbacks: A patient who tapers off opioids in order to be maintained on bupe is substituting one addictive drug for another. But for many, there is no alternative. It's bupe, or an untimely death.

Although bupe makes it harder to overdose, its side effects, which include constipation, dizziness, drowsiness, feeling drunk, and the inability to concentrate, have not been well studied and ultimately may turn out to be just as detrimental as those that accompany OxyContin. There is a distinct possibility that ten years from now—unless it is far more regulated than opioid prescribing has ever been—medication-assisted treatment will produce its own unintended consequences. To date, it remains unclear whether buprenorphine offers the best solution or whether it will trigger another opioid-driven pharmaceutical gold rush, leaving addiction and death in its wake.

IN THE DAYS after the CDC laid down the law in March 2016, other agencies, professional societies, and associations rushed to get on board, to avoid appearing to be moneygrubbing and out of step. The FDA had its tail between its legs. Under Robert M. Califf, its new top official, the agency did its best to distance itself from the pharmaceutical industry. The FDA was primed, its leaders wrote in the *New England Journal of Medicine*, "to comprehensively review our portfolio of activities, reassess our strategy, and take aggressive actions when there is good reason to believe that doing so will make a positive difference." A year later with President Trump in office, and a newly appointed FDA commissioner who looked kindly upon Wall Street, the agency would once again be best friends with Big Pharma and the device industry.

Still, various parties insisted that the Joint Commission should take responsibility. The organization refused to accept the blame and explained, accurately, that it had never endorsed pain as the fifth vital sign. "The standards DO NOT require the use of drugs to manage a patient's pain; and when a drug is appropriate, the standards do not specify which drug should be prescribed," a high-level executive explained. Apparently, there had been a gross misunderstanding back in 2001, when the Joint Commission endorsed "compassionate treatments," costing thousands of lives and hundreds of millions of dollars.

Interestingly, throughout this orgy of finger-pointing, Russell Portenoy's name was rarely invoked. Searching Google, I saw that Beth Israel Hospital had merged with Mount Sinai, causing a great deal of staff reshuffling. When I checked Beth Israel's website, I saw that Portenoy, who had long served as the highly visible chair of the department of pain medicine and palliative care, was nowhere to be seen. He hadn't disappeared: He remained a professor of neurology at the Albert Einstein College of Medicine, and the editor in chief of the journal *Pain*. But as a physician, he had a discreet new posting as chief medical officer of a hospice facility in Brooklyn, a place far removed from public scrutiny, where he could see to it that patients didn't suffer pain in the final days of their lives.

PART II

SOLUTIONS

I'M CERTAIN THAT what you've just read has left you feeling painfully cynical. The good news is that the bad news is finally behind us.

After studying the supermarket of options for treatment, I set out to try the most promising ones myself. By the time I got started on the hands-on stuff, I was fifty-five years old, deconditioned from adhering to the standard back pain victim's list of things to avoid. As so many of us are, I was convinced that my spine was fragile, even on the verge of shattering beyond repair.

In the process, I realized that I was wrong about that. On my team of back pain wizards were rehabilitation, postural, and ergonomic specialists; exercise physiologists; cognitive psychologists; and experts in meditation and kinesiology. Some took me on as a client, parsing my musculoskeletal failings as I sweated, groused, and worried that I was doing myself permanent damage. In other cases, my role was to observe, as the best of the best put clients through their paces.

I cannot count the number of people who admitted that they chose injections, surgery, and pharmaceutical pain management over rehab, simply because those medical interventions were covered by their insurance (and seemed quick and easy), while cognitive behavioral psychology sessions and intensive exercise were difficult to find, had to be paid for out of pocket, and took lots of time.

But with ample evidence that spinal fusion can send a patient into a costly tailspin, and that neither spinal injections nor long-term opioid therapy is evidence-based, new coverage approaches are emerging. Some HMOs, Accountable Care Organizations, and other self-insured enterprises have begun to offer free classes in back-healthy disciplines like Tai Chi and Feldenkrais. How this might change in the future, if the Trump administration follows through on its promise to disband the Affordable Care Act is hard to know. As we will see, a few prescient groups have contracted with specialized back pain rehabilitation facilities, insisting that patients undergo intensive exercise programs before other interventions are even contemplated.

For the time being, this means that in order to get the type of care we really need, most of us will have to ante up cold cash. The prospect of spending even more money horrified me. But as I talked to patients who had "saved" a few thousand dollars by having surgery or injections, and were still incapacitated, I understood what was meant by "opportunity cost." They had lost months or years of their lives.

There are exceptions, of course, but most people who find their way out of the abyss—and most days, I can count myself among them—make it a priority to set aside the time and the money required to rebuild their bodies. It's worth being insistent with your health insurance provider: If the employee you get on the phone when you call to check on your coverage says he has never heard of an intensive exercise rehab program, but assures you that the provider will pay $100,000 for surgery, let me know and I'll send out a copy of this book, with the relevant studies highlighted in yellow.

In the following chapters, you'll encounter people who thought they were lost but finally found a way out. You'll also meet the experts who helped them break free. Whether you seek out these options and experts personally, or take advantage of what you've learned to find yourself an equally adept and educated practitioner, I congratulate you in advance for your gumption.

Now, onward, to the realms where solutions dwell.

9

Head Case

WHAT YOUR BRAIN HAS TO DO
WITH YOUR BACK

As CHRONIC BACK pain patients, we like to think we are well versed in the specifics of our conditions. We speak knowledgeably of our herniated discs, sciatica, and spinal stenosis. But you never hear people describe their "central sensitization," or their struggles with "guarding," or "fear-avoidant behavior," or "pain catastrophizing," because these terms exist outside the medical vocabulary.

I was attending a meeting for epidemiologists when I first encountered those terms. When I asked one of the participants to tell me what they meant, she pointed out that I had just gone into an exaggeratedly deep knee bend to set my briefcase on the ground; then I'd groaned. The former, she explained, was an example of guarding. That deep squat did not protect my back. Neither did the groaning. I was broadcasting my feelings, to be sure that the people around me recognized the gravity of my situation.

My doctor had told me that I could cause permanent damage, I told the epidemiologist. I was just following his orders. I was afraid to lift groceries out of the car trunk, or to unload the dishwasher, or even to make the bed. In fact, by telling me to avoid such activities, she said, my physician had done me a gross disservice. He had invited me to become a "pain catastrophizer," fixated on a supposedly inevitable worst-case scenario. Furthermore, by bending so awkwardly, I avoided using my weakened back muscles, making sure they became even less competent. The epidemiologist asked if I'd ever heard of the phenomenon of "central sensitization," a condition in which the central nervous system essentially blew a gasket, generating back pain in the absence of an actual injury. Yet again, I hadn't.

BEFORE I COULD begin to understand what could go profoundly wrong with the central nervous system, I had a lot to learn about the neurobiology of pain. More than three centuries ago, French philosopher René Descartes had proposed a theory that neatly separated the mind from the body, in an effort to dispel the idea that pain and sickness were evidence of diabolical possession. Cartesian theory, as it has come to be called, held that the brain was a passive recipient of pain information and that pain intensity rose in synchrony with the amount of actual tissue damage. The corollary was problematic, because it suggested that in the absence of a wound, a burn, or a shattered bone, pain ought not to be a factor.

It was not until 1965, when Canadian psychologist Ronald Melzack and British neurobiologist Patrick Wall set out to explain how pain could persist in the absence of an injury, that this understanding began to change. (A literal interpretation of the mind-body split would continue to be taught in medical school classrooms well into the 1970s.) Challenging the established understanding, Melzack and Wall referred to the "gate control theory of pain," hypothesizing that nerve cells in the spinal cord acted like gates, flipping open to allow pain messages to pass through, or closing to prevent such messages from reaching the brain. They realized that by electrically stimulating the painful area, or applying heat or cold, it was possible to interrupt synaptic impulses and "fool" the brain into thinking the pain had stopped.

Melzack and Wall's research was entirely theoretical; it would be years before there were MRI machines that allowed neuroscientists to see what was happening in real time. But what they posited opened the door to further examination of the key role of the central nervous system (CNS) in generating pain signals. Clifford J. Woolf, a young anesthesiologist with a PhD in neurobiology, had worked in Patrick

Wall's laboratory at University College London. In 1983, he was the first to describe the phenomenon of "central sensitization," a condition in which injury to peripheral nerves—those outside the spinal cord and the brain, in the skin, muscle, and connective tissue—lead to an inflammatory response. Over time, the central nervous system—the anatomical term for the spinal cord and the brain—was afflicted, becoming persistently reactive to stimuli and undergoing cellular and molecular changes that resulted in chronic pain. Later, with the development of high-powered functional magnetic resonance imaging (fMRI), Woolf explored the ways in which neurons in different brain regions communicate, how they form a greater number of synapses, and how that leads to the perception of pain.

A simplified explanation of this highly complex neurobiological process is that, when an injury has afflicted one or more of the nerves and the ganglia outside the brain and the spinal cord, neurons in the central nervous system can also become agitated. This bumped-up signal-to-noise ratio may result in increased activation of calcium channels, which boosts the number of chemical messages traveling between nerve cells. Certain vulnerable neurons also get a dose of NMDA (N-methyl-D-aspartate), another brain chemical that exacerbates the process, again increasing the production of calcium ions and sending even more messages whirling around the CNS. Scientists believe that this process may be what causes central sensitization.

A hypothesis has emerged that suggests that central sensitization in fact reflects a type of neurobiological learning disorder; in essence, the brain has misinterpreted and registered messages and is unable to change course. Some researchers have remarked that central sensitization may be seen as a form of classical conditioning: Just as Pavlov's dogs learned to salivate in response to a bell, the body "learns" to experience chronic pain in response to inconsequential stimuli.

As I've noted, many injuries or conditions that lead to central sensitization result from what ought to be only fleeting insults to the peripheral nervous system—twisting the "wrong" way, for instance. Although no causative link has been established, it is clear that there are predisposing factors, such as a tendency to suffer from stress, anxiety, or depression. Once pain has started, factors such as guarding, social isolation, and sleep deprivation—all associated with ongoing pain—may lower pain thresholds even further, thus making the brain more susceptible to central sensitization. Recent research has revealed what many patients know all too well: Chronic back pain is often accompanied by other types of pain, including headaches, other musculoskeletal disorders, temporomandibular joint disorders, fibromyalgia, irritable bowel syndrome, and chronic fatigue syndrome. People who develop central sensitization may also find light, noise, or smells unusually disturbing.

A. Vania Apkarian, a prominent neuroscientist at Northwestern University's Feinberg School of Medicine, has made important inroads into studying central sensitization. In the provocatively named Pain and Passions Lab, which Apkarian runs, his team uses an advanced form of MRI to elucidate how, and where, pain arises, and to evaluate its cognitive consequences.

"When we started this research in 1999," the scientist said, "very few people believed that pain was more than nerves sending a signal into one part of the brain." With grants from the National Institute of Neurological Disorders and Stroke—part of the National Institutes of Health, NIH—Apkarian demonstrated that, instead of simply responding to externally generated discomfort, under siege, the brain itself would begin to generate the pain. Beyond that, in the presence of chronic pain lasting five years, Apkarian found the brain was structurally transformed, sacrificing 5 to 11 percent of its gray matter density. The hippocampus, a region of the brain that is integral to multiple cognitive processes, including the consolidation of memory, is composed mostly of gray matter, and Apkarian found that in patients who had suffered through years of chronic pain, this region was markedly smaller in size. (And in what may turn out to be the most important discovery yet, as reported in the *Journal of Pain*, in less than three months of treatment, cognitive behavioral therapy has been shown to have the potential to enhance the density and volume of gray matter in a chronic pain patient's prefrontal cortex, representing an actual reversal of pain-induced changes in brain structure.)

Apkarian's team also observed that in a group of people who had experienced chronic pain for ten years, there was a noticeable change in the way the hippocampus and medial prefrontal cortex communicated. The nucleus accumbens, involved in the cognitive processing of motivation and pleasure, also behaved aberrantly, chatting up a storm with the prefrontal cortex.

When Apkarian's researchers studied this phenomenon further, using state-of-the-art analysis of neuronal genes and proteins, they found that this "chattiness" represented a profound reorganization of the neuronal connections between the nucleus accumbens and the medial prefrontal cortex. (The former is involved in the cognitive processing of motivation and pleasure, while, among its many tasks, the latter processes sensory information, like what hurts, how much, and how threatening it is.) In the absence of chronic pain, Apkarian's lab revealed, the medial prefrontal cortex is only mildly influenced by the nucleus accumbens. But in the presence of continuous discomfort, that balance shifts. In response, a person's motivation and capacity for decision-making—such as the grit required to get out of bed or off the couch in the presence of pain—may dim. That was important news, because it meant that the nucleus accumbens could be studied as an effective target for pharmaceutical intervention, perhaps one that could limit or entirely avoid the development of chronic pain syndromes.

Apkarian has found relevant neurological underpinnings for depression; isolation; and decline of motivation, empathy, and trust—as well as for the inclination to dash from one doctor to the next, opting for interventions for which clinical evidence is negligible or absent. Other research teams are also studying how genetics affects the way a person experiences pain, but it will be years before we understand how all the pieces fit together.

What we know now is that there are gene variations that may "wire" certain people for suffering while leaving others unscathed. The enzyme catechol-O-methyltransferase (COMT) is essential to the production of several stress-related neurotransmitters, including dopamine, norepinephrine, and epinephrine, each of which is involved in modulating mood and cognition. One variant of COMT produces a slower-acting enzyme that leaves a flood of dopamine intact within the synapse, a condition that is associated with a very high level of stress.

People who inherit that slow-acting COMT variant may be especially emotional and pain-sensitive. Intriguingly, unless they choose more even-keeled partners, it's likely that their progeny will share their tendency toward pain sensitivity. Research on the topic is still limited, but scientists suspect that this shared genetic background, rather than any identifiable pathology, is the reason that pain hypersensitivity often runs in families. In contrast, about 15 percent of the population carry the "bulletproof" polymorphism on the GCH1 gene, which leaves them remarkably impervious to pain. At least one study has shown that patients with this polymorphism recover much more successfully from spine surgery than their ultrasensitive COMT-positive brethren.

Because the painkiller business has been so lucrative, pharmaceutical companies have not yet developed a drug that can prevent peripheral nerve pain from edging toward central sensitization. The prescription drugs gabapentin and pregabalin, both of which put the brakes on calcium ions, are often used successfully to treat neuropathic pain such as sciatica, but there is no evidence to suggest that they can stop the shift to central sensitization, or turn back the tide.

Other pharmaceuticals, called NMDA antagonists, have also been evaluated in laboratory studies. Shown to block the excess "chatter" that occurs between overwhelmed neurons, these drugs are just beginning to be studied in humans in the treatment of chronic pain. Almost everyone who suffers from back pain has taken non-steroidal anti-inflammatory drugs, known as "NSAIDs." Among conventional NSAIDs, ibuprofen (Advil) and naproxen (Aleve) are the most popular. NSAIDs work by blocking the production of hormone-like prostaglandins, which trigger inflammation and pain. But prostaglandins also protect the gastrointestinal lining and the heart, and blocking them is a recipe for damage.

In the mid-2000s, several major pharmaceutical companies came out with a new type of NSAID, intended to treat chronic pain in patients with rheumatoid arthritis and osteoarthritis. The COX-2 inhibitors, sold under the brand names Celebrex, Vioxx, and Bextra, diminished the production of pain-producing prostaglandins, but did not block the production of the protective ones, thereby producing fewer gastrointestinal side effects. Physicians prescribed the COX-2 drugs, which manufacturers hailed as "ten times safer than NSAIDS," to about 100 million people. They cost ten times as much as conventional NSAIDs, but given the improved safety profile, most physicians automatically prescribed COX-2 drugs for the treatment of chronic musculoskeletal pain.

In 2004, new studies that pitted COX-2 drugs against conventional NSAIDs showed that, in fact, the former appeared to almost double the risk of heart attacks and strokes. At the FDA's behest, Vioxx and Bextra came off the shelves. Perhaps so that a comparator drug would stay on the market, Celebrex, manufactured by Pfizer, was allowed to remain, equipped with the FDA's black box warning, alerting patients to serious cardiovascular risks. Soon after, the FDA expanded the black box warning to cover all NSAIDs, including ibuprofen and naproxen. That federal decision opened a handsome new opportunity for opioid manufacturers, who could claim, without mentioning the risk of addiction, overdose and death, that their drugs offered superior gastrointestinal and cardiovascular safety profiles.

Pfizer manufactured Celebrex, which is the brand name for celecoxib. In an effort to demonstrate "non-inferiority" to conventional NSAIDs, which would allow Celebrex to regain center stage, the company funded the PRECISION trial, recruiting 24,000 patients, all of whom were at risk for cardiac events. Patients were randomly assigned to 100 milligrams of celexcocib twice daily, or 600 milligrams of ibuprofen three times daily, or 375 milligrams of naproxen twice daily, with the option to increase therapy for unrelieved symptoms.

To everyone's surprise, when the outcomes were published in the *New England Journal of Medicine* in 2016, it appeared that, in patients who were at risk of strokes or heart attacks, using celecoxib for at least

six months presented no greater risk than using naproxen or ibuprofen. In terms of gastrointestinal events and kidney failure, celecoxib
was modestly safer than either of the other drugs. To many experts,
these outcomes seemed a little too predictable. Many experts questioned the PRECISION trial's legitimacy. They pointed out that, over
twelve years, 68 percent of the recruited patients had dropped out of
the trial. Beyond that, like any company that funded a trial of its own
product, Pfizer had shaped the outcomes to suit its own needs. Car-
diologists who wrote in to the *NEJM* were not persuaded that their
patients should be on NSAIDs of any kind.

But, in the midst of all the PRECISION trial hoopla, an important question had not been asked or answered. Millions of patients
who had once been maintained on opioids for chronic arthritis pain
were no longer on them, and their quality of life had suffered. Baby
boomers and even members of Gen X would be looking for relief
from common inflammatory conditions. Should physicians prescribe conventional NSAIDs, at moderate doses, for those patients?
Should they prescribe Celebrex, or any new COX-2 inhibitors that
were surely on their way to market, now that non-inferiority had
been established?

Other studies had shown that, in patients with no other cardiovascular risk factors, the *relative risk* of heart attack or stroke was low
for all three drugs. The risk was much lower, in fact, than the risk of
heart attack or stroke due to smoking or obesity or uncontrolled high
blood pressure. Surely, among patients whose quality of life was slipping away, and for whom gastrointestinal side effects were a problem,
COX-2 inhibitors were worth considering. But most experts believed
that far more analysis was required. Other prospects under investigation for pain relief include harnessing antibodies that neutralize
inflammation-causing chemicals, and most recently, using powerful
extracts from specific strains of cannabis.

Recent reports show that people who use marijuana for pain relief
require lower doses of opioids, suggesting that the effect is considerable. The safety factor is important: A study published in *JAMA Internal Medicine* in October 2014 revealed that the fatal opioid overdose

rate in states that permit marijuana to be prescribed for medical use (twenty-three states at this writing), is one-quarter the mortality rate of states in which this is illegal.

But the real hope for treating pain does not rest in smoking, inhaling, or eating marijuana. It involves extracting cannabidiol, the active, and non-psychotropic, ingredient in *Cannabis sativa*, and studying its properties. This is easier said than done. Because the FDA classifies marijuana as a Schedule I drug—in the same category as heroin and LSD (lysergic acid diethylamide), with no current indication for pharmaceutical use—it's been next to impossible for scientists to get permission to research its possibilities.

For any drug development team that wants to send a cannabidiol-based drug through clinical trials and then into the FDA's regulatory pipeline, the hurdles remain imposing. (In contrast, opioids, recognized as highly addictive, are on Schedule II, and plans for clinical trials are approved readily.) In two decades, the pharmacology department at the University of Mississippi—the single entity that the U.S. government allows to produce research-grade cannabis—has provided just enough of the plant for the National Institute on Drug Abuse to give the go-ahead for sixteen studies, only a few of which have investigated pain-relieving properties.

Some prominent scientists have asserted that cannabinoid-based drugs could offer a better risk/benefit profile than opioids. They also think that NIDA, an agency that works closely with the FDA, has intentionally avoided supporting studies that might show that these drugs are useful in treating pain and reducing inflammation. Because restrictions are fewer in Europe, at least one company, the United Kingdom's GW Pharmaceuticals, managed to produce a drug that combines two cannabis extracts, cannabidiol and THC (delta-9-tetrahydrocannabinol), packaged in the form of a nose spray. Sativex is already on the market in the UK, Spain, Germany, Denmark, Czech Republic, Canada, and New Zealand for the treatment of the spasticity that accompanies multiple sclerosis. In the United States, when Sativex was tested in Phase III clinical trials for the treatment of very severe cancer pain, it was no more effective than a placebo.

Now that the prescription of opioid medications for the treatment of chronic pain is severely limited, cannabinoid research has started to attract considerable attention from pharmaceutical companies, and regulatory requirements for clinical trials have already been eased. In a regulatory environment that may become even more supportive of Big Pharma, it's hard to predict cannabidiol's prospects.

LONG BEFORE SCIENTISTS had access to the imaging technology that allowed them to visualize neuronal activity, physiatrist John Sarno grasped the relationship between chronic pain and emotional distress. Every time I told anyone I was writing about back pain, I learned to expect questions about whether I knew Sarno's work. Almost everyone had run into someone who had been cured by Sarno, often after years of discomfort. I was happy to be able to inform his many admirers that, yes, I had actually spoken with the rock star of the back world. By the time we talked on the phone, Sarno was well up in years—and perhaps less guarded about expressing his feelings than he would have been in his younger days.

After medical school at Columbia University College of Physicians and Surgeons, John Sarno worked for a decade as a family practitioner in a small town in upstate New York, making house calls and delivering babies on kitchen tables. He returned to Manhattan for further training in the medical specialty of physiatry, at NYU Langone Medical Center's Rusk Institute of Rehabilitation Medicine.

At first, Sarno treated hospitalized patients who had suffered strokes and spinal cord injuries or lost limbs to amputation. They worked hard in physical therapy, and according to him most succeeded in regaining significant function. But when Sarno was reassigned in 1965 to the outpatient department at the Rusk Institute of Rehabilitation Medicine, where he became director of the back pain clinic, his patients did not respond well to standard physical therapy protocols. Instead, like migrating birds, they flitted from practitioner to practitioner, fruitlessly trying to find someone who could fix them.

One of John Sarno's senior colleagues at NYU, physiatrist Hans Kraus, had treated John F. Kennedy's intractable back pain with an intensive exercise protocol. The president had already undergone decades of treatment, including several spine surgeries. The young and reputedly vigorous president was actually so weak, Kraus found, that he couldn't do a single sit-up. When he was directed to touch his toes, his fingers did not even reach to his knees. In October 1961, JFK started the Kraus program, a rigorous routine including aerobic, strength, and flexibility exercises performed twice a day, three days a week. Within a year, the president was able to lift his small children, pull on his own socks, and swing a golf club.

Kraus diagnosed what he called a "muscle tension syndrome," common among people who were exposed to significant stress, with no ready escape by means of physical action. "Your muscles, your mind, your heart and all your organs prepare to act, but you do nothing," Kraus wrote in his book, *Backache, Stress and Tension*. "You may wish to fight, you may wish to flee, but modern civilization prevents you from carrying out your natural impulses. . . . You race your engines without going anywhere."

Chronic muscle tension, Kraus hypothesized, created a cycle that continually generated more pain. He recognized that, without sufficient exercise, oxygen-deprived muscles undergo a process called anaerobic glycolysis, through which lactic acid and other wastes accumulate in the body. Although many other specialists had failed with JFK, Kraus succeeded.

John Sarno saw the wisdom in exercise, but he recognized that workouts three times a week were not in the cards for most of his patients. Nor was Sarno convinced that exercise would resolve their back problems, which he viewed as manifestations of emotional turmoil. Although Sarno was neither psychoanalytically trained, nor well acquainted with the works of Sigmund Freud, he attributed the pent-up rage to an unruly subconscious process rather than a physiological one. If he could convince a patient that his subconscious was kicking up a fuss in order to distract him from personal issues, and that this fuss was manifested in reduced blood flow to the postural muscles, the patient would relinquish the notion that something was structurally wrong and shortly return to a functional life. He called the condition "tension myositis syndrome," or "TMS."

Sarno found that the patients who had the most success with his approach were hardworking perfectionists, driven by self-imposed pressure that left them feeling stretched to the breaking point. Often, they'd had a chaotic childhood, when they'd struggled to gain control over unpredictable and toxic environments. Although the specifics would not come to light for a couple of decades, in time, research would show that people (especially women) who experience significant physical and psychological adversity in childhood are at greater risk for chronic pain than those whose early days were less challenging.

SARNO PUBLISHED HIS first book in 1982, but it was not until *Healing Back Pain: The Mind-Body Connection* came out in 1991, eventually selling over a million copies, that he became a household name. In 1998, when Sarno published *The Mindbody Prescription: Healing the Body, Healing the Pain*, *20/20* coanchor John Stossel was in the midst of his own struggle. After Stossel sat down with Sarno for a chat, he realized that his back felt better for the first time in months. As he planned a TV special on Sarno, Stossel requested permission to call twenty of his patients, randomly chosen from the doctor's medical charts. The patients that Stossel's team interviewed all reported being "better," or even "much better." Roughly fifteen million people watched that segment, and Sarno became "America's back doctor."

But there was a problem. Sarno was unmistakably bad for business. He did not endear himself to the medical community when he announced that physicians were "chiefly responsible for the pain epidemic that now exists in this country."

Once patients became Sarnoites, they lost their appetite for serial interventions. They canceled long-scheduled surgical procedures, usually at the eleventh hour, citing a new perception that their problems were emotional, rather than orthopedic. They stopped getting

MRIs and spinal injections, and didn't show up for physical therapy appointments.

At the peak of his popularity, John Sarno charged up to $1,500 for in-person consultations. But each week he set aside several days when he spoke, gratis, to prospective or current patients, regardless of whether they were celebrities, housewives, or truck drivers. He exorcised author and business pundit Tony Schwartz's spinal demons in forty-eight hours. In our phone interview, Schwartz outlined why he thought Sarno's approach was so successful: "He takes the fear out of the equation—the fear of 'Uh-oh, something must really be wrong with me,'" he explained. "And the impact on symptoms is dramatic."

Most of Sarno's patients never actually saw him. Renn Kaminski, a retired New Jersey police officer, struggled with back pain and sciatica for thirty years—from the time he was nineteen until he reached the age of forty-nine. "Three or four times a year," he said, "I'd be out of commission for a week. It might be because I'd been involved in a foot chase, or because I'd twisted the wrong way when I was putting on my pants."

In the middle of a six-month episode of recurrent sciatica, Kaminski limped down the hallway of a local elementary school, where he was teaching kids about drug safety. The school's principal, familiar with the symptoms, handed him his own dog-eared copy of *Healing Back Pain*. "I took it home," Kaminski said, "but I was in too much pain to read it, so I tossed it on the coffee table, where it gathered dust for a couple of months."

When he finally mustered the energy, Kaminski read the book straight through—several times. "Suddenly, I realized that my problem was that my mind was messing with me," he said. Two weeks later, he was better. "I haven't had serious pain since," he said, "which is not to say that I haven't felt that threatening twinge, where you go, 'Now, I've done it.' But when that happens, I just shake my hips like a hula dancer—like Stan Musial on the Cardinals used to—and then I stand up straight and walk away. I don't obsess. I didn't change my circumstances. I just changed the way my body reacted to the circumstances."

FOR YEARS, KEN MALLOY was hired to develop patient training videos for New York University's medical facilities. He also video-taped John Sarno's lectures, presented to audiences filled with back pain patients. Malloy, who later would become a coach for people with chronic pain, admired Sarno greatly, but whenever he mentioned him to hospital administrators, doctors, or nurses, "they rolled their eyes, as if to say, 'That wacko over at Rusk,'" he recalled, because they could not abide his insistence on the existence of a mind-body connection. "I remember sitting with him in his office, on the ground floor level of the NYU hospital, with the light streaming in, hitting the side of his craggy face. And I said, 'John, do you think the world will ever catch on?' And he said, 'Ken, honestly, not in my lifetime, and likely not in your lifetime.'"

When, in one of our conversations, I asked Sarno—eighty-eight years old and contemplating his accomplishments and failures, what he thought back pain specialists were doing wrong, he answered readily. "They're thinking like mechanics," he said. "They want to find out what's wrong with the machine and fix it. They treat the symptoms. They should know better. Symptomatic treatment is not good medicine. What's going on right now is a disgrace." It bugged him to no end that his colleagues ignored him or, worse, made fun of him. By his count he'd treated, conservatively, ten thousand patients, which was nothing to sneeze at. He'd published volumes that, decades later, still topped Amazon's list of back pain books. But he was never asked to speak at professional meetings, or invited, as most eminent specialists are, to lecture to professional groups about tension myositis syndrome or to deliver hospital grand rounds. "Of the medical profession," he told me, "99.999 percent will not accept this diagnosis of TMS. I do not get flak; I just get ignored. I've always wanted the approval of my peers, and I haven't gotten it."

John Sarno's yearning for acceptance got to me. I felt like calling all those I knew in the back pain industry, and insisting that, finally—before it was too late—they acknowledge his contribution. He sounded deeply tired; I suspected this would be our final conversation. I had one last question to ask: Did he recognize that the insights he'd developed in the 1980s were now making waves in the most elite academic circles? That multimillion-dollar brain imaging equipment had irretrievably linked body and mind? "No," he said quietly. "I was not aware." I could send him medical journal articles to prove it, I said, if he'd like to see them. "I don't read the journals," he said. "I don't care about the fancy machines. I just see that patients get better, and that's all that matters, really." And then we said good-bye and Sarno hung up the receiver with a clatter.

I did not expect to hear from John Sarno again, but a year and a half later, America's back doctor did have his day in the sun. At the invitation of Senator Tom Harkin (D-Iowa) and Philip A. Pizzo, the IOM committee chairman, he testified at a hearing of the U.S. Senate Committee on Health, Education, Labor, and Pensions titled "Pain in America: Exploring Challenges to Relief." As is standard at such events, pharmaceutical manufacturers and industry experts spoke about the importance of maintaining patients' access to prescribed painkillers. When his turn came, the ninety-year-old Sarno, five foot two, owl-like and sage in oversize round horn-rimmed glasses, delivered his message with great clarity, as if he'd been waiting all his years to present this summary.

"The bias that common pain must be the result of structural abnormalities of the spine, or chemically or mechanically induced deficiencies of muscle, coupled with the belief that emotions do not induce physiological change, [has] contributed to the exponential increase in the incidence of these now common pain disorders," he told the assembled group. The frequent diagnosis of such pain disorders was "an iatrogenic disaster," he added, and one for which, as a society, "we are paying dearly."

Soon after his moment on Capitol Hill, patients who phoned the Rusk Institute heard a recorded message from his secretary announcing that Dr. Sarno had stopped seeing patients. He wished them good luck. Prospective and long-standing patients called the hospital switchboard, to no avail. For months, no one picked up Sarno's mantle. Finally, physician Ira Rashbaum, who had worked alongside Sarno since 1991. began taking phone calls from Sarno's frantic patients. But unlike Sarno, who diagnosed thousands of patients over the phone, Rashbaum, a physical medicine and rehab specialist, insisted on seeing his patients in the clinic. "What if I just talked to a patient on the phone and missed something important, like cancer, or ankylosing spondylitis, or rheumatoid arthritis, or arthritic psoriasis, or diabetic neuropathy?" Rashbaum asked, when we spoke. "It would not be a good idea at all, just to call that tension myositis syndrome, or TMS."

With just the power of persuasion at his disposal, John Sarno convinced tens of thousands of people to reject symptoms that had incapacitated them for months or even years. With words alone, he helped people relinquish the belief that their functional lives had ended prematurely. For one man, working out of a tiny office, he had been remarkably influential, providing a cheap and fast way to go forward. As Tony Schwartz said, he took the fear out of the equation.

JOHN SARNO'S CONVICTION that the mind and the body were inextricably connected was definitely not fashionable in his heyday. But today, the best chronic pain rehabilitation programs (CPRPs) focus on dealing with psychological roadblocks. Sent into hiding for many years, the enemy in chronic back pain has once again been identified. It is not a herniated disc or a gnarly facet joint, but fear-avoidant behavior, pain catastrophizing, and guarding.

Typically, in a CPRP, physicians, psychologists, physical therapists, occupational therapists, and nurses are actively involved in treatment, which includes physical reconditioning and cognitive behavioral interventions, and occurs over a period of three or four weeks in a five-day-a-week program. The best patient outcomes are produced in about one hundred hours of intensive therapy over about twenty days. Research shows that part-time programs and programs that occur a couple of days a week do not work nearly as efficiently. Depending on the program, the attitude toward opioid prescription varies. Some programs do not wean patients from opioids, while others insist that they taper before they are admitted. Still others have in-house detox facilities, where withdrawal is "medically-assisted," as described in chapter 8.

Whether the patient's focus is getting back on the factory floor, summoning the strength and confidence to lift a grandchild, or being able to click back into ski bindings, a top-flight CPRP emphasizes a program of active rather than passive care. Although several important and widely published studies have now shown that chronic pain rehabilitation programs are the optimal approach to treating nonspecific back pain of long duration, few physicians are up to speed on this subject.

When I informally surveyed primary care doctors, spine surgeons, interventional pain physicians, and pain medicine experts, asking whether they sent their patients with persistent back pain to chronic pain rehab programs, several misunderstood the question and thought I was asking whether they sent painkiller-addicted patients to drug rehab programs. In general, if the physicians I queried were under the age of sixty, the term "chronic pain rehab" didn't ring a bell. Only retired physicians could remember that, in the middle of the twentieth century, chronic pain rehabilitation programs were present in nearly every teaching hospital. They were popular at a time when spine surgery was understood to pose unacceptable risks, and opioids were reserved for terminal cancer patients. For many years, health care plans readily picked up the tab for these comprehensive programs, which even in the 1960s cost about $20,000.

In 1961, the University of Washington School of Medicine established the first monthlong, ten-hour-a-day CPRP. For years, that program flourished, spawning a throng of kindred ones around the country. The protocol included diagnosis, treatment, and vocational training, with strengthening, stretching, aerobics, swimming, relaxation therapy, and stress management. Physicians from all over the world visited the University of Washington to study the American model. Patients dependent on "happy pills," like the widely prescribed barbiturate Miltown, and muscle relaxants like Soma, were required to hand over their drugs before they could start the program; sometimes they dropped off shopping bags filled with medications.

FOR YEARS, CHRONIC back pain rehab programs quietly accomplished their goals, sending large numbers of patients back to work. Few were judged to be permanently disabled by unspecific on-the-job back pain, a diagnosis that, back in those days, would not hold water with an administrative court judge, but today is commonly accepted.

As I noted in chapter 1, in 1984, when Congress enacted reforms that liberalized the disability screening process, back pain patients became far more likely to qualify for permanent disability on SSDI. The percentage of claims listing "musculoskeletal disease" as the cause of disability would double—and then nearly triple. Medical interventions—chiropractic, physical therapy, injections, surgery, pain management on opioids—did little to benefit the patient, but lawyers, practitioners, clinics, hospitals, and device manufacturers made out like bandits, because every single intervention could be billed, and paid for, separately, racking up profits in multiple departments. The thicker a patient's chart—and the more invasive the list of interventions—the more likely that patient was to gain the sympathy of an administrative court judge, and a ruling of permanent disability. The new regulations did not work in favor of chronic pain rehab programs, which bundled everything together, rather than billing piecemeal for individual services, and instead of being profit centers, often cost their hospitals money.

Observing this change, behavioral psychologist Wilbert E. Fordyce, a faculty member at the University of Washington, forecast that skyrocketing disability-related costs would not only manufacture disabled patients, but also permanently drain the Social Security trust fund. To study the matter, Fordyce chaired the Task Force on Pain in the Workplace.

When Fordyce's committee published its findings in 1995, its timing could not have been worse. The FDA had just approved the BAK interbody fusion cage. Device manufacturers anticipated doing high-volume business, as many more surgical procedures were performed on workers' compensation patients. The task force report went so far as to challenge the very concept of "back pain–related disability, concluding that "non-specific low back pain" was a "problem of activity intolerance," rather than a problem requiring medical attention.

The committee warned against relying on subjective pain assessment tools in determining who should get disability payments. Such tools as the "smiling-to-crying" pain scale that Purdue Pharma had introduced to hospitals, or the American Medical Association's metric of range of motion (ROM) assessment, weren't accurate. Anyone could claim 10 out of 10 on the pain scale, or choose to move with as little fluidity as the Tin Man in *The Wizard of Oz*, especially if he was a plaintiff following his attorney's instructions.

Fordyce's committee instead advocated quantitative measurements of weakness and strength, followed by what Fordyce described as "functional restoration." Mostly, that involved progressively increasing levels of exercise, until the patient could lift, push, sit, and stand in a way that would allow him to carry out his job. Within six weeks, the worker would either return to active employment, with function fully restored, or be "reclassified"—this time, as unemployed. People would have tremendous impetus to get better and get back to work.

Within days after the task force released its report, workers' compensation insurers, plaintiffs' attorneys, independent medical examiners, device manufacturers, physicians' professional societies, and pharmaceutical manufacturers' front groups were up in arms. They fought tenaciously, crushing the task force's recommendations, and in some cases, ruining earnest individuals' career prospects. Just as Fordyce had predicted, between 1980 and 2010, the number of disabled worker beneficiaries increased by 187 percent, draining the Social Security trust fund of its assets.

When hospitals understood how profitable surgical procedures and interventional pain management programs could be, many of them shut down their chronic pain rehab programs, and invested instead in flashy new spine surgery centers and interventional pain management clinics. Patients whose attorneys had advised them to undergo lumbar spinal fusion in order to assure themselves (and their lawyers) of the most lucrative settlement, were in fact often permanently disabled by the surgery. They wound up on long-term, high-dose opioid treatment.

A few programs managed to stay in business because their sponsoring hospitals were willing to absorb their losses. Others went private, leaving the teaching hospital environment behind. The Cleveland Clinic and Mayo Clinic stayed the course. So did Dartmouth-Hitchcock's Functional Restoration Program, which in 2002 moved from the University of Vermont to Dartmouth-Hitchcock hospital in Lebanon, New Hampshire; and PRIDE (Productive Rehabilitation Institute of Dallas for Ergonomics), which, under the leadership of its founder and medical director, orthopedic surgeon Tom Mayer (who coined the term "functional restoration"), settled into its facility in Dallas, Texas, in 1983. Today, with the cost of a multilevel spinal fusion tipping the scales at $125,000, and long-term opioid treatment on the no-go list, these legacy programs, marginalized for decades, serve as models for the development of promising new approaches to treating chronic pain. Chronic pain rehabilitation programs, which cost $20,000 to $30,000, are opening in private facilities and in teaching and community hospitals around the country. A study at the University of Washington revealed that the CPRP approach is approximately twenty-six times more cost-effective in terms of returning patients to work than spine surgery, while an analysis of costs at the three-week, eight-and-a-half-hour-a-day, five-day-a-week program at the Jacksonville, Florida, Mayo Clinic chronic pain rehabilitation program showed as much as a 90 percent reduction in costs when the periods before and after care were compared.

But no matter what they promise, it's important to realize that scams abound. Quality differs markedly from center to center. Many so-called "chronic pain clinics" are no more than "buzzword" fronts for interventional pain physicians, who dole out painkillers and perform epidural spinal injections. Although more will certainly make the grade in the next several years, in 2015, only sixty-six CPRP programs were certified by CARF, the Commission on Accreditation of Rehabilitation Facilities. Many centers function without accreditation, but even those with CARF's blessing should be examined carefully to make sure that intensive exercise and cognitive behavioral therapy, rather than invasive procedures, are the focus.

IN 2008, WITH an eye to the future, the Rehabilitation Institute of Chicago (RIC), which had puttered along since it opened in 1954, opted to expand its program, moving its CPRP, colloquially called "Chronic Pain Boot Camp," to a twelve-thousand-square-foot facility in the Gold Coast neighborhood on the border of Lake Michigan, where it occupies two floors of high-end commercial real estate.

A year later, the American Pain Society designated RIC's chronic pain program a "Center of Excellence" for its work in interdisciplinary care. The program is set up to treat ten patients a week. Before entering, patients undergo a stringent three-hour evaluation process. Patients with conditions that preclude intensive exercise are not accepted, and about a fifth of those who enter do not graduate.

When I visited physiatrist Steven Stanos, anxious to have a look at what went on in "boot camp," he was the director of RIC's Center for Pain Management, a position he'd held for almost a decade. His office window offered a fine view of Lake Michigan, and the crescent of the Oak Street beach. The moniker "boot camp" made sense, he said, "because just as military boot camp [was] training for battle, this [was] training for life." Patients worked hard—five days a week, eight hours a day, for four weeks. They might begin the day with an eight a.m. Feldenkrais class, followed by a cardio conditioning session. Then came a pool workout, followed by lunch. In the afternoon, a group counseling meeting was followed by individual physical therapy. Patients engaged in four or five exercise classes each day, but there were also slots in the schedule devoted to learning relaxation techniques, including biofeedback and meditation. No absences were permitted, and there was always weekend homework.

This was an expensive program to run. RIC employed four psychologists, two relaxation specialists, three occupational therapists, four physical therapists, two full-time physicians, four part-time physicians, three nurses, and a patient-care tech. The facility maintained twenty memberships at the large private Equinox gym next door, where patients worked out with therapists several times a week.

Typically, patients' health insurance covered some or most of the program. There were administrators at RIC whose entire job consisted of negotiating with health insurance and workers' compensation providers. When I asked how much the program cost, if a patient paid out of pocket, one administrator calculated it at a staggering $45,000. But no one ever paid that way.

"We've seen some patients come into the program who have had seven back surgeries in ten years," Steven Stanos said, adding that one spinal fusion surgery—never mind the revisions that often follow—can cost more than the time spent at RIC, with far less certainty of a good outcome. RIC's challenging job is to educate insurance providers so that they know why chronic pain rehabilitation programs both are cost-effective and have better outcomes than shots, opioid therapy, and surgery. But it's rough sledding. "They can't think beyond a list of individual services provided by individual disciplines, which they cover or do not cover, when we are talking about multiple therapies, in multiple disciplines, multiple times a week," said Stanos.

I WAS SO engaged in Steve Stanos's description of the struggle that I was a few minutes late for Caryn Feldman's group cognitive behavioral therapy session. Feldman, an assistant professor at Northwestern University's Feinberg School of Medicine, specializes in behavioral medicine. Her academic research focuses on the benefits of meditation in the treatment of chronic pain.

She wore a necklace with a medallion bearing a circle with a slash through the word "pain." Peering over cherry-colored eyeglass frames from her seat at the end of the table, Feldman was surrounded by patients who were set to graduate from the program that afternoon. I'd agreed to assign pseudonyms to the boot camp patients I'd meet that day, in order to maintain HIPAA (Health Insurance Portability and Accountability Act of 1996) confidentiality requirements.

Until his neck pain put him out of commission, Karl,* in his mid-

fifties, had been a big-shot tech executive for three decades. Donald*
had worked as a pastry chef for thirty-three years, until his enduring sciatica made that impossible. Pale, quiet Patricia,* was a fibromyalgia sufferer. Then there was Julio,* in his mid-twenties, whose
crushed pelvis (he was sandwiched between a bulldozer and a front-
end loader on a construction site), had landed him in the hospital for
eight months. He'd been told he would never walk unassisted again,
but that afternoon, he'd leave RIC on his own two feet, wearing just
an ankle brace.

Since it was graduation day, Feldman asked people to comment on
what aspect of the program had helped them the most. "I've gotten
a lot better at positive self-talk," Donald said, "which I use when the
pain level ratchets up." On weekends off from the program, he'd begun to meditate at the Shambhala Meditation Center near his house
in Rogers Park. Meditation, he explained, helped him accept feelings
and perceptions as they arose, without dwelling on their long-term
implications. Patricia said she found the most help in biofeedback.
"You can go to Shangri-la," she murmured, "and just forget everything." Julio liked biofeedback, too, because it helped him get control
over muscular tension. That's where he was headed, for one last session, before the program would be over.

Karl, who used to run, hike, and go on backpacking trips, admitted that even with graduation scheduled for that afternoon, it was
hard for him to imagine a different future. "Pain really screwed me
up. I lost my dream job, and all my outlets for stress relief, like running three and a half miles a day, and most of my social stuff," he said.
"If I could go back to functioning in a semi-normal way, even without
work, I would be so ecstatic. I have seen six surgeons. I've been to
three pain clinics, including here. I feel like all the bullets in the gun
have been fired." Although they left him feeling nauseated and dizzy,
he expected to stay on the high-dose, extended-release opioids that
he'd been taking for several years. He could not see how he would
manage without them.

Feldman did not sugarcoat how difficult the road ahead would be
for these patients. "It's really hard," she emphasized, "to go it alone.

Support is essential—support and understanding." They must not allow themselves to backslide, or to lapse into thinking they could find a miracle fix out there that could take the pain away. They would succeed or fail based on their own hard work.

When the meeting ended, I followed Julio to the biofeedback room. Speaking softly, Eugénie Pabst, his instructor, spritzed lavender and ginger aromatherapy spray around the room. By observing his own breathing patterns on a monitor, and intentionally quieting them, she explained, Julio could learn to relax and reduce his muscular tension. After he settled into a comfortable chair, electrodes were attached to his shoulders and neck. "The upper trapezius muscles are a good overall indication of his tension level," Pabst explained. "It tells me how much guarding and bracing he's doing." To get a baseline reading, she asked Julio to shrug his shoulders up to his ears. Optimum relaxed breathing occurs at six to eight breaths per minute, she said, but Julio's respiration was much faster.

Three weeks earlier, Julio's muscle tension level had measured at level six, out of a possible high of ten. Activating muscles that did not need to be activated had become a habit for him, one that Pabst would help him break. Now, said Pabst, glancing at the spiky red caterpillar tracings as they crawled across the monitor, the reading was at two. Before this session was over, the goal was to get it to zero.

"Allow the chair to completely support your body," Pabst said soothingly. Julio studied the tracings on the monitor and adjusted his breathing. "Gain control of your shoulders, upper back, then lower back, gluteal muscles . . . feel the bones in contact with the chair," Pabst said. Slowly, the red line on the monitor flattened.

He looked so peaceful that I wanted to ask for my own turn in the biofeedback chair, but I was headed for the physical and occupational therapy department, where RIC had built a mini-apartment. This was smart: In this residential space, patients who had long since abandoned domestic chores could once again take charge of their own lives, practicing tasks like changing the sheets, putting away groceries, taking out the trash, and loading and unloading the dishwasher.

WHEN MY TOUR was finished, I settled down with Caryn Feldman in her office for a debriefing. I could see why patients were so drawn to her; she was maternal but not saccharine, kind but not at all condescending. "I try to help present people with a more realistic and hopeful perspective," she said. "Every patient who comes to RIC has been contending with infinite, long-standing problems. This is where they come last, when they are at the end of their rope. They're grieving for the months or years they've lost to practitioners who wanted to sell them cures."

Although therapists and patients discuss pain during cognitive behavioral therapy sessions, they are not encouraged "to aimlessly, mindlessly dwell on it," Feldman explained. They are discouraged from using the words that back pain patients often employ, like "agonizing," "unbearable," and "hellish." It's a delicate balance, said Feldman, but when the patient has a sense of mastery over his own body and mind, and no longer feels like a helpless victim, the pain catastrophizing and fear-avoidant behavior come to an end, and healing can begin.

"We are not overly empathetic, nor do we pull a 'We're the experts and you know nothing,' routine," she said. "Instead, we ask, 'What techniques are you going to use to deal with that pain?'" The program worked so well, Feldman added, because all parts of the team were under the same roof and meeting weekly to discuss each patient's progress. There were near-constant interactions among staff members in different disciplines. This was rare in the world of chronic pain rehabilitation; and it was practically unknown in conventional medicine's approach to musculoskeletal disorders. "There's no other way you're going to get a pain psychologist, a physiatrist, a PT, and a biofeedback specialist to sit down and have a conversation together about your case," she observed. Such briefings took a lot of time, and insurance providers balked at paying for that time, she added.

The group dynamic was equally important. "There's something magical that happens when folks who have long felt incredibly alone and isolated and misunderstood get to meet each other and to see what it's like to chat with someone who gets what they are going through," Feldman said. "They will take advice from long-suffering peers more readily than they will accept it from a therapist." The group environment also helps patients conquer feelings of social isolation. Beyond that, the camaraderie of the group was keenly important. Studies in humans and other mammals have shown that the brain perceives social isolation as a type of stress, leading to impaired thinking and other stress-related medical problems, including heart disease, diabetes, and obesity.

In boot camp, patients learn how to get through a tough day where they face powerful emotions without collapsing into helplessness, Feldman explained. Sex is an important topic. How to have sex without getting hurt—and how to get back on the horse after a miscalculated move that leaves you groaning for the wrong reasons—is rarely discussed in physicians' exam rooms. But in boot camp, the important technicalities of pacing and positioning during sex, and how to reignite desire, are subjects that Feldman addresses. "Feelings of guilt can compound the patient's already weak self-esteem," she explained. "But as patients emerge from depression and anxiety, and start to feel more hopeful about life, their libidos frequently return."

My forty-five minutes with Caryn Feldman went fast. I wished I'd had someone with her skill set and kindness in my life, as I struggled through the worst of my back pain. Although the need for qualified pain psychologists' services is exploding, they are very hard to find, except on the staff of chronic pain rehabilitation programs. A psychologist who is not specially trained in cognitive behavioral therapy for chronic pain may actually make things worse, by encouraging the patient to "talk it through," and dwell on the pain, rather than to find ways to manage it.

In Steve Stanos's office, we went over a few final things.

First up was sleep deprivation. About half of lower back pain sufferers report clinical insomnia; in a control group of patients without back pain, only 7 percent reported poor sleep quality. It was essential that a patient who was slated to enter the boot camp program could get a full night's rest. "There's no way patients are going to manage to actively exercise for hours a day unless they can sleep at night," Stanos said. Although they have side effects, and are not a long-term solution, said Stanos, drugs like Ambien can work wonders. "It's amazing the gigantic difference a pain patient can feel when he's had a couple of nights when he doesn't wake up five times, but only once or twice," he said.

Not everyone succeeds at boot camp, Steve Stanos acknowledged. The challenge, he said, was "to change people's maladaptive thinking, including the entrenched idea that hurt means harm." This month's graduating class was particularly small, about half the size it was at matriculation. Some of those absent patients, he said, did not want to do the hard work involved. Or they may have behaved in ways that did not contribute to the success of the others.

"Some patients just don't fit into the group, and others fail to set concrete goals, or they refuse to participate in some vital part of the program," he said. "Some of them really like their painkillers, and the attention they get for being in pain, and the lifestyle of not having to do anything, and they're not giving it up. This is not necessarily something we can ascertain in advance."

AFTER MY MORNING at RIC, Caryn Feldman connected me with two boot camp graduates. Gayle Parseghian permitted her real name to be used; while Melinda Wilson* requested a pseudonym. The RIC chronic pain rehabilitation program had saved them, they agreed—but still, they'd endured some very rough times.

Parseghian was from Toledo, Ohio, but I reached her by phone at her family's ski cabin near Bozeman, Montana. Several years earlier, when she was fifty-three and teaching dance to college students, Parseghian and her husband, Tom, attempted to move a new acquisition, a heavy church pew, down a long flight of stairs to its new home in the family room. The pew, which came from Tom's alma mater, Notre Dame, proved too much for Parseghian. The week after Thanksgiving, she checked into the community hospital, with severe back pain, coupled with numbness and tingling in her left leg. With the local spine surgeon out of town on his own holiday, Parseghian was scheduled seven days hence for a three-level spinal fusion.

With a week to think things over, Parseghian decided to delay the surgery. In the year and a half that followed, she hobbled from one doctor to the next, trying, as she put it, "to create some semblance of organized treatment." She collected notes in a huge binder, detailing her appointments with seven physical therapists, several chiropractors, interventional pain physicians, and two other spine surgeons. Several spinal injections provided only the most fleeting relief. She tried traditional Chinese medicine–style acupuncture, and laid out $1,000 for herbal medicine patches and vitamin shots, still to no avail. Emotionally, she was in a very dark place.

"I had been a dancer; my body was my instrument," Parseghian said. "And now I was in so much pain I couldn't go out. I didn't want my husband to leave for work in the morning, because I was so afraid of sitting in my house, depressed and feeling like it was the end." For her family, she tried to put on a happy face. Her son was planning a wedding, and she certainly didn't want to be a killjoy.

Painkillers brought some relief, but she found that she didn't care about anything. "Opioids are not a fix, and that wasn't a road I wanted to follow," she said, "but the pain got so bad I found myself breaking the tablets into little pieces to control it." When she accidentally overdosed, Parseghian chucked the pills and visited several psychotherapists, hoping to find one who could help. "They didn't seem to understand how terribly I missed the life I'd had," Parseghian said. "One wanted me to bring a picture of myself as a little girl. Another told me to suck it up and go get another injection, although the others hadn't worked. After I left, I cried in the parking lot."

In a neurosurgeon's waiting room at the Cleveland Clinic, Parseghian came upon a magazine article describing how a woman who suffered a severe accident had recovered in the chronic pain program at RIC. "It was like I was reading about myself," Parseghian said. "I ripped it out and put it in my purse, thinking that if the neurosurgeon didn't work out, boot camp might be my last-ditch effort."

The neurosurgeon didn't work out. So back at home in Toledo, she studied RIC's website, appreciating the fact that cognitive behavioral therapy was considered as crucial to a successful outcome as exercise. To participate, she would need to stay in Chicago for a month. Her health care plan, she learned, was prepared to fork out $150,000 for a three-level spinal fusion requiring a ten-day hospital stay. But the insurance provider would not say how much, if anything, it would pay for a chronic pain rehab program. Aware that her family could be in the hole for thousands, Parseghian and her husband recognized that, after her two years in pain, this was probably her last chance, and signed up.

At the beginning of her first meeting with psychologist Caryn Feldman, Gail Parseghian burst into tears. "I knew right away that she was wonderful," she said. "Finally, I could let my guard down."

"You get a daily schedule," Parseghian said, "just as if you are going to work. You can't be late. You start at eight a.m. and you go to five p.m., and after that, you have reading and homework and a journal to keep, which the staff checks. It was rigorous, but that was part of my healing. For the first time in a couple of years, I felt like I was being productive. With meditation and biofeedback, you learn how to teach yourself to relax, to remain calm, and that's really an important component. You learn that if the pain comes back—if you have a relapse—you will not be at sea, floundering and drowning."

Nine people entered the boot camp program when she did, but after three weeks, only five remained. Some participants were asked to leave, Parseghian said, because "they came in thinking someone else could cure them. The program is about changing how you react to things, and how you live your life, and you can't do that with a negative attitude. You have to work that out of your system."

She learned how to better monitor her stress level. "There's that saying, 'It's all in your head,' but for me, it really was. I'm very type A. I work very hard and I say yes to too many things. I'd been through a very difficult period caring for my mother, and the stars just lined up. Stress affects different people in different ways, and unrelenting back pain was how it affected me."

Ultimately, the Parseghians' health plan paid most of her bill at

RIC. "We owed RIC a little money," Parseghian said. "But we would have found a way to pay for it all if we had to; it was that important."

The next winter, when she returned to the slopes, she joined a group of advanced skiers in a master class, grateful to once again be engaged in the sport she loved. Her back felt fine. Then—just a few weeks before we spoke on the phone—she had finished her last run of the day, and was quietly poling her way to the parking lot, when she tumbled off a ledge, crashed onto an unforgiving catwalk, and fractured her shoulder.

The shoulder was painful, but her main concern was how her back would handle her physical limitations, as she healed. She knew she couldn't afford the luxury of taking it easy. If an exercise was impossible, she found a substitute. And she had every intention of rejoining her advanced ski group. "I'm getting on that mountain again," she assured me. "I'll go back to RIC if I have to, for a refresher course. But I want to live life, and I'm going to do what gives me joy."

Melinda Wilson,* the other person to whom Caryn Feldman introduced me, was a fifty-two-year-old freelance copywriter who lived about seventy miles outside Chicago. In September 2009, she and her husband, Dan,* an army engineer who had served in Afghanistan and Iraq, adopted the second of two Ethiopian children. On the fourteen-hour flight from Addis Ababa, the infant slept soundly in her arms, but Wilson's back was in a vise. At home, the pain did not relent. Because she could not manage to sit at her desk, she resigned from her job after ten years as the executive assistant of the chairman of a technology company.

Two months after the couple brought the new baby home, a local orthopedic surgeon ordered an MRI, and diagnosed the aching Wilson with degenerative disc disease, a bulging disc, a herniated disc, and spinal stenosis at two levels. "I had all sorts of epidurals and nerve blocks, and trigger point injections, without benefit," she said. She agreed to have a minimally invasive spinal decompression procedure, which helped for only a couple of weeks.

After the procedure, her surgeon prescribed Norco, a drug similar to Vicodin, but containing slightly less acetaminophen. She began with four tablets a day; soon she was up to twelve. "For two and a half years, most of the time I just lay in bed, trying to handle the pain," Wilson said. "I was completely dependent on the Norco, but I had to time how I took it, so I could drive the kids, do the laundry, and take the dishes out of the dishwasher." Five out of seven days a week, the family existed on frozen meals because she couldn't go to the supermarket.

She entered RIC's boot camp in March 2011 along with nine other people. For months before the program began, Wilson had barely moved. "The schedule they handed me the first day would have tried the endurance of an Olympic athlete," she said. "They push you to your limits, and if you don't try your hardest, believe me, you are going to feel bad about it. My muscles were like Jell-O. I was so weak I didn't think I'd make it."

That first morning, drenched in sweat, with her heart racing, she managed to stay on the treadmill for six minutes. For the first week, "everyone in the group was in shock," Wilson reflected. "I remember thinking, 'If I get down on that floor to exercise, I'll never get up. If I get in that pool, I'll never hoist myself out.' Some part of me was going to have to push or pull, and I didn't think I had what it took."

With Caryn Feldman, she talked about her deepest fear—that she would always be a disabled parent and a burden to her children. "I knew the acetaminophen was going to ruin my liver," Wilson said, "and I had two small kids I needed to get to adulthood. With the amount of medication I was on, I wondered if I would be around long enough to get them out of the house.

"This back issue had sucked the life out of my dreams," she told Feldman. "We talked about how to cope with my grief and guilt," Wilson said. "You alienate a lot of people when you have chronic pain. Things were not right with my husband. There was a lot of disappointment on his part—that I might be disabled for our entire lives. It wouldn't be the life we'd planned. I wasn't the daughter my mother needed or the mother my children needed."

For the first two and a half weeks of boot camp, Wilson felt as if she was on a roller coaster, up and down from hour to hour. But

quickly, Wilson noticed a change in herself—and in the other participants. By the third week, almost everyone could fully engage in every
activity. "I had the tools in my pocket to maintain my improvement,"
she said, "and the numbness in my leg was starting to subside."

After graduation, for the first few weeks at home, she kept up the
good work. She started shopping and cooking again, reveling in her
ability to walk through the market, picking out fruits and vegetables
for her family, rather than, as she described it, "limping painfully
through the store as fast as I could to grab Libby's stir-fry in a pouch."

But in the outside world, it was hard to maintain what she had
learned. "You get used to living on a schedule for four weeks, and you
feel great because you've been exercising and taking care of yourself,"
she said. "You convince yourself that you'll do fine without all that
exercise and therapy. But then you have your life to deal with—all the
things you didn't have to do before. I went down that path and fell on
my face."

When Wilson completed boot camp at RIC, most patients arrived
on opioids, and opioid therapy continued to be a standard part of
the program's protocol. When Stanos switched Wilson from twelve
Norco a day to a 50-microgram Duragesic transdermal patch coated
with the opioid fentanyl, she asked no questions. Fentanyl was a
powerhouse of a drug; it was one hundred times more potent than
morphine, and posed a mortal risk to pets, infants, and toddlers who
might accidentally come in contact with the patch, or ingest it. Wilson would never know why Stanos prescribed such a risky drug. He
had financial relationships with several painkiller manufacturers, but
not with Janssen, which makes the Duragesic patch.

Briefly, Wilson felt much better than she had while on Norco. "I
was able to get around, and my head was not as fuzzy," she said. But
within weeks, as her body acclimated to the fentanyl, the transdermal patch no longer provided adequate pain relief. Stanos added one
Norco tablet a day to her drug cocktail, but Wilson soon increased
that to four, hoping she could cover her breakthrough pain.

"You think you are functioning on these drugs, but you are not,"
she said. "I was tired of having to time my interactions with my

kids—driving, playtime, shopping—around the patches and the pain pills, which by that point did not seem to actually help the pain. What scared me into drug rehab was the thought that maybe the meds could be causing my pain, and I was going to be stuck on this stuff forever. I wanted off them, whatever it took."

Since at that time, RIC's protocol did not incorporate a drug treatment program, Wilson admitted herself to a local detox program at Alexian Brothers Behavioral Health's Center for Addiction Medicine. There, she detoxed over three miserable inpatient days—a very short taper schedule, especially for fentanyl, which can linger for weeks in the body. She got started on a maintenance dose of buprenorphine, which cooled her cravings, but did not assuage her pain. Fresh out of detox, she enrolled in a six-hour-per-day, monthlong Alexian outpatient program. Determined not to be dependent on any opioid, Wilson did what very few individuals with severe opioid use disorders can do: She weaned herself off buprenorphine completely.

When I checked in with Wilson more than three years after she finished the RIC program, her e-mail response brimmed with energy and humor. "Life's bumps" still left her in pain, she acknowledged. Stress and anxiety went straight to her back and her legs. But if she adhered religiously to her boot camp routine—walking on the treadmill for twenty minutes, using the rowing machine for fifteen, stretching, and strength training—she was good, she said. "Sometimes I get cocky and let it slide," she reflected, "and that always bites me in the ass."

She had been out kicking a soccer ball with her kids the other day, she reported. "At the end of this long ordeal with my back, I've come to the conclusion that the things that helped and continue to help are exercise, meditation, and good old-fashioned massage therapy. There is no other way to explain how it is that I am still afflicted with the same measured and documented conditions—spinal stenosis, degenerative disc disease, and a couple of bulging discs, and yet my life has returned almost to normal."

Wilson sent me a holiday photo of the family of four cuddling on their red leather sofa, an extravagantly decorated Christmas tree in the background. Her husband was traveling less—just one or two weeks a month—and the kids were doing pretty well, she wrote. "As I got better, the kids got happier," she said. "The dogs are still hobbling around, and the parrot still kicks up a ruckus, but it's all good—and I wouldn't trade it for anything in the world."

THE BOOT CAMP program at RIC attracts patients of all ages, from every walk of life. The next chronic pain rehabilitation program I visited, the Functional Restoration Program at Dartmouth-Hitchcock Spine Center in Lebanon, New Hampshire, focused primarily on returning younger and middle-aged patients to the workforce. Nearly half were workers' compensation claimants. If you ask spine surgeons or busy primary care doctors to tell you about their most challenging cases, work comp claimants with back pain will usually top the list. Disturbing as it is, the common medical wisdom is that no matter what you do for such patients, they will not get better. In lives rife with financial, domestic, and psychological problems, the premise is, the incentive for them to remain disabled outweighs the incentive to recover.

Rowland G. Hazard, the director of the Functional Restoration Program at Dartmouth-Hitchcock, is tall and lanky, with a thoughtful and congenial manner. An internist, he's also professor of orthopedics and medicine at the Geisel School of Medicine at Dartmouth. His goal, he explained, is to transform small groups of back pain patients who have long been disabled into productive and active individuals. That feat is accomplished in thirteen eight-hour sessions, held Monday through Friday, over a period of three weeks.

When spine surgeons and pain management experts visit the program in Lebanon, New Hampshire, said Hazard, "frankly, their jaws drop. What they see here does not fit their medical model. They're always hunting for something they can fix surgically, or treat with medications. And here we have a model that does not rely on pills and shots and surgery but is a matter of people helping each other, through fairly simple training techniques." Any patient who does not suffer from a limiting health condition, such as heart disease, who is willing to work hard—and to deal with the pain that is standard for nearly everyone in the first couple of weeks—is a candidate for the Functional Restoration Program.

While I was on-site I planned to shadow seven patients, most of whom were dependent on high-dose opioid treatment, and many of whom had been out of work for months or years. They ranged in age from twenty-five to forty-five. Four had already failed surgical procedures. The previous day, all had undergone three-and-a-half-hour physical evaluations, during which they also answered questions about anxiety levels, clinical depression, and sleep deprivation. They set targets for their return to work, as well as benchmarks for getting back to recreational and daily activities. On the day I showed up, they were about to tackle their first active program day. Some had barely moved in years.

As Eric Hartmann, the chief physical therapist, walked me down the hall, he warned that there would be some emotional moments. "People cry," he assured me, "both men and women; the person who doesn't shed a tear is the exception." For these patients, he explained, "everything is new. The movements are unfamiliar, and they are afraid they will not survive. What they're about to experience—the eight-hour days, the quantity of activity—that is something that no one has been doing."

Those who lived more than an hour and a half away had already moved into a local motel for the program's duration. Those who lived within ninety minutes were expected to drive home each night and return in the morning, admittedly a tall order for people with debilitating back pain.

As we entered the small sunny gym where the group had gathered, Hartmann described the tricky psychological milieu of functional restoration. "When people come to us," he said, "they have fear. That's expected. But we really want to hear that they are committing to a meaningful physical target. We set a specific lifting goal, a certain level for running and walking. And if they are not moving toward that goal—if their functional ability has hit a plateau and is just kind of hovering in the same zone—then we have to acknowledge that the program is not working, and it may be best for that patient to leave. We don't want to keep torturing people for no reason."

Standing beside an exercise machine, physical therapist Raynee Carlson spoke with this session's participants. There were four men—Matt, Wayne, Jacob, and Clifford—and three women: Polly, Shauna and Lianne.* The oldest person in the room by a long shot, and fit enough to be inspiring but not intimidating, Carlson demonstrated the morning's routine. Soon, men who that morning had been reluctant to carry a bag of groceries egged one another on toward doing more reps, lifting free weights and pedaling stationary bikes. "Try to pace yourself," Hartmann said in mock exasperation, "so you're not dead tired before noon." The program's motto, he noted, is, "Go hard, but go safely."

Weights down, the next exercise involved spinal extension—lying prone on a physical therapy table while raising the shoulders and chest in a "cobra pose." For several of the group members, just getting onto the table posed a challenge. "It's already killing me, before I start," Matt announced, red-faced and grimacing. Polly said she was getting light-headed and swayed a little. Neither physical therapist suggested taking it easy. Functional restoration is about leaping the hurdle of fear avoidance, and unavoidably, there will be some discomfort—even some pain. I noticed that a framed, handwritten quote—a gift from a long-ago graduated patient—hung on the wall: "Once you get it through your head that you are not going to harm yourself—[but] it is going to hurt—you'll make it." Knowing you will survive is the goal.

"The people who get well understand that this is not something we can do in a few weeks," Carlson told me. "This is actually for the rest of your life, and it's going to take up a lot of your time." She cut our discussion short when she noticed that her patients had gathered at the far end of the room, where they were reviewing their injuries, the details of their drug cocktails, and the particulars of their disability settlements. This was exactly the behavior that FRP sought to extinguish. It was high time for the carton lift, which was Hartmann's purview. "For the last hour," he told the group, "we've been working the small muscles. Now, we're going to do some real-life movement. You'll learn a smart way to lift really heavy things."

Along the gym's far wall, there were multiple rows of industrial shelving, each level stocked with plastic milk crates containing steel bricks. "We always hear the right way to lift is to bend the knees, and to be slow and cautious in your movements," Hartmann said, "but as I'm sure you're all aware, that's not always possible."

Polly and Shauna, both of whom who hurt their backs while lifting patients in assisted living facilities, nodded in agreement. Hartmann encouraged the group to lift the heavy milk crates at moderate speed, without any of the standard precautions. He explained that lifting slowly and gingerly, as back pain patients are often taught, only increases the time span during which the back muscles must endure the extra load.

The sounds of thumping, clunking crates and groaning patients filled the center. "Jeezus," said Polly, her flame-red pigtails flying as she bobbed up and down. "Hoo-wee," said Wayne. "This is exactly the kind of work I was doing when I hurt myself."

"This is putting a lot of pressure on my low back," Matt announced doubtfully. The next day, he said, he intended to wear his industrial lifting belt—an idea that Hartmann nixed as counterproductive. The FRP doesn't allow braces or supports, or distractions like earbuds and personal music. "The point is to use your back and to get it strong," Hartmann told Matt. "That's what you're doing now, properly, and you aren't hurting yourself, are you?"

In the second week, Hartmann told me, participants' pain typically flared, provoking all manner of catastrophizing, guarding, and fear-avoidant behavior. Patients came up with dozens of reasons why they absolutely had to sit out the next round, but this was not permitted. "In week three, the turnaround begins," Hartmann said, "as they start to reach their goals. They deal with the pain because they can see that nothing they do makes it permanently worse."

People were still gasping for breath when Raynee Carlson hauled out the industrial sled, an aluminum rectangle equipped with sliders on its base and sturdy handles on either end. For the next half hour, participants took turns pushing the sled back and forth across the floor, with arms thrust forward, spine extended, and chin jutting, as other team members cheered them on. The competitive aspect was important: No one wanted to be the one who stopped halfway through. At this early stage, the sled was bare. But over the next two weeks, the load would increase to about fifty pounds, to be pushed across the floor ten times, akin to the workload anticipated in an industrial setting.

After lunch, when everyone felt drowsy, it was time for an high-energy game of beach ball volleyball. Earlier that morning, most had questioned the safety of bending over to tie their shoelaces. By afternoon, the same crowd was whooping and leaping and ducking and stretching, determined to keep the ball aloft for as long as possible. In less than six hours, fear-avoidant behavior and guarding had vanished. Physical therapists Carlson and Hartmann joined in the game, advertising the fact that the best-ever score was 708 sequential taps—achieved without letting the ball touch the ground. When the game ended—after a respectable 312 taps—Clifford proclaimed, grinning: "So, this is how you start doing things without thinking about whether or not it's going to hurt you. You find out you're still alive and kicking. You had a little pain—and that's all." Carlson and Hartmann nodded approvingly. The activity was so fast that the players reacted without thinking; they were unguarded and unguided. They reached, they jumped, they bent and stepped without thinking. Instead of getting hurt, they found themselves having fun in a social environment.

Later that afternoon, Rowland Hazard invited me to join him in the small conference room where he would meet individually with each patient. With his white coat hanging on a peg behind him, he went through the details of each person's assessment, writ large on a pull-down projection screen. Hazard confirmed existing activity restrictions, surgeries, drug cocktails, and especially, the patient's future goals.

Patients had been trained to dwell on their pain and limitations; to focus on what they could not do, rather than what was possible, as they proceeded through serial medical interventions. For them to make it through the program, that would have to stop. At first, they'd need the constant encouragement and supervision of a staff including a doctor, occupational and physical therapists, and a nurse-practitioner, but the plan was to learn how to make it all work in real life.

Even if they recovered, in a struggling New England economy, Hazard's patients, most of whom had been employed as laborers in industrial settings, could not expect to find their original jobs waiting for them. Matt would never go back to being a stonemason; that was over. Nor would Wayne lift twelve-hundred-pound sheets of window glass off a truck. But as their physical abilities were restored, FRP's next move was to help them find jobs that once again would make them productive members of society. Otherwise, they could quickly relapse into old habits.

WHEN I LEFT New Hampshire in 2009, insurance providers were ready to pay for surgery, shots, and painkillers. Functional restoration was still regarded as an archaic treatment approach, a leftover that was inconvenient for workers and employers. Getting patients to agree to sign up for three weeks of grueling exercise was a problem.

Then, in November 2015, the *Wall Street Journal* published an article that extolled the innovations of Rowland Hazard's program at Dartmouth-Hitchcock Medical Center. Since Hazard's program—and others like it—had been around for more than four decades, the title of the article, "New Help for Back Pain," wasn't quite accurate. The real news was buried: The program cost about $17,000, the article explained, and some health care plans were willing to cover it; beyond that, Dartmouth-Hitchcock Medical Center could provide financial assistance as necessary. In the wake of the *Wall Street Journal* article, CEOs and chief financial officers, tired of ever-burgeoning workers' compensation costs, started asking their insurers to consider similar functional restoration programs, not only for laborers, but for all employees.

For me, that article served as a harbinger: The time had arrived for programs such as RIC's boot camp and the Dartmouth-Hitchcock FRP, flat-fee and nearly risk free, to supplant more dicey interventions.

There is a tendency among health care professionals to blame the patient when things do not go well. Although all patients are vulnerable, workers' comp patients are most subject to this type of shaming. It is easy to declare that patients are invested in staying in pain, that there are emotional problems and addiction problems; and this is often true. But what is left unsaid is that typically, a tag team of doctors, lawyers, and work comp insurers have shepherded such patients down the road to disability; the patients are victims rather than the perpetrators. I watched as supposedly incorrigible workers' comp patients made the transition from being unable to tie their own shoes to playing enthusiastic beach ball volleyball. In a very short time, I saw the light come back into their eyes, as the glimmer of a productive future unfolded before them.

10

The Back Whisperers

HOW TO FIND A REHABILITATION PARTNER

All parts of the body which have a function, if used in moderation and exercised in labors in which each is accustomed, become thereby healthy, well developed and age more slowly, but if unused and left idle, they become liable to disease, defective in growth and age quickly.

—Hippocrates

I WAS PERFORMING MY usual daily routine at the gym when a middle-aged man joined me on the mat. His back was feeling creaky again, he told his personal trainer. He'd barely moved all weekend, because his doctor had warned him to take it easy.

"Pain is a warning sign," the trainer responded rather robotically. "If it hurts, we stop." He had no idea that he was echoing a three-decades-old sentiment, one that back pain experts had long ago consigned to the garbage heap.

In 1982, steeped in the zeitgeist of the period, *New York Times* health columnist Jane Brody wrote that "the guiding principle of all exercise should be: If it causes back pain or makes it worse, don't do it." Although made with the best of intentions, that statement persuaded tens of thousands of people that even mild exercise that provoked pain could cause permanent damage. Fourteen years later, when Brody updated her comments—observing, perfectly accurately, that it was the "lack of exercise that can lead to further deterioration, invalidism and pain"—doctors continued to cling to the old ways, ordering painkillers, rest, ice, gentle walking, and physical therapy. It was rare for a physician to refer a patient to a pain rehab expert who concentrated on intensive, spine-focused exercise, and it still is. Many MDs—including spine surgeons—don't know that back pain rehab specialists exist.

More than two hundred thousand people search Google each month for "back pain," and another thirty-five thousand seek information on spine surgery. Forty-four thousand go to Google to seek information on painkillers, but only forty individuals type in the search word "rehab."

It can be challenging to track them down, but such experts—I call them "back whisperers"—are definitely out there. Choosing can be challenging: Typically, the kind and sympathetic trainer who responds to every grimace and groan (very possibly out of concern that if he hurts you, you'll never book another session) is not going to be the one who guides you to recovery. For that, you will need a fearless leader—someone who is not afraid to challenge you, who has seen it all before, and who knows that, although what you are about to do may be uncomfortable, it will not put you in harm's way.

Back whisperers are not profession-specific: In their ranks, you will find physiatrists, orthopedic surgeons, physical therapists, personal trainers, disenchanted chiropractors, and exercise scientists. Here's what they have in common: They are able to observe how you walk and sit and stand, and grasp what your posture and gait say about your muscles, tendons, and ligaments. Generally, they focus on functional training, prescribing exercise regimens that are "non-pain-contingent" (whining will get you nowhere), "quantitative" (you will not be allowed to quit until you hit your "number"), and "high-dose" (you will do this routine on a schedule rather than when the spirit moves you). Although they agree on the basics—for instance, the value of non-pain-contingent, quantitative exercise—back whisperers often diverge on the specifics.

For instance, although some back whisperers put great stock in stretching, human biomechanist Stuart McGill, a professor of kinesiology at University of Waterloo in Ontario, Canada, is not a fan. In fact, he's against the practice, calling it a waste of time, and observing that it can make recovery harder. In contrast, Massachusetts physiatrist James Rainville, renowned for his esteemed back pain rehab program at New England Baptist Hospital in suburban Boston, integrates stretching exercises into every patient's protocol. At Physicians Neck and Back Center, Brian Nelson (who you met in chapter 3 and will get to know better in the next chapter) swears by the Roman chair (a platform that supports your weight at a slight angle while you strengthen your back and glutes) for building strength and endurance. In comparison, Stuart McGill, who works with some of the world's most valuable athletes, dislikes any exercise that calls for such extreme spinal extension. Physical therapist Joe Zarett, who runs a state-of-the-art, intensive exercise-focused program in Philadelphia, views manual therapy—including mobilization and deep tissue massage—as important to recovery; at the end of almost every session, patients undergo bodywork. But neither Rainville, McGill, nor Nelson subscribes to these passive approaches to care. When such different viewpoints are held by very experienced people, it can certainly be confusing.

Despite their differences, as I spent time with this diverse group, I recognized that they shared the knack of being able to inspire confidence and the desire to work hard in people who might otherwise be disinclined to get off the couch. They knew how to get people over the hump of delayed onset muscle soreness (DOMS) that came on a couple of days after a workout. They knew how to avoid injuring them, without ever babying them. They did not give a hoot about building vanity muscles—biceps, the superficial rectus abdominis (also known as the "six-pack"). But they understood how to repair dysfunctional movement patterns that engendered pain and incapacity.

Because I couldn't recognize my own aberrant movement patterns (most of us can't), I needed a trainer who would correct me relentlessly, until new ones were successfully "grooved." Of my shortcomings, physical therapist Brian Beaudoin considered "gluteal amnesia" to be the most serious. I'd been stuck in my desk chair for so many years that two muscles, called the iliopsoas, that meet in the groin and stretch from mid-spine to pelvis, flexing and externally rotating the hip joint, were far too short, interfering with the hip adductors, which stretch from the pubic bone to the thigh. Like most other women in my family, I had a flat backside. But this, I would learn, was by no means an asset: When the gluteus maximus lacks a nice melon shape, it means that there is not enough muscle on board to support the pelvis and the spine. My hamstrings were tight, and the multifidi—a series of small, paired muscles that stabilize the entire length of the spine—were extremely weak. Brian Beaudoin showed me how my belly button pointed slightly to the right, evidence that my spine was slightly twisted, contributing to muscular tension.

Not just anyone in possession of a business card with the title "personal trainer" on it would be right for me, Beaudoin said. Far too many of his patients came to him after they were hurt in the gym, by trainers who somehow mistook a person in late middle age for a twenty-something. Some franchised extreme fitness programs, he noted, hurt their clients so predictably that wily physical therapists and chiropractors opened clinics within hobbling distance.

For as little as $60, private companies, few of them accredited by the National Commission for Certifying Agencies, issued cheap and meaningless "certified personal trainer" credentials to aspiring coaches, after the completion of an online test. The enthusiastic trainer who pinned a business card to the bulletin board in the neighborhood juice bar, or gave you a "complimentary" coaching session on the first day of your new gym membership, might have very little experience with back pain patients.

As noted in chapter 2, a better way to get a referral is to ask for one from a physical therapist who has the letters OCS, for orthopedic clinical specialist, after his or her name. The website of the American College of Sports Medicine is also an excellent resource. Type in the words "clinical exercise specialist," and the search engine will return data filtered by level of certification, city, and zip code. The National Strength and Conditioning Association (NSCA), based in Colorado Springs, Colorado, also turns out "certified strength and conditioning specialists," most of whom have degrees in exercise science, as well as the specialized knowledge it takes to deal with bad backs.

As you search the Internet, look for candidates with backgrounds in "orthopedic sports medicine," "corrective exercise," "non-pain-contingent exercise," "functional rehabilitation," and "strength training." It's a plus to have undertaken coursework with rehab's big guns, among them Stuart McGill, Craig Liebenson, Gray Cook, Joseph Heller, and Karel Lewit, but ask questions: Did your prospective trainer read a book, or study with the expert for a weekend, a month, or several years? Avoid personal trainers who prioritize vague, "holistic" terms in their bios, like "fitness," "weight loss," "nutrition," "toning," and "wellness," because that expertise does not require specific coursework or certification, and is unlikely to help you resolve your back pain.

Before we parted ways after that first visit to his physical therapy clinic, Brian Beaudoin picked up the phone and left Diana Williams a message. Twice a week, he wanted me to travel twenty minutes each way to the gym in San Francisco's Presidio where she saw clients, paying the toll for the Golden Gate bridge. I thought he had to be kidding: Where would I find the time? Couldn't I just follow a video instead? Given my lack of motor awareness, he said, I could not. Besides, back pain patients were notorious for cheating, avoiding the use of painful muscles and joints, to the point where the exercises they performed were worthless, or even destructive.

When I spoke with Diana Williams later that afternoon, I manufactured every excuse in the book. I described the electrical shocks, muscle spasms, sudden weakness, a grinding toothache in my hip, and pins and needles in my feet. What I liked, I said, was swimming, and everyone knew that this was great for bad backs. (Later, I'd discover that although swimming is fine cardiovascular exercise and good for stress reduction, when you swim on your belly, your spine, from tailbone to neck, is positioned in a slight back bend, a position that's not helpful for people whose spine is intolerant of extension. Beyond that, because swimming is not a weight-bearing exercise, it doesn't help build bone density as efficiently as, say, training with free weights.)

Ignoring my chatter, she said she'd see me on Monday at two p.m. The following week, she looked me over carefully and then asked, just as she would ask twice a week for three years to come, "So, Cathryn—what's going on today with your body?" I looked her over just as carefully—this fiftyish, buff, blond, green-eyed mother of two teenage boys, who—from the stories she told while I sweated—were apparently just as rambunctious as my own. We couldn't have been more different: I was all brains, and she was a dedicated athlete. But we were destined to become great friends.

Within the first ten minutes of our workout together, it was clear, as Beaudoin had already pointed out, that I could not stand on one leg, because the muscles designed to keep me upright were so weak. My squats were malformed. In a plank, I looked like a warped board, my stomach bowing deeply toward the floor. My shoulders would not roll open, and my bony scapulae did not know their job. When Diana ordered a set of biceps curls with light free weights, I nearly conked myself in the head. She didn't laugh: Instead, she observed, quite correctly, that I seemed to have trouble using my brain and my body at the same time. No matter how attentively I watched as she demonstrated an exercise, I forgot what I was supposed to be doing. Beyond that, I cheated like mad. Diana had to physically move my limbs and trunk and alter my stance. As Brian Beaudoin had indicated, I was a motor moron. This was clearly not "mindless" exercise: I needed to use my brain if I wanted to fix my back. She made sure I wasn't bored, or in unreasonable pain—and about halfway through my first session, I realized that I was actually enjoying myself.

If I promised to come in fifteen minutes early to get on the elliptical trainer, and remain for fifteen minutes after the session ended to independently exercise whatever part of my body we'd neglected that day, this effort at physical redemption was going to cost me $100 a week—$400 a month, nearly $5,000 a year. I'd never dreamed I'd spend that on exercise. But if I didn't do it, the opportunity costs would be staggering. My back could put me out of business.

The next few weeks would be rough, Diana said, but I would soon recognize that this was a different kind of pain: a welcome sign that I was getting stronger. Between my twice-a-week sessions, I was forbidden to indulge my inclination to sit at my desk for eight hours straight; no exercise could compensate for such indolence. Nor should I expect to "store up" exercise time. If I stopped working out, the pain would return within days, and each time that happened, it would take longer to recover. We shook hands on the deal, and my physical education officially began.

Twice a week, I left my desk around noon and headed for the gym, eating sliced cold chicken or hard-boiled eggs as I drove, so that I'd have sufficient energy to survive what Diana would dish out. For a month, I was in pitiful condition.

And then, I started to see a change. I abandoned the ancient T-shirts and gym shorts I'd had since college. The day I showed up in a new tank top and yoga pants, I spotted Diana grinning in the mirror behind me. "Look at yourself, lady," she said. My jutting collarbone, the bony strut between the sternum and the scapulae, had been replaced with something I could barely identify: a wide expanse of chest. My shoulders were no longer up around my ears, and my neck was less like a No. 2 pencil. There were neat little caps of muscle on my shoulders, and the bony bird wings were barely visible on my back. "I'm an Amazon," I announced, coining what would become my nickname around the gym. I named Diana the "Goddess of Exercise."

After a year, the physical changes were obvious: For the first time since the age of thirteen, when I'd achieved the height of five foot eight, I'd abandoned the classic tall-girl, chin-poking, slouched posture that had become my hallmark. I'd replaced the pancake-flat posterior with frankly perky glutes meant to support my pelvis. My routine with Diana varied, but most days we started with lunges, planks, squats, and bridges and then moved on to weight resistance training, using free weights, pulleys, and my favorite, the TRX setup, a pair of long black and yellow straps with handles, which allowed me to lift my own body weight at precipitous angles.

The resistance training made me feel energetic, smart, and strong—and no wonder: Studies show that it's a helpful therapy for osteoporosis and osteoarthritis. It also improves glucose metabolism and insulin sensitivity, while lowering blood pressure. Recent studies of older adults show that moderate-intensity strength training increases the production of new neurons in the brain, improving central nervous system processing, decreasing anxiety, and improving memory and sleep hygiene.

I trusted Diana to push me as far as I could go but never further—and some days, she had a lot of convincing to do. When my elderly little dog (the predecessor of the one who insisted that I get out of my chair every two hours), became too ill to manage the stairs, I picked up a twenty-pound restaurant-sized sack of rice at Costco, and took it to the gym. Under Diana's watchful eye, I practiced squatting to scoop that inert bag off the floor and into my arms, so that I might do the same for the ailing animal at home.

Not every problem could be resolved. Seats on planes, saggy soft beds, chairs built for short people, and hellish rental cars continued to cause considerable pain. But every time I arrived in a new city, I used the opportunity to visit a top trainer to learn some new tricks.

ON A REPORTING trip that took me around the country and eventually back to Philadelphia, I realized that I had not exercised in a week. My excuses were stellar: I'd had no space, no yoga mat, no free weights, and no time. (And once, when I had time, I thought the motel room carpet was too dirty.) Just as Diana had warned, once again, I was limping along. On a cool autumn day, as I creaked toward Tenth and Chestnut, where two world-class spine surgeons at Rothman Institute Orthopaedics awaited me, I felt a familiar unease: What if this particular back pain episode was not temporary? What if it were instead the blow from which I would not recover?

Todd J. Albert and Alexander Vaccaro were known for performing the most complex spine procedures on patients with congenital deformities, trauma, and cancer. Although I didn't know it at the time, Todd Albert would soon take up the post of surgeon in chief and medical director at the Hospital for Special Surgery in New York City. But when the two men, dressed in scrubs after a full morning in the OR, met me in their office in the hospital, we spoke of an even more difficult type of patient; the one who had nonspecific back pain and insisted that he needed surgery.

"There's this faulty logic we hear all the time," said Vaccaro, his thick dark hair still plastered to his scalp from sweating under the tie-back scrub cap he'd just removed. "The thinking is generally that the patient has tried everything else—physical therapy, injections, you name it—and it hasn't been effective, and therefore the obvious next step is surgery." But despite what patients think, Vaccaro said, surgery was *never* the "obvious next step." If it were that simple, he said, "then we would have solved the challenge of back pain, which we certainly haven't."

"Patients come in to see me," added Todd Albert, "and there is literally no reason for them to be sitting there. We try to avoid this: Before they get through the door, we try to refer them to an in-house physiatrist or physical therapist, but they get huffy. They say they don't want to see a physiatrist; they want to see me." By the time they make it into his exam room, Albert explained, they've fought so hard to get there that they're absolutely committed to surgical intervention. "They've waited weeks for the evaluation," he said, "and they've valet-parked, and they've spent an hour in the reception area, and they think they are going to talk me into surgery. And then I—a person who makes a living doing surgery—walk into the room and say, 'Hey, sorry, you're not a candidate.'"

"Patients get furious," Albert reflected. "They look at me like I'm their last hope in the world. And then they ask the question we dread: 'Well, then, Doctor, what am I to do?'"

I understood that feeling of desperation, I told the two of them—the sense that you would do anything to rid yourself of the pain. Todd Albert studied me for a moment before he spoke again. "If you're prepared to really sweat, I know someone who can help you," Albert said. "He's a physical therapist; there is no one better. I'll call over there for you right now." And within a few minutes, one of the top spine surgeons in the world had made a late afternoon date for me with Joe Zarett at Zarett Rehab.

THE BUILDING'S PLAIN exterior gave no hint of what I was going to find inside. The elevator doors opened onto a modern foyer decorated with pale wooden furniture, upholstered in soft butter-colored leather. Built into one wall, a saltwater aquarium housed a large school of iridescent blue fish. A couple of attentive young women dressed in polo shirts embroidered with the Zarett logo—a superhero-style Z— invited me to thumb through a binder filled with articles about Zarett and his clientele.

Seconds later, Zarett himself appeared. Although his face could have belonged to a tough and grizzled prizefighter, he was dressed to impress, in wool trousers, designer loafers, and an elegant shirt, the French cuffs rolled back to reveal his powerful forearms.

He and his family had emigrated from Ukraine when he was fifteen, he told me as we settled into his office. After earning his BA in the United States, he went on to get a degree in physical therapy, specializing in gross anatomy and dissection. In 1995, he opened his own orthopedic rehab facility, in the dark, dingy, and showerless basement of the building in which we currently sat. He eventually built the multi-floor gym of his dreams, large enough for six trainers and six clients to work together without tripping over one another.

The typical client at Zarett Rehab visited two or three times a week, usually for ninety minutes each time. The cost varied, depending on the treatment delivered, but the average session ran to $95 and included forty-five minutes of exercise, followed by manual manipulation and deep tissue massage, all overseen by the man everyone called "Joe." There was absolutely no downtime, as I was about to see for myself.

"This process is not about feeling good or relaxed," Zarett said. "When clients come here, they will not be walking on a treadmill while reading the newspaper. The goal is not just to recover but to maintain that recovery, in regular supervised workouts."

When people first come in, it's usually to treat a musculoskeletal injury, often acquired in an ill-fated attempt to shape up in a gym. "People go to a gym," Zarett said, "because they're getting a divorce, and they have twenty-five pounds to lose, and then they mess themselves up. The gym doesn't care what happens to you. The trainers they have on hand are undereducated. You're supposed to do the circuit, following the little pictures on the machines. There are plenty of ways to cheat, and people try to outdo each other on machines they have no business being on."

Zarett wanted to know about my own situation. He had a pretty good idea of what was wrong with me, he said. People tended to think that their problems were unique, but he'd been at it so long that he could quickly identify familiar patterns. We agreed to meet the next morning. "Be sure you eat breakfast, at least an hour before," Zarett said as he showed me to the elevator. "You're going to need it."

At dawn, a couple of boiled eggs sitting heavily in my stomach, I rolled my suitcase and laptop down Philly's cobbled lanes. Joe Zarett was waiting for me, and immediately took a case history. The trauma of that fall off a horse onto my hip when I was sixteen, he explained, had likely initiated a pattern of guarding from which I'd never recovered. The trip to LSI for surgery, he suspected, had done me more harm than good. In a treatment area between flowing striped drapes, he instructed me to remove my clothing. In over three decades as an investigative reporter, this would be the first time (but not the last) I'd try to take notes and maintain a professional demeanor, while I was dressed only in my undergarments.

As I walked back and forth at his behest, Zarett scrutinized my spine. "Okay," he said, "you have a little bit of scoliosis, a little bit of asymmetry between the left shoulder and the right, which means you're always tilted slightly to the right." He asked me to bend forward to touch my toes, and then backward, arching my spine. "The sacroiliac joint on the right is moving too much," he observed, "but the one on the left isn't moving at all." That condition, he acknowledged, might be the outcome of overzealous chiropractic treatment, which sometimes can stretch out the ligaments surrounding the sacroiliac joint.

Even before he touched my lower back, Zarett predicted that the erector spinae would be weak, especially on the right side. As he manipulated my trunk and limbs with his enormous meaty hands, he zeroed in on my most painful spots, as if someone had drawn him a road map in advance.

He palpated a rock-hard zone on the right side of my lower abdomen, near my hipbone. The muscle in question was the same one that Brian Beaudoin had incriminated earlier, my iliopsoas. "It's very important that this muscle is released," Zarett said. Usually, this took three or four sessions of rigorous manual treatment, he explained. "So if we're going to do it all in one day," he said, "we'd better get busy."

The muscles on the right side of my body, throughout my pelvis, thigh, calf, ankle, and foot, were generally dysfunctional, he said. Instead of having a balanced gait, I walked on the instep of my right foot, disturbing the function of everything up the chain. (The foot, which absorbs tremendous weight with every step, is one of the most complex structures of the human anatomy: It contains one-eighth of the bones in the body; thirty-five joints; and more than one hundred ligaments, tendons, and muscles.) "It's amazing how people ignore the feet, as if the back and the rest of the body have nothing to do with them," Zarett said. "How your foot hits the ground will affect everything the whole way up, including, of course, your low back." Without warning, he seized me by the Achilles tendon, making me yelp. "When this ankle starts to move properly again," he said, "you will feel considerably better." The part that hurt, he advised, was rarely the perpetrator, but nevertheless, it was almost always the part that was prepped for surgery.

Therapists always blamed my troubles on my hamstrings, I told Zarett. "Well, they're wrong," he said emphatically. "There's no problem with your hamstrings. You have a problem with your hip extensors, which control the backward movement of your thighs. They're much too tight, from sitting at your desk all day. And I don't like what I see in your upper thoracic area, which is developing such a curve forward that your spine cannot correctly support your weight."

We were scheduled to meet his lead trainer, who would work with me, he said, for "forty-five take-no-prisoners minutes." He promised me that Trey was going to make me work as I had never worked before.

"Right now, you're all about internal rotators in your shoulders, also the result of sitting so much," Zarett said. "That's why your upper spine curls forward like that. We're going to focus on your external rotators, the ones that are supposed to draw your shoulders back. This will never happen by itself. You must have a specific exercise routine to address it. But if you work effectively on your lumbar stabilizers, you are going to be *perfect.*" I thought about how often Diana begged me to stand up straight. I could maintain that posture only briefly. If I was tired, my shoulders slouched. If I could just get those lumbar stabilizers in gear, maybe I could make strides.

In Zarett's gym, a dozen or so people were deep into their morning workouts. Most were middle-aged or older, soaked in sweat and panting. Frankly, it was terrifying. Trey warned me that he would not ask me if anything hurt, because everything would. He made me promise that if I had serious, sharp pain, I would tell him; otherwise, in this gym, I was expected to work to exhaustion, without excessive griping. Form was important, but so was attitude. Joe Zarett did not like slackers, and those who refused would be released from his care.

First up was the UltraSlide, a laminated ten-foot strip emblazoned with the familiar superhero Z logo. Trey handed me a pair of black booties to slip on over my sneakers, which made the strip as slippery as a skating rink, and directed me to assume a plank position. On a rubber mat, a plank is mildly challenging. On the UltraSlide, when Trey instructed me to move my hands and feet as if I were running in place, I collapsed like a drunken platypus. I'd had enough, I told Trey. "Do I mark that on the chart as an outright refusal, then?" he asked. "Yes," I said. "Absolutely."

Trey guided me through a series of abdominal exercises, a few of which seemed familiar. "You are a cheater," he announced, loudly enough for everyone in the gym to hear, explaining that every crunch or leg raise I'd done in the previous half-century had been a waste of time. "Every time you try to perform an abdominal contraction," he said, "instead you're using your hip flexors, which are already too tight. You're making them tighter." In the future, Trey explained, I would execute my abdominal exercises with my back resting on a big exercise ball. "In that position," he said, "you will not be able to recruit your hip flexors, and you will get somewhere."

Next up were clamshell exercises. "Easy," I thought. I'd been doing those for years. Lying on my side on a therapy table, legs bent, I lifted the top knee, much as a male dog would do at a hydrant. Trey scowled. I had allowed the hip on top to roll forward. "If your hip does not remain vertical," said Trey, "you are using your back to create momentum, and the exercise is worthless." I wondered how many hours I'd spent, and how much money I'd wasted, doing exercises that looked vaguely like the ones I was supposed to be doing, but which did not actually help me at all.

Another challenge lay ahead: the Saunders Total Back. This apparatus, a first cousin of the Roman chair, a tilted platform designed to stabilize the pelvis and isolate the lumbar extensors, looked like a good place to grab a quick nap. Then Trey directed me to elevate my upper body for "the Blackburns." From a front-lying position on the Saunders Total Back, he instructed me to raise my arms and lower them at various angles. As I wheezed my way through this routine, uncertain about whether I would survive, Joe Zarett materialized nearby, castigating a distinguished-looking gentleman for both his form and his attitude. "I don't care if you only do it once," he scolded. "Do it right. And get here on time."

Then he turned his attention to me. "Yeah," he said, placing a hand on my right hip, "this is absolutely weak. You've done no work on it. It has never been addressed." Diana and I had been working on that hip for months, apparently without perceptible results. He handed me a yellow Thera-Band—a resilient latex loop—and told me to take it home and slip it around my legs when I practiced clamshells. It would help me rebuild the muscles around my right hip joint. "Better idea," he mused; "you should just cancel your plans and stay for two weeks. In two weeks, I could really do something with you."

I didn't doubt him. But this was not the first time—nor would it be the last—that a practitioner or trainer had told me that his (or hers) was the right way, that a predecessor had it all wrong, and yet again, depressingly, I had wasted both my money and my time. From the trainer's perspective, I understood the importance of gaining trust and fealty. As a client, unless you developed a bit of Stockholm syndrome, bonding with a person who made you do uncomfortable things, you would not stay with the program.

Zarett introduced me to several of his clients before I left the gym floor. There was Jay Federman, a seventy-two-year-old retinal ophthalmologist, whose hair flopped rhythmically as he tackled the Blackburns, displaying far more alacrity than I'd mustered. Two years earlier, he'd taken his bad back to several spine surgeon colleagues, who'd agreed that he needed an operation. But a neurologist friend, recognizing that Federman's career as an eye surgeon depended on maintaining perfect control of his hands, sent him to see Zarett. There had been no spine operation. He'd been coming to the gym three times a week for sixteen months. The workouts permitted him to continue to operate, for three or four hours straight, Federman said. Joe Zarett had sentenced him to this routine, for the rest of his life. "When you go on vacation and stop doing it, it's amazing how fast you can lose ground," he said.

As Zarett and I stepped out of the elevator, we ran into seventy-four-year-old Jerry Muchnik, who had just completed his workout. He'd barely survived Rosh Hashanah services, he explained, when it was already time to attend those for Yom Kippur. "That's four hours, each day, on hard benches," Muchnik reported. He'd developed a brutal case of sciatica, and was using two canes to get around. "I need an ice massage on Mr. Muchnik," Zarett bellowed. "I need him frozen, now." About a minute later, Muchnik was on a therapy table, coated in Biofreeze and snoring loudly.

It was time for my own therapy, Zarett said, and he was issuing me his best weapon. That would be Marlena, a massage therapist with a kind, shy smile and a broad and powerful physique. Zarett gave Marlena her orders: She was to do battle with my psoas and glutes, not stopping until the enemy raised the white flag. She took on the psoas first, her fingers disappearing up to the second knuckle in the folds of my lower abdominal region, where she assaulted that knotted, spasming muscle. I was crying, but I also couldn't stop laughing: Two treatment rooms away, Joe was seeing the mother of one of his high-level executive clients, and the woman had made the notable error of trying to boss Zarett around. "This may be the first referral I've ever made to a chiropractor in my entire career," he announced, so that we could all hear. "But, madam, that's what I recommend for you."

Marlena flipped me over, and, as if there were a pot of gold to be unearthed beneath my right glute, she went after the buried piriformis muscle. Zarett recommended that, unless I was willing to tolerate some very concerned looks, for the next week, I stay clear of locker rooms and bathing suits, since I would be bruised purple, maroon, and blue. When I came back to Philly, he would use *gua sha*, a muscle-scraping technique that has its origins in traditional Chinese medicine. Specifically, he planned to use *gua sha* to address my tight right Achilles tendon and the fascial sheath surrounding the muscles of my thoracic spine. By starting an inflammatory cycle, he explained, this would break down the peripheral capillaries, just under the skin, encouraging new cells to multiply and new tissue to form.

I told Zarett I'd be back soon. I could already feel the difference in my leg and hip. As I headed down the hall to the shower, I ran into Jerry Muchnik, who had a big smile on his face. He was on his own two feet, having discarded the canes. "I'm a new man," he said, merrily waving good-bye.

I rushed to Philadelphia's Union Station, just in time for my train. When a young man, probably a college student, attempted to toss his book-filled backpack onto the overhead rack, it fell short and tumbled to the ground. Fresh from my experience with Trey, I lifted my roll-aboard and, like a stevedore, I heaved it onto the shelf. The kid's eyebrows shot up and his face flushed with embarrassment. "I should probably start working out," he said, as he took his seat.

FROM THE FIRST, I'd wanted to spend some time with biomechanist Stuart McGill, who has made a career of studying why it is that bones, muscles, and ligaments of the spine function, or fail. But McGill was a hard guy to nail down. He dealt mostly with elite athletes and what he called "basket case backs." At times, in a single day, he received three hundred e-mails from patients, requiring him, out of self-preservation, to "select all" and do a mass delete. Those who were serious about being in touch with him would write a second time, or a third, until they finally made the cut.

My best chance to meet with him, McGill said, was to show up when he was leading a California seminar, as he did several times each year. So that I'd be prepared, I studied his YouTube videos, textbooks, and scientific papers. Then I got the word: In two weeks, he'd be in Long Beach, to run a training session for exercise and rehab specialists.

At the University of Waterloo, McGill was in command of two laboratories. In the in vitro lab, pig cadaver spines (obtained from a local slaughterhouse) were tested to see how intervertebral discs and endplates respond under high-stress conditions. In the in vivo lab, with the goal of determining which movements were harmless and which caused pain, McGill's research team recorded and evaluated muscle activation patterns in active human beings who were wired to a computerized "virtual spine."

McGill explained that the notion that back pain is caused by an inciting event—a bad lift, or too many hours in the car, for instance—failed to account for the role of cumulative trauma, the result of sustained mechanical dysfunction. As long as poor body mechanics are a problem, it's difficult to heal muscles or ligaments: Standard strengthening exercises won't do the job. "The biggest mistake that trainers make is failing to address the movement flaws that created the problem in the first place," said McGill. "If you start strength training when there is a broken motor pattern, you will end up strengthening the dysfunction. And of course, the pain will return."

Because they concentrate on isolating individual muscle groups, exercise machines—despite being found in gyms across America, where they are continually updated with even more complicated whiz-bang equipment—don't correct the problem, McGill explained.

Most are worthless, except to build vanity muscles. As an example, as Brian Beaudoin had, he mentioned the leg press machine. "Since neither workers nor athletes perform tasks this way, that type of training isn't transferable and, worse, may cause inappropriate grooving of motor/motion patterns," McGill said.

The better approach, McGill believed, is to correct movement patterns with exercise, carefully matching the exercise dose to the tolerance of the client. When that's achieved, it's time to build endurance in the muscle groups responsible for producing what he described as "quality of movement"—breaking bad habits and teaching the body to recruit the appropriate muscles for a particular task. "When all of those things have been accomplished, and not before," McGill cautioned, "we work on developing speed, power, and agility."

BY THE TIME I arrived at his room in the Long Beach Hyatt Regency, McGill had already spent twenty minutes in an evaluation with Rick, who squirmed in a faux Louis XIV armchair, and asked me not to use his last name. "Our job today," McGill announced to the two of us, "is to begin to understand Rick's back."

Rick, who like me, had flown in from the Bay Area, was a very tall guy in his early forties, with a broad, high forehead and an aquiline nose. His back had bothered him since he was a teenager, and he'd begun seeing a chiropractor at around the age of fifteen. That afternoon, he carried himself in a military posture until the moment he started talking, when he forgot and slumped. He was an optical engineer in the semiconductor industry, who spent very long hours at the computer. There was barely a half-inch of clearance between Rick's six-foot-five frame and his car's roof, which meant that throughout his two-hour daily commute, he sat in a shrimplike curl. His mattress, McGill discovered, was nine years old. Every few months, Rick took a long flight to Asia for work, remaining only a couple of days before he turned around and flew back.

After eighteen months of attending a "flow" yoga class with his girlfriend, he'd obediently followed the instructor into a warrior pose variation, raising his back leg until it was parallel to the ground. The result was an unrelenting case of sciatica. He was "gimping along," Rick said, when he first discovered McGill in a *New York Times* article, accompanied by a video. In the piece, called "Core Myths," the biomechanist explained that the technique being taught in virtually every gym in America—the practice of sucking in, or "hollowing" your belly, while tightening your abs—would not support or in any way strengthen your back. Instead, hollowing the belly pulled the spine out of alignment, weakening the entire structure. "The idea has reached trainers and through them, the public, that the core means only the abs. There's no science behind that idea," McGill told the *Times*.

Rick was so impressed with what he'd read that he ordered McGill's textbook, *Low Back Disorders: Evidence-Based Prevention and Rehabilitation*. He presented this weighty tome to his physical therapist, who had long been telling him to hollow his belly and tighten his abdominal muscles. She had never heard of McGill or his exercises, she told Rick, and besides, she had a standard protocol she employed for lumbar spine patients. "I went home from that appointment extremely discouraged," Rick said. "I wanted to be able to follow McGill's plan, but I had no idea where my psoas muscle was. I didn't know there was a sacroiliac joint. I thought the hip structure was just one big bone, not three with two joints." That's when Rick wrote to McGill, seeking a consultation. He was willing to fly to Toronto, rent a car, and then make the hour-long drive to Waterloo, remaining as long as necessary. Instead, McGill asked him to come to Long Beach, to see what could be done for him in a brief afternoon.

Some months before, Rick's orthopedist had diagnosed spinal facet arthritis, a condition in which arthritic changes and inflammation develop in the tiny joints, and the spidery nerves that infiltrate those joints convey severe and diffuse pain. After McGill examined Rick's radiology report, he asked him to lie facedown on the hotel room bed, raising his straightened legs off the bed by a few inches, which he did without a problem. "If you had facet arthritis," McGill announced, "you would be screaming. And you don't present in any other way as an arthritic guy." The more likely source of the problem, McGill proposed, and one that the radiology report had failed to identify, was retrolisthesis, a posterior displacement where one vertebra slips backward over the adjacent one, irritating the spinal nerves.

McGill was not surprised by the omission. "When people come in with their scans and their long medical histories, I see all kinds of things that the radiologists have missed," he said. "And what the radiologist missed, the orthopedic surgeon, focused on the skeleton, never notices. Most clinicians do not have the expertise or tools to diagnose back troubles at a tissue-based level." This sent patients to surgery for no reason. "When medical personnel hand out those 'unspecific back pain' diagnoses, it means that they have reached the end of their expertise," he added. "Effectively, they blame the owner of the bad back for not trying hard enough, or being mentally weak. That's quite a dishonorable thing, for the doctor to blame the patient for the doctor's failure."

Rehabilitating a very bad back, said McGill, was typically a "whole-body, even whole-person endeavor." McGill observed that much of the advice that doctors and physical therapists offer back pain patients every day is incorrect and therefore doomed to exacerbate the symptoms. For instance, for lifting tasks, most clinicians advise patients to bend the knees and keep the back straight. "This forms the foundation for virtually every set of ergonomic guidelines provided to reduce the risk of work-related injury," McGill said. "But very few jobs can be performed this way—nearly all require either a stooping posture or a squat."

He trained patients in that squat, until they could do it perfectly. He discouraged forward bending—toe touching, sit-ups, forward bends such as are commonly performed in yoga classes. "The idea is to spare the spinal discs, which have only so many bends in them before they are damaged." Genetics largely determines how tough spinal discs are, he said, "but there's no need to exacerbate what heredity has dished out."

Tracking down the mechanical problem, and cutting out what he calls "perturbed movement patterns," makes a big difference. McGill described a young woman patient who had been evaluated by at least twelve specialists in five years, among them, physical therapists, chiropractors, psychologists, physiatrists, neurologists, and orthopedists. Eventually, her troubles had been attributed to clinical depression.

McGill doubted that diagnosis. He observed that the woman could bend backward with no problem. But any activity that involved flexion—that shrimplike curl of the spine—caused her pain. For five years, she had dutifully performed pelvic tilts, knee-to-chest stretches, and sit-ups, usually early in the morning, when her intervertebral discs were engorged with fluid and therefore at their most vulnerable. When they were out walking, her large, strong, and ill-mannered dog jerked her this way and that. "These activities were poorly chosen," said McGill, "because every one of them taxed her already-sensitized lumbar spine." When the patient changed her exercise routine, and found a dog walker, her pain relented.

McGill noted that there were people who "choose to give themselves bad backs." One of his patients, a software engineer who sat in front of a computer all day, wore skintight jeans when she came to see him. "I told her that her hips were frozen, thanks to her choice of attire," he said. "She couldn't flex them, so her back was flattened. I suggested a pair of pleated pants to give her sufficient mobility." She did not like the fashion implications of pleated pants, and chose to stick with the skinny jeans. (People who wear cowboy boots and high heels suffer from similar problems.)

Other patients engaged in far too much stretching, he said. This felt good, because it stimulated the erector spinae's receptors, sending reward messages to the brain. Stretches that physical therapists and personal trainers frequently suggested to back pain patients, such as pulling the knees to the chest, might give the perception of relief, McGill explained. But they do not resolve the problem, because the underlying tissues constantly sustain more damage, which guarantees more pain and stiffness and can cause joint laxity—which in turn could lead to instability, resulting in more damage and pain. The whole idea of "flexibility," said McGill, is generally misguided, because people who have extensive range of motion in the spinal column often have little muscle, putting them at great risk of injury. "The muscles in our legs, arms, and hips are designed to do the work of bending and twisting; the muscles around the spine are designed to stabilize," he said. Once the spine has been stabilized and strengthened, flexibility can be addressed—but there is no scientific evidence that being as limber as Gumby, the bendable toy, improves back health.

In McGill's regimen, he replaced stretching exercises with isometric torso challenges, such as the front and side plank, which allowed the patient to focus on building muscle endurance while minimizing the demand on the spine. "Too many exercises are prescribed for back pain sufferers that exceed the tolerance of their compromised tissues," he asserted. "That guarantees that the patient will stay a patient. Every time you do a traditional crunch, you're flexing the lumbar spine and stressing the posterior part of the annulus. I see far too many people who have six-pack abs and a ruined back."

As you may have discovered, there are still physicians who tell their low back pain patients to do sit-ups to strengthen their abdominal muscles. While I was studying McGill's textbook, I came upon this ill-considered advice from Mehmet Oz and Michael Roizen, in their best-selling book *You: Staying Young—The Owner's Manual for Looking Good and Feeling Great*. In the "Myth or Fact" section, the doctors assure the reader that doing sit-ups will save his back. "Not only will abdominal exercises strengthen your bones and the muscles of the back," they write, "but they will also strengthen your entire midsection—which takes weight and pressure off your back. So add crunches to your routine, as well as leg lifts and bent-over back rows." Not one of those recommendations, said McGill, should be considered safe or effective.

AS MCGILL OUTLINED his philosophy, Rick spontaneously curved into the yoga asana known as Child's Pose, with his trunk folded over his thighs. It was one of his favorites. "Child's Pose is killing you," McGill said curtly. "You have to stop doing it."

There were other forbidden activities. "Sitting in the car for two hours each day is not helping you recover, nor are those plane trips to the Far East," McGill told him. Rick had not anticipated a complete lifestyle change—but if he wanted to leave the back pain behind, said McGill, he would have to remove the offending stimuli—the micro-car, the commute, the ancient mattress, the yoga class (and, as it turned out, the committed yogi girlfriend).

Over the next half hour, McGill put Rick through a series of ex-ercises. Rick warmed up with some back bridges, where the pelvis comes off the floor. Instantly, McGill stopped him, observing that, to push his hips into the air, Rick had recruited his hamstrings, instead of contracting his gluteus muscles. The hamstrings had to be left out of the exercise or the effort would be wasted. "Doing this right is essential," McGill emphasized, "because it establishes gluteal domi-nance in everything else you do." I could relate. Like mine, Rick's hip extensors were far too tight from sitting all day. His glutes were unde-veloped, McGill remarked, eyeing his client's flat backside. Without the glutes' strong support while walking, sitting, and standing, Rick put a crushing load on his spine. "Remember," McGill instructed, "the glutes are the motor. They do the work."

In a YouTube video that is posted in the back pain resources sec-tion of my website, McGill offers an overview of the exercises he rec-ommends for most people with painful lumbar spines. In five years, I have sent perhaps three dozen people—including my husband, my brother, and my son's middle-aged boss, all of them decked with recent-onset back pain—to watch that video and to practice what Mc-Gill preached. Predictably, they e-mailed me to report the miracle: Within a period ranging from a few hours to a few days, they were back on their feet. Many continued to do those exercises every day.

Rick and McGill started with the cat-camel stretch, and then moved on to lunges. Next came McGill's famous lumbar stability ex-ercises, called the "Big Three," designed to impose the lowest possible load on the lumbar spine while increasing muscle endurance. With McGill beside him on his hands and knees on the carpet, Rick tried the curl-up, the side bridge (there are several variations), and the bird dog.

"It is not enough to simply perform an exercise," McGill reminded Rick. "It must be performed to perfection." A hiked-up hip, a flaccid belly, or an unstable shoulder could nix the value of the exercise. No position should be held for too long: More reps were better than longer holds, which could generate oxygen starvation and acid buildup in the muscles.

Although for months Rick had been doing these exercises on his own, he'd been doing them improperly. His shoulders sank, the thoracic region of his spine and his scapulae protruded, and the lumbar region sank toward the floor. "Strong, strong, strong," McGill said, scowling and squeezing Rick's shoulder. "Man up now." Under McGill's tutelage, Rick adjusted the uncooperative body parts until he looked as substantial and motionless as a museum bronze.

It would take Rick about three months of performing the Big Three daily before he saw a difference. But this was a fifteen-minute-a-day lifetime commitment. "Your back will be bulletproof after a while," McGill said, handing over a page of drawings of stick figures illustrating his exercise protocol. Three hours after the session began, Rick and McGill exchanged handshakes and promised to stay in touch.

LATER, AS WE dug into platters of fish and chips at a restaurant down the street from the Hyatt, McGill recommended keeping a journal of daily activities, documenting the ebb and flow of pain and stiffness. "Then, when you have a series of setbacks," he said, "you can probably identify the task or activity that causes you the trouble." The journal's other important role was to document progress, which could be so slow that you might fail to recognize it.

While keeping that journal, McGill said, a patient might realize that sexual intercourse was one of the pain-provoking activities. The pelvic thrust demands enthusiastic lumbar flexion and extension. Over several years, McGill and his clinical investigator, Natalie Sidorkewicz, used biomechanical analysis to study what McGill discreetly referred to as "the midnight movement." It was difficult, if not impossible, to focus on maintaining good body mechanics, McGill acknowledged, when endorphins were flooding your brain, temporarily obliterating sensations of pain. But the next day, the back pain sufferer often paid dearly, and this resulted in "marked reduction in coital frequency."

In the spine biomechanics lab, McGill and Sidorkewicz initially recruited ten heterosexual couples with healthy spines and asked them to have sex in situ, using five randomly assigned intercourse positions, to see how pelvic thrusting affected the *male* spine. Eight infrared motion capture cameras kept track of the movement of reflective dots, strategically placed on the participants' bodies. Among the variations were two approaches to the missionary position, with the man on top of the woman and facing her; two approaches to the "quadruped," or "doggy" position, with the man situated behind the woman on all fours; and the "spoon," or "side-lying position," in which the man and woman rested on their sides, with the woman's back against the man's chest.

The researchers learned that for men whose pain is brought on by spinal flexion, spooning is the worst choice. The missionary position is better, and one of the doggy variations also had merit. For men whose pain derived from spinal extension, however, spooning was more successful than either of the other options.

The next study, McGill promised, would focus on better positions for women with back pain. (Don't hold me to it, but the word is that the "cowgirl" arrangement, with the woman sitting astride a man lying on his back, ranks pretty high.) Side-lying, scissor-leg positions, while not exactly *Cosmo* stuff, limit spinal flexion and extension, and get the job done, without provoking pain. Whether McGill will be able to arrive at an arrangement that would satisfy the complex requirements of a "double back pain" heterosexual couple remains to be seen, and as yet, no study is planned to evaluate how same-sex couples, one or both of whom suffer from low back pain, might best proceed.

Before we parted, I vowed to hit those spine stabilization exercises, and I kept my promise. The Big Three—the curl-up, the side bridge, and the bird dog—would become as much a part of my daily routine as brushing my teeth. I would do them anywhere I could find a reasonably clean piece of floor—even in the airport lounge at LAX, where having commenced the exercises myself, I found myself running an impromptu McGill Big Three class. After first informing everyone that I was an investigative reporter, rather than a physician or any kind of therapist, I nudged a shoulder, ordered a belly to be contracted, and questioned the position of hips that were so out of kilter they could have belonged to the Old Gray Mare. Then I sent everyone the link to McGill's video.

THE NEXT BACK whisperer on my list, James Rainville, was chief of physical medicine and rehabilitation at New England Baptist Hospital in Boston. He'd treated thousands of patients at the NEBH spine program, which he'd started in 1997. Rowland Hazard, the medical director of the Functional Restoration Program at Dartmouth-Hitchcock's Medical Center, had called the physiatrist to tell him I wanted to interview him. Mark Schoene, who edits the monthly, and often disruptive-of-the-status-quo *Back Letter*, had sent his seventy-five-year-old mother to be treated by "Jim" Rainville. "To my amazement," Schoene wrote in an e-mail, "she was lifting 60-pound boxes within a few weeks. Her pain went away completely and never really came back."

Rainville focused on what he called "non-pain-contingent, quota-based exercise." Translated, that meant exercises that were performed, under supervision, at a prescribed dose, without dwelling on associated discomfort. Although rigorous exercise was his tool, the goal was to eliminate kinesiophobia—the fear of movement. The grimacing, the groaning, the odd body mechanics—these have to go, said Rainville, and they do, as soon as patients are confident that, rather than threatening the sanctity of life and limb, such normal activity is safe and healthy.

On a bright September afternoon, I traveled out to NEBH, to meet Rainville and his colleagues, physician Carol Hartigan and lead physical therapist Lisa Childs. Like Stu McGill, Brian Nelson, and Joe Zarett, Rainville oozed nonnegotiable authority. A tall, strong, square-jawed man with bushy eyebrows and the august demeanor of a mature lion, he ushered me toward his office, down a hallway lined with pictures of high-profile patients. "People believe that they have no alternative except to come to a kind of a truce with their pain, doing only those activities that are absolutely essential, while giving up almost everything else," he said as we walked. "Back patients are afraid they will make things worse if they do anything strenuous, which is a natural conclusion—but it's not a correct one in the vast majority of patients."

In contrast to Stu McGill's biomechanical orientation, Rainville believed that back pain was usually unrelated to anomalies in spinal anatomy. Instead, it reflected a nervous system malfunction, in which normal sensations of movement were misinterpreted as pain messages. "That process," said Rainville, "is what drives people with back pain completely crazy, because it means that so many things produce discomfort."

Over the past couple of decades, while the neuroscientists worked out their hypotheses regarding central sensitization, Rainville and his team investigated ways in which exercise could train the brain to respond differently, thus raising the pain threshold. "We're still studying this hypersensitivity of the nervous system," Rainville said, "but we recognize that patients who engage in regular strenuous exercise are just not as pain-sensitive."

Rainville didn't buy McGill's premise that "perturbed," or dysfunctional motor patterns had to be remedied before building strength and endurance. Nor did he believe that a particular combination of exercises—his or anyone else's—provided the ideal solution. "Although patients are often convinced that they need to get rid of pain before they can start exercising," he said, "that is generally impossible."

What was really important for the spine, he explained, is that the intervertebral discs are squeezed and released ("loaded and unloaded") regularly, so that oxygen and nutrients could be properly diffused through the vertebral end plates. Once patients figured out that "they can move and they can do things they were afraid to do before, and that nothing bad will happen," Rainville said, "they shed a lot of the anxiety that hovers around back pain patients all the time."

DURING THE 1980S, the NEBH spine program was set up like Rowland Hazard's at Dartmouth-Hitchcock, with groups of patients meeting daily, five days a week, over four weeks. But as health plans dumped functional restoration in favor of lumbar spinal fusion surgery, epidural steroid injections, and opioids, Rainville found that insurers were reimbursing at about fifteen dollars per patient training session.

"We began to simplify a lot," Lisa Childs, NEBH's head physical therapist, told me, "so that we could survive." In 2009, Rainville's program moved from a group orientation to a one-on-one approach. On average, patients make nine visits of forty-five minutes each, at a total cost of about $900. Depending on the patient's health care plan coverage, some or most of it may be picked up by the provider.

Today, after receiving a physician's order for physical therapy, NEBH's physical therapists work twice a week with the patients who live in the area. Those who come in from out of town have longer and more intensive sessions, but fewer of them. When insurance reimbursement runs out, patients either stop treatment or elect to pay out of pocket. It takes three or four weeks for a patient to get a slot for an evaluation with physiatrists Rainville and Hartigan, but when the assessment is completed, he or she can enter the program immediately.

Increasingly, patients come to NEBH from out of town. Some remain in Boston for weeks, staying in a hotel or a short-term rental, while others require only a few sessions before they manage on their own. After patients go home, Rainville helps them connect with a physiatrist who was trained at NEBH, or with an established physical therapist or MD who is well versed in Rainville's treatment philosophy.

After we finished talking in his office, Rainville walked me down the hall to the gym, where Lisa Childs's patient was draped over the

Roman chair, her hips and thighs resting on thick pads, as she raised and lowered her upper body to strengthen the erector spinae. "A lot of it is trust-building," Childs said. "Getting patients' trust is huge. I ask them to start at a quarter or half of what I believe their potential is. It's important for them to see that they are progressing. Once they get that, we move on to the next phase, which is very goal-oriented and progressive. You engage them, you educate them, you take them through the process slowly. And after they leave, you [continue to] check in [with them] by phone."

In the corner of the gym, an older gentleman stacked milk crates, filled with five-pound steel bricks—the same task I'd seen performed by much younger patients at Dartmouth-Hitchcock. Was it effective to have a person who was in his seventies pursue such a demanding task? The act of lifting was part of most people's daily activity, Rainville explained. This man would not be afraid to lift his groceries out of the trunk of the car.

In order to effectively manage the requirements of everyday life, Rainville said, a sixty-year-old woman ought to be able to raise just over a third of her body weight from the floor to waist height, ten times in a row. She should also be able to lift a quarter of her body weight from waist to shoulder height, ten times. A man, he said, needs to be able to lift half of his body weight from floor to waist height and 40 percent his body weight from waist to shoulder. I calculated that given my weight of 143, I should be able to lift roughly 45 pounds from floor to table and 35 pounds from table to shoulder height.

I told James Rainville that I doubted I could manage that assignment twice, never mind ten times in a row. He wasn't surprised: Typically, chronic low back pain patients could lift just one-third to one-half the weight that individuals with healthy backs could manage. In part, health care practitioners were responsible, because they advised patients that lifting was dangerous and should be avoided. Without exercise, muscles weakened and lost function. At the Spine Center, said Rainville, patients got moving again. "You lift the crates filled with metal bricks without anything terrible happening. . . . And then, when your grandchild comes running to you, you just pick that child up, because it's nothing compared to what you have been doing in therapy."

No one admired James Rainville more than Jerome Groopman, chief of experimental medicine at Beth Israel Deaconess Medical Center in Boston, professor at Harvard Medical School, author of five books, and staff writer for the *New Yorker*. Despite his extraordinary achievements in medicine, science, and literature, back pain had nearly felled him early in his career. In a *New Yorker* article called "A Knife in the Back," and also in his book *The Anatomy of Hope*, published in 2003, he described his experience. In his late twenties, he'd just completed his medical training at Massachusetts General Hospital when he decided to prepare to run the Boston Marathon. When back and leg pain set in, his surgeon identified a bulging lumbar disc, and performed a microdiscectomy. Six months later—it was on a Sunday morning—Groopman stood up after breakfast and collapsed, as what felt to him like electric shocks raced down his buttocks and into his legs.

He moved to Los Angeles to take up a high-pressure fellowship in hematology and oncology at UCLA, but he was in enormous pain. Desperate to feel better, he consulted a rheumatologist, a neurosurgeon, and a sports medicine doctor, none of whom believed he was a candidate for surgery. Groopman continued to hunt for a willing orthopedic surgeon, until he found one in Beverly Hills, who recommended a lumbar fusion, and who advised him that, within a few weeks, he'd be able to start running again. In retrospect, given his medical training, Groopman said, he should have known that it would be impossible to recover so quickly from major surgery. But he was panicked about his professional and personal future. "The desire to be healed will trump common sense," he said, observing that when it comes to their own personal health, even physicians who should know better can make bad decisions. His wife (also a physician) tried to restrain him. "She tried to caution me," he said. "But I became convinced this guy in Beverly Hills had the answer."

After the procedure, as soon as Groopman awoke from anesthesia, he knew that something had gone wrong. In his book, *The Anatomy of Hope,* he explained that "the orthopedist postulated that the blood spilled during surgery had inflamed my nerve roots, causing the severe pain and preventing my legs from functioning normally." He returned home in a body brace. He could not stand or sit. "I was in bed all day and all night, with my torso packed in ice," he remembered, "sleeping a few scant hours only with large doses of painkillers." The surgeon found nothing wrong on new X-rays (MRIs were not yet available). He told Groopman that it was likely that scar tissue was strangling his spinal nerves, so that every time he twisted his body, those nerves were tugged, igniting firecrackers of pain. The surgeon was willing to try again, but Groopman declined the offer.

Instead, he kept a hospital gurney in his lab, so that he could lie down on his back to read and hold meetings. It was a struggle to walk, but he worked out a way to look through the eyepiece of the microscope without bending over, he said, "because quick flexion was risky." When he began physical therapy, he found the clinic's staff to be kind and encouraging, but the other patients had different goals. They were elderly, "with severely arthritic hips and knees that had been replaced," he explained, and the therapy was passive. "I would lie on my back, and the therapists would slowly move my legs up and down."

Two years after the surgery, he could walk several blocks, swim five laps, and use a stationary bicycle for a few minutes, but every movement, even getting out of bed, was fraught with the potential for pain. "I would shift my legs over the side of the bed and cautiously lift my trunk, using the force of my forearms to avoid a pull on my back," Groopman said. He vowed to stay away from doctors. "One had badly hurt me, and none could help me," he said. "I had a narrative in my head that permanent damage had been done and that I would have to live with [those] restrictions."

In 1999, after Groopman had spent nineteen years trying to make the best of a bad situation, a massage therapist triggered a muscle spasm that lasted for weeks, gripping him from neck to hip. A rheumatologist colleague told him to make an appointment to see Jim Rainville at NEBH.

Rainville performed a detailed physical examination, evaluating each muscle and joint for strength. Then he applied an inclinometer, an instrument that resembled a protractor, "and took exact measurements of the range of rotation of my hips, spine, and neck as I moved forward, bent backward, and turned to each side," Groopman said. In every case, the assessment demanded that he move in ways that he had avoided for years. When he was finished, Rainville studied Groopman's MRI on a light box. Then he told his patient that there was nothing wrong with his spine, nor were there any concurrent or undiagnosed illnesses that might be causing his pain.

Rainville had an "incredibly forceful personality. He was like a bomb attack, totally in your face," Groopman said. "You are worshipping the volcano god of pain," the physiatrist told his patient. "The volcano god of pain is your master. You've sacrificed things you love, activities that give your life joy, to be kept free from pain. You say to the volcano god: 'I will give up walking long distances if you keep me out of pain. I will give up lifting my children if you keep me out of pain. I will give up travel, because long trips stress my spine. Just keep me from pain.'"

The dilemma, Rainville observed, was that this god could be appeased only briefly; it was never fully satisfied with any offering, and over time, the volcano god worshipper's life contracted into "a very, very narrow space." Groopman, who by then wondered if he might have wandered into the hands of a quack, remained mute. He was "unsure how to respond to this barrage." His thoughts raced: "He doesn't understand my condition, the immutable scars from the surgery. He is dangerous, threatening to upset even the little equilibrium I've established over the years."

"You think what I am saying is complete bullshit," Rainville retorted, sensing his patient's reluctance. "You've lived all these years without any real hope, and it's hard to open that door and glimpse another kind of life. You can walk out of my office right now and believe everything you've believed for the past nineteen years, and live the way you have. Or you can test me. And I'll tell you now, I'm right." Rainville dared him to ignore the pain. "It doesn't mean anything serious," he said. "As your mind reorients its beliefs, the pain will lessen." His low back muscles were functioning at 30 percent of normal capacity, the physiatrist warned him. His tendons and ligaments had also contracted from lack of use. In the program that he would soon begin, if he stuck around, he'd do cardiovascular work, stretching, and weight training. He could expect to have those familiar jolts of pain in his buttocks and thighs, and unusually intense muscle spasms. But the exercise routine would rewire his brain so that instead of perceiving pain as a threat, he'd experience it as a sensation. And when the pain no longer had his rapt attention, said Rainville, it would begin to fade.

When Rainville walked him over to the gym, Groopman balked. "To my mind, it looked like a Roman torture chamber. Every single thing I'd been told not to do, patients in there were doing," he said. He watched "a little five foot one elderly Italian woman . . . from Boston, and she was schlepping a milk crate full of steel bricks around," Groopman said. He figured that if she could do it, he—at half her age and at the height of six foot five—should be able to manage.

BEFORE HE COULD get started in the formal rehabilitation program, Rainville directed him to do three weeks of stretching exercises at home. "My body was so feeble," Groopman recounted, "that even lifting my legs up against gravity broke a sweat." Pain shot from his buttocks down his legs, all the way to his feet. Despite his complaints, the NEBH therapists did not relent. "I'd leave the sessions depleted, and need to rest for hours, lying in bed on ice packs to numb the protesting nerves and muscles," Groopman said.

He thought about quitting, but the possibility of regaining a much bigger life, no longer under the thumb of the volcano god of pain, stayed with him. After several months, what Groopman described as the "cacophony of pain" went silent. Occasionally, when he attempted a new activity, he'd suffer a setback, but then he'd quickly regain his ground. "What happened in there," he said, "was absolutely amazing. Basically, it showed that the vast body of conventional thinking was just wrong."

When I caught up with Groopman, he had entered his sixties. He swam or biked six days a week; on his "day off," he stretched; and he rarely thought about his back. He followed a restorative yoga program on a DVD, called *Yoga for the Rest of Us*, led by Peggy Cappy, a middle-aged woman whose demeanor he appreciated, because, as he put it, she didn't look as if she was "about to scale Mount Everest."

Not all patients were as responsive to Rainville's program as Jerome Groopman. The most challenging rehabilitation patients, Rainville said, could not relinquish the belief that the pain existed to alert them to some unhealed and dangerous injury. Within that group, Rainville explained, there are subgroups for whom chronic back pain comes with financial and personal benefits. Claiming debilitating back pain is a socially acceptable way, for instance, to avoid household chores, work, family duties, or sexual and emotional intimacy. Some people use it as a way to ensure a supply of opioids. When fear-avoidant behavior persists, suggesting underlying emotional issues, Rainville may recommend that the patient seek psychological help, with a therapist who understands the significance of what appears on a radiology report, and can comfortably repudiate physicians' directives. Over many years, he'd referred patients to a number of therapists, but the one I got to know was psychologist Ron Siegel.

Early in my research, Siegel's 2001 book, *Back Sense: A Revolutionary Approach to Halting the Cycle of Chronic Back Pain*, had caught my attention on a bookstore shelf. In the 1980s, Siegel, who has taught at Harvard Medical School for more than thirty years, spent four and a half months wrestling with back pain he thought might disable him for life. After talking on Skype for a few hours, we met at his brother's bungalow in Sacramento, California. Twenty-three years earlier, in this very house, Siegel remarked, he'd decided to try to work off some anxiety on his brother's NordicTrack exercise machine. That's when the pain struck.

When Siegel was a teenager, his mother's back had "gone out." As was standard practice at the time, she'd been ordered to bed rest for several months. From that moment on, there were always cautions and restrictions about what she could do. "So when I started having pain down my leg," Siegel said, "the scenario felt familiar. It was a big 'uh-oh.' I thought it was very serious. I was terrified." Siegel's orthopedic surgeon identified a herniated disc at L5-S1. He ordered the young psychologist, who was struggling to build his practice, to remain flat on his back, except when he had to walk to the bathroom. In what Siegel described as "a bizarre parody of the classic psychoanalytic situation," he ordered a raised platform to be constructed in his office, so that he could comply with his doctor's orders while, from a chair, his patients revisited their deepest fears.

He'd been in pain for a couple of months when his wife, also a psychologist, mentioned that his condition appeared to worsen noticeably whenever the couple argued. After that contretemps, his back hurt more than ever, and he was scheduled for surgery. But before he went ahead, a colleague recommended that he talk to a friend who, within hours of reading John Sarno's book *Healing Back Pain,* had fully recovered. Siegel, by profession an introspective sort, thought that Sarno worked only for people who were oblivious to their own feelings.

The woman, who was indeed back on her feet, asked Siegel what he was doing right then. "What I always do," he said. "I'm lying here." She told him to go out to buy some groceries; she thought his wife would appreciate it. He couldn't walk a block, he told her, and he certainly couldn't carry groceries, but he reasoned that there was little to lose since he already had a date in the OR.

The first block was torture. His left leg burned and cramped, the consequence, he assumed, of the herniated disc. But after he managed another block, he noticed that pain also shot down his right leg. That was peculiar—because a herniated disc did not normally cause pain in both legs. "I thought that maybe I'd shattered my spine altogether," he said. Then, he considered whether anxiety might be causing the physiological symptoms. Ignoring his doctor's orders, he started to move and sit normally. Two weeks later, he canceled his date in the OR. He was driving, exercising, and doing yoga again. A year after his recovery, he explained, he started to think about how he might help back pain patients "avoid going down unproductive paths and having back pain ruin their lives."

Initially, he accepted John Sarno's hypothesis that the unconscious was running the show. But in time, he recognized that "the central emotional issue is simply the fear of the back pain, fear of being disabled by the pain, fear of having your life interrupted. Pain causes distress, which causes muscles to tighten, which causes more pain." From his perspective, which was similar to that of JFK's physiatrist, Hans Kraus, the problem was a fight-or-flight response gone awry. In the presence of a threat, and in preparation for taking action, Siegel explained, our hearts beat faster, and we become more alert. This works to protect us from peril, but the fight-or-flight response can be activated too frequently, in ways that cause all sorts of problems. If a person stays continually in a state of threatened arousal, research showed, tension accumulates and muscles start to hurt. Feeling trapped and powerless stimulates prolonged activation of the stress regulation system, flooding the body with the hormone cortisol.

His patients considered their troubles to be relatively minor, Siegel recognized, until they read their radiology reports or viewed the scans, at which point the pain that had been merely annoying became severe and disabling. "There's nothing like an image of your spine, with bulging discs, to scare the heck out of you," Siegel said. "It's like, 'Oh my God, what is that?' Patients have been told that the discs in their spine are like torn jelly doughnuts, and the jelly has leaked out. They come to feel that their backs are extremely fragile and they are afraid of squishing out more 'jelly,' or rupturing another doughnut. They've been told that their spines are chronically unstable, or arthritic, or like that of a seventy-year-old person, or that they have a curvature, or a short leg or flat feet." With that scary information in mind, they view everything through the lens of "how will this affect my back," said Siegel, "and this alone generates tons of anxiety, including the fear that no matter what you do now, you're going to pay for it later."

WHEN SIEGEL MET Rainville in the mid-1990s, the physiatrist's spine program was already established at NEBH. It worked, Siegel thought, not only because patients got physically strong, but also because "it would be impossible to lift those heavy milk crates and still be afraid of normal activity," Siegel said.

When a surgeon told a patient never to arch his back; always to bend his knees; to avoid lifting, stop jogging; sit in special chairs, avoid sleeping on his stomach, skip the breast stroke, stay off bicycles, and prop himself up with pillows when having sex—Siegel instructed that patient to ask a question. Were there good reasons, from the surgeon's perspective, to believe that if the patient were to move completely normally—while incrementally developing strength, flexibility, and endurance—that he would cause irreversible damage to his spine? Faced with that query, nearly all physicians agreed that irreversible damage was unlikely. Some warned that exercise, although not specifically dangerous, would cause more pain. When a patient reported that his surgeon said that moving would make him hurt more, Siegel encouraged him to take the risk of living a rich, full life *in pain*. The other option was to be disabled and without prospects— while still living in pain.

"Most people thought it would be better to have their lives back," said Siegel, "and so they would begin moving normally—opening windows and taking out the garbage and loading the washer, just like everybody else. And then they started feeling better. Most people aren't actually afraid of the pain," Siegel said thoughtfully, as our visit came to a close. "You can be raised from your bed at two a.m. in the grip of a severe cramp in your calf, without being thrown into the same kind of existential funk that much milder back pain will cause. Patients are afraid of the disability, of the prospect of not being able to live their lives, to do their jobs. That's what scares the bejeebers out of them. They need reassurance that it is safe to do this, that it is a healthy and a good idea. And that reassurance is most trusted when it comes from both a physician and a psychologist."

AS DESIRABLE AS it would be to sign on with a top-flight back whisperer like Joe Zarett, James Rainville, or Stuart McGill, for many of us the logistics of leaving home for weeks at a time are too challenging and the price is too high. This makes finding local champions a necessity. Two long-standing chronic pain sufferers, Bruce Kaiser and Kim Greenberg, whom we met briefly in chapter 8, where their physician-prescribed opioid-use disorders were discussed, were convinced that their functional lives were over, until they found exercise specialists who revised their thinking.

Greenberg's stepdaughter reported that her beautiful and charming stepmother had been on a steep decline. Half a decade earlier, she had survived a serious automobile accident. When two spine operations failed, her surgeon sent her to pain management. Under the care of an aggressive prescriber of painkillers, she worked her way up to a very high daily dose of OxyContin. She also had a medicine cabinet full of Vicodin, antianxiety drugs, sleeping pills, antidepressants, and neuropathic drugs meant to calm her nervous system. Each year, her interventional pain physician gave her four epidural steroid injections; twice a year, she underwent radiofrequency ablation of the facet joints.

None of it helped. In pain, and distressed to discover that her doctor would no longer increase her opioid dose, in May 2012 Greenberg decided to taper the drugs, join a gym, and start working with a trainer. She got lucky: The guy, assigned randomly, had talent. Never one to do things halfway, she trekked to the gym four times a week; on the other days, she did squats and weight training at home. A couple of years after this routine had become entrenched, she said, "I'm doing things I never dreamed I'd do. I'm like an animal—the way I was when I was younger. I'm bulking up and getting muscle mass back. There are days when I have pain, but I'm not worried about it. When people ask me how I am, it's so nice to be able to say I feel great. I don't have to put on my pain face."

Bruce Kaiser, in his fifties, had also managed to escape. As the director of the wine department at a major auction house, for years he'd regularly lifted forty-pound boxes full of precious vintages. After a two-level lumbar fusion, intended to get him back to work, lifting anything became impossible. "First, I took tons of Vicodin," he said. "Then I moved on to OxyContin, until the dose was up to 160 milligrams every eight hours—and I still needed more opioids for 'breakthrough' pain."

Instead of putting Kaiser back on the job, the opioids left him unable to concentrate or sustain a train of thought. Under the circumstances, he could no longer work as an auctioneer. He decided to quit the drugs cold turkey, but what he expected to be an awful few weeks turned into nine months of misery. Like Olivier Laude, he was beside himself. "I had terrible shortness of breath, as if a huge weight was on my chest, coupled with despair, exhaustion, and the shakes," he said.

In 2012, at a friend's house, Bruce spotted a flyer from personal trainer Krista Durbin, who had made a specialty of working with chronic pain patients. She made house calls, charging $75 an hour. "It was very hard stuff," he said. "I hadn't used those muscles in years. Every time I worked with her, I'd sweat through two shirts. But Krista said I had no choice; I had to get my quads and glutes and internal obliques working again. The minute I said I wasn't sore, she'd take it as a signal to make the workout harder."

By the summer of 2012, Kaiser was off the drugs and feeling more fit than he had in decades. Out of self-preservation, three or four times a week, he did his exercises on his own. "I knew if I didn't, I'd never survive it when Krista came over," he said. Still, he could not have done it without her. "It's delusional to think that this is something you can do by yourself, or that the pain is just going to go away," he said, "or that in the absence of your own hard work, someone else can make it go away."

Both Greenberg and Kaiser said that from time to time, they had flare-ups. But they were no longer scared that a flare-up marked the beginning of the end. Kaiser's wife was gratified when her husband stopped limping and groaning, and agreed to plan some long-delayed travel. Greenberg's stepdaughter told me that she loved being with her stepmother, who was once again engaged, energetic, and lively.

Greenberg and Kaiser had every intention of sticking with their workouts indefinitely. But we're all human, and we all have the inclination—if we're feeling pretty good, or we get sick, or work gets tough, or family comes to visit, or it rains—to give ourselves a break from a time-consuming and exacting routine. When I followed up with them about a year after our initial interviews, I discovered that both Greenberg and Kaiser had cut back on their workouts with their trainers. They had their reasons: Neither wanted to pay for exercise indefinitely; both felt that they perhaps could devote fewer hours to exercise without losing ground. Bruce Kaiser thought he'd plateaued and could maintain his gains on his own. But within a few weeks, both Kaiser and Greenberg reported, they went sharply downhill. Both were surprised by how quickly their fitness levels declined and by how fast their pain had returned.

I understood exactly how they felt. I had not intended to stop my sessions with Diana. I assumed that we were and would be exercise partners for life, creaking through push-ups together when we were eighty-five. But in April 2014, after a couple of years of flying back and forth across the country to tend to the needs of aging parents, my husband and I pulled up stakes and shifted our base to the east coast, where we would remain until both my parents passed away in 2015.

I swore I would find myself a trainer and devote at least twenty minutes each morning to the McGill Big Three. Frankly, I was mentally and physically exhausted: If I had a few free minutes, I opted for the couch rather than my exercise mat. In a matter of weeks, the pain came back. As my days grew more frantic with caregiving, and my own life shrank, I bubbled over with resentment. John Sarno would have had a field day. Now, both my hips felt as if ice picks had been jammed in the joints. The muscle spasms in my buttocks were so bad that I muttered four-letter words as I struggled to walk down the street, and of course my lower back ached. I ordered myself to move, but I didn't listen.

After hobbling around for weeks, I tried some exercise classes near my dad's place. Most classes meant for reasonably fit people don't work for patients who are in the middle of a bad back pain episode. These were no exception: Among the overly rigorous and unstructured options I tried were chair Pilates, CrossFit, competitive and sweaty yoga, a gymnastic routine involving a fruitless attempt to lift my body off the floor by pulling myself up on rings, and a class that involved exercises performed on a vibrating platform, resulting in a peculiar feeling in my bones and innards but no evident reduction in discomfort. Until I found a new back whisperer in New York, I resigned myself to being trapped, like so many other people I'd encountered, in a cycle of inactivity and pain.

One day, luck finally smiled on me. I was waiting to pick up a salad for lunch when I happened to see a neatly printed card on a bulletin board. Someone was offering one-on-one training at a small private gym. I blinked: The address on the card was immediately adjacent to the apartment building I was temporarily calling home. Skeptically, I made an appointment for the next morning. Vinnie LaSpina, in his late twenties, was waiting for me. A competitive weight lifter, he was built like a refrigerator. I worried that he might be one of those trainers who mistook me for someone who aspired to compete in Ironman triathlons.

But Vinnie understood how to help me and, more important, how not to hurt me. He had read Stuart McGill. He had anatomy posters pinned up all over the gym and a therapy table next to the elliptical trainer. His price for a half-hour session was $50, which, by New York standards, was very reasonable.

With the attitude of someone who liked a challenge, he pointed out that my latissimus dorsi—the broad swaths of muscles that cover the rib cage—were not working worth a damn. Given that my daily tasks—among them, helping older people to extricate themselves from cars and beds, pushing a wheelchair, and carrying groceries—put so much strain on my upper body, I needed to "get those babies working, fast," Vinnie said. My squatting and hip hinging techniques also left a lot to be desired. When I got those important motor patterns under control, my body would automatically recruit the correct muscle groups, removing the burden from my sore hips. Starting that morning, I was in Vinnie's gym three times a week. Occasionally, I'd climb onto the therapy table, and he'd have a heart-to-heart with my right hamstring, which was behaving like worn elastic: Stretch it out, and it lay there limply; it did not snap back. Mornings, I woke up with a hamstring that felt hopelessly bruised, until one day I ran for a bus. As I leaped aboard, I realized that I'd done a block in record time, and I had no pain. I was back in fighting trim.

11

The Right Kind of Hurt

HOW A MUCH-MALIGNED MACHINE MAY
STILL CHANGE EVERYTHING

I N THE LATE 1980s, after ten years in practice, Brian Nelson, the disenchanted Minnesota orthopedic surgeon we first met in chapter 3, realized that much of the spine surgery he did wasn't working. "None of us enjoys treating patients we can't help," he said. "I used traditional approaches, and I had the traditional poor success rate." After much soul-searching, he quit the OR and started Physicians Neck and Back Clinic (PNBC), dedicated exclusively to the nonoperative care of back and neck pain patients. Over the next twenty-two years, Nelson expanded the practice until he presided over six clinics, a team of sixteen physicians, and about twenty physical therapists.

Over the quarter century that Brian Nelson ran PNBC's program, practitioners treated 120,000 patients. Although many said it could not be done, Nelson figured out how to deliver consistently excellent and cost-effective back pain treatment to 115 new patients each week. Patients spent $2,500 for twenty-four individual sessions of forty-five minutes each. In 2009, HealthPartners, the largest consumer-governed, nonprofit health care delivery organization in the United States, with $3 billion in revenues, acquired PNBC, dropped "Clinic" in favor of "Center," and made Nelson's program available to its 1.5 million members. Six years later, Nelson retired, confident that PNBC was in good hands.

From the beginning, PNBC's approach to rehab was quantitative and non-pain-contingent, terms that meant, essentially, "You're going to do more reps today than you did last week." Nelson's many research papers backed up his theories. A *Journal of Orthopaedics* study of 895 patients, nearly all of whom had failed six other treatments before starting at PNBC, showed that 76 percent reported their outcomes as good or excellent after going through rehab at Nelson's clinic.

BRIAN NELSON, THE distinguished midwestern physician, has the erect bearing and serious demeanor of the Air Force officer he was. I thought Brian Nelson was one of a kind, until I discovered that he had a philosophical doppelganger in Zurich, Switzerland.

That would be Werner Kieser, who with his wife, Gabriela, runs Kieser Training, with nearly three hundred thousand members and 138 rehab-oriented gyms in Europe, Asia, and Australia.

In their younger days, I discovered, both men were the protégés of exercise titan Arthur Jones. A swashbuckling gunslinger who dropped out of school before he finished ninth grade, Jones spent his teenage years riding the rails. In his early twenties, with nary a prospect, he moved into the Tulsa, Oklahoma, YMCA and, in an effort to put muscle on his puny frame, he began to lift the clumsy barbells in the gym. "I ended up with the arms and legs of a gorilla, on the body of a spider monkey," he recalled later, in a *Forbes* magazine interview. "I figured there was something wrong with the exercise tool."

To correct this failure, Jones invented a nautilus shell–shaped pulley that varied the resistance imposed throughout the range of motion of a particular exercise, and integrated the technology into a series of twenty machines. In 1970, he founded Nautilus Sports/Medical Industries, a company that, at its peak, would gross more than $300 million annually.

Unapologetically eccentric, Jones was also a great raconteur; this made him a popular, larger-than-life guest on late night talk shows. How much of his autobiography is apocryphal, no one can say. But, as he told the story, by the end of World War II, he owned a fleet of surplus B-25 medium bombers, in which he transported unspecified cargo from several Latin American countries, attracting the scrutiny of both the Central Intelligence Agency and the Federal Bureau of Investigation. He filmed and produced wildlife movies, and engaged illicitly in what he referred to as the "animal business," importing hundreds of thousands of Rhodesian monkeys, thousands of tons of snakes, and millions of tropical fish. When he was no longer welcome in Africa, he returned to live on a large farm in Ocala, Florida, transporting sixty-three baby elephants (average weight, 750 pounds), in a stripped-down American Airlines commercial passenger jet he'd bought for that purpose. In time, to that menagerie he added three rhinoceroses and a gorilla named Mickey, who would serve as a model in the Nautilus advertising campaign.

Jones recognized that even in the strongest bodybuilders, the muscles that supported the lumbar spine—the psoas major, quadratus lumborum, multifidus, and erector spinae—were under-developed. When he invented a Nautilus back machine, specifically intended to strengthen these muscles, other gym equipment manufacturers rushed to copy it. The joke was on them, Jones said, because almost as soon as he put the new machine on the market, he realized that it didn't do what it was supposed to do. Using it, bodybuilders developed powerful gluteus maximus and quadriceps (thigh muscles), but their lumbar extensor muscles remained as weak and atrophied as ever.

Jones recognized that this first effort had failed because his weight lifters could cheat. They rotated the pelvis and harnessed the glutes, thighs, and knees to perform the exercise, leaving the back muscles out of the equation.

The mammoth MedX lumbar extension machine was Jones's answer to this problem. It locked down the pelvis and the thighs, making cheating impossible. Then, utilizing a complicated arrangement of straps, cinches, and buckles, it isolated the lumbar extensor muscles, forcing them into action. Jones equipped his invention with a rudimentary computer and software package that could produce a quantitative assessment of lumbar strength. If sessions were prescribed in a specific dose, with the expectation of specific improvement, the machine would not only work for bodybuilders, but would also cure patients with back pain. He wanted to eliminate the vague language of physical therapists, who spoke of "patient progress," without providing useful metrics. With the computer turned on, set to track what happened in every session, outcomes would be clear. Either a person was getting stronger, or he wasn't.

In June 1986, persuaded as he was that MedX was the future for rehabbing back pain patients, Arthur Jones sold his controlling interest in Nautilus for $23 million. For the machine to be used in health care, it would need to go through clinical trials and receive FDA approval as a Class II device. (That rating is given to products that present minor risks, like powered wheelchairs.) Realizing that the FDA would demand clinical evidence, he joined forces with the University of Florida Center for Exercise Science, donating about $8 million to the school to pay the salaries of the staff that would run MedX research. Later, there would be lots of questions about conflicts of interest, and how these might have affected MedX outcomes, but University of Florida president Marshall Criser was enthusiastic. "Arthur Jones has a reputation as a man who gets things done and never does anything halfway," he said, adding that the school welcomed "the opportunity to join in his crusade against lower back problems."

In the preliminary tests on people who trained on the MedX once a week for ten weeks, the lumbar extensor machine more than doubled lower back muscle strength, recalled the center's director, Michael Pollock. "It was like these muscles had never been trained before," he said, "even though most of the fifteen study participants were physically active, and at least half of them had been working out on Nautilus equipment, including the [original] back machine."

The machines, which weighed a couple of tons, were built "like German tanks," observed researcher Dave Carpenter, who ran many of the professional training sessions. Eventually, he'd help Brian Nelson manage Physicians Neck and Back Clinic. "Arthur Jones could have done it faster, cheaper, or in a less effective way, and made just as much money," Carpenter said. "The engineers were after him to use a lesser gauge of steel, but he refused." When a hurricane struck a chiropractor's office in Homestead, Florida, the entire structure was torn from its foundation, but the MedX remained just where it had been, on the missing building's cement pad.

THREE YEARS AFTER Jones started testing the MedX lumbar extension machine at the University of Florida, the company received the FDA's approval. At training seminars, Arthur Jones told prospective clients—among them physicians, chiropractors, and physical therapists—that "as soon as you flipped the switch," MedX became "a license to print money." With the FDA approval in place, he promised, Medicare and private health insurance providers would reimburse for sessions on the $100,000 MedX machine.

Within months, it was evident that MedX was effective. Anywhere that a MedX lumbar extensor machine was up and running, spine surgeons complained bitterly that their surgery volume was declining. Physical therapists thought that chiropractors who bought or leased the MedX were walking off with their patients. Both physicians and PTs requested that Medicare make a special effort to scrutinize MedX billings and reimbursement requests.

Designed to serve as a stand-alone therapy, the machine was never meant to be a profit-generating "add-on" to other protocols. But chiropractors were double- and triple-billing, tacking MedX training onto bills for adjustments, ultrasound, and electrical stimulation. In 1996, Carpenter and the other researchers were worried. "More and more third-party payers were denying payment," said Dave Carpenter, "and we knew that if we couldn't stop it, it would be the end of MedX. Third-party payers had no way of knowing which providers were legitimate and which were gouging." They assembled a utilization steering committee, and issued guidelines that set out rules for billing.

Unfortunately, it was already too late. Although MedX served a completely different purpose, it was still a back therapy machine intended for spine care, and as such, Medicare lumped it into the same category as the spinal decompression unit I discussed in chapter 2, and called it experimental, declining to pay for treatments. Large private health insurance providers and self-insuring entities like Washington State's Department of Labor and Industries followed suit. From that moment, in many states, MedX therapy would be reimbursed at the same rate as a session of exercise on a $25 inflated plastic Swiss ball. Over the next several years, many MedX machines were relegated to dusty, dark corners, with sheets thrown over them. In 1996, because Medicare was not going to pay, and therefore it was unlikely that MedX would ever fulfill its inventor's dream of "printing money," Arthur Jones announced that he would put MedX on the auction block.

Even as insurers left MedX out in the cold, Brian Nelson had great faith in the future of the machine, which was an important part of the protocol at PNBC. Worried about MedX's future, he assembled a group of investors who were willing to pay $12.5 million for the company. But Nelson's offer arrived too late: Jones had already agreed to sell MedX for $3 million to a group from Singapore. Werner Kieser and his wife, Gabi, bought the European manufacturing license for MedX equipment, as well as the right to use the technology, and they hired one of the engineers who had developed the machine under Arthur Jones. The Kiesers began to manufacture the lumbar extensor machines in Dieburg, Germany, under the brand name Delphenex; this gave them a ready supply of equipment for their gyms.

Within a few years, the German magazine *Der Spiegel* would refer to Werner Kieser as "the deadly enemy of orthopedists."

WHILE KIESER BUILT his gyms in Europe, Brian Nelson worked on his program at PNBC. About 15 percent of the people who came to the clinic for help had already undergone at least one spine surgery that had failed, Nelson told me. One of his goals was to prevent those unsuccessful procedures. "I always tell people, when we're talking about surgery, that there are three things that can happen to you— you can be better, you can be the same, or you can be worse. But that's not what most people understand. They get that they could be better, and they also seem to intuitively understand that it might not work, but that's where they stop. They never think that they could actually be worse. They don't factor that in, because I can tell you that over the last twenty years, I've seen hundreds and hundreds—probably thousands—of people who have had surgery and are worse after it. There are more failures in back surgery than in any other kind of surgery. When you do a hip replacement, you hear from the patient: Boy, I wish I'd done this years ago—thank you. But you don't hear that a lot for back pain."

His real job at PNBC, Nelson explained, was to gain the trust of patients, by explaining the benefits of the right kind of exercise, and the shortcomings of MRIs and other diagnostic tests. What passed for "conservative treatment" was far too vague, Nelson said. "Nobody has ever defined it, so it is whatever you want it to be—PT or massage or acupuncture.

"One of the things we ask when evaluating patients is, 'Have you ever had formal physical therapy or exercise treatment?' and about 90 percent of patients have had it—and it failed. What failed? You can't say that exercise doesn't work unless you've failed an aggressive exercise program." With his exercise program, Nelson found, he could shrink the pool of people getting MRIs and other diagnostic tests by 75 percent.

BRIAN NELSON AND I had spent hours talking before we managed to schedule a time to meet in person. "Back pain is an incurable disease, for which you need a regime that you will stay on for the rest of your life," he told me on the phone. "If you're not willing to give me five to eight minutes a day, then I can't help you. I use the metaphor of brushing your teeth to explain it to patients. If you were meticulous about your dental care for a year, and you went to see your dentist who told you that your teeth and gums looked wonderful, would you say, 'Well, I've got that one covered, and I don't need to brush or floss ever again?' It's exactly the same with back pain. You are never cured. You are controlled because of your behavior. Whether you succeed in our program depends, more than anything, on your own self-discipline."

With that philosophy in mind, I checked into my motel on the out-skirts of Minneapolis and went immediately to the tiny gym, to run through the Stuart McGill exercises. At nine thirty the next morning, Nelson, well over six feet tall, with a thick shock of pure silver hair, big square hands, and the physique of someone younger than sixty-seven, rolled into the driveway in his station wagon. A military guy, he'd piloted fighter planes, F-4 Phantoms, in Southeast Asia, flying 238 combat missions in 1971 and 1972. He was too modest to mention it, but one of his colleagues would tell me that Nelson's plane had been hit by a surface-to-air missile over enemy territory. He survived after crash-landing back at Da Nang Air Base. And the next morning, as if nothing had happened, Nelson got up and flew his next mission.

As soon as we pulled into the clinic parking lot in Woodbury, Min-nesota, the trip down memory lane ended. Suddenly all business, Nel-son hustled me out of the car, into the clinic, and down a corridor, past a busy gym. Once I was in the conference room, he fetched coffee for both of us. Even though we'd discussed the machine's complicated backstory for months, he remarked that he'd rather that I never men-tion MedX and his name in the same sentence. "I prefer to say that we use an aggressive exercise approach, in a spinal conditioning program meant to improve strength, flexibility, and endurance," he said. "The brand of equipment we use is not important." He'd already provided so much of the history of the machine, and his involvement with its development, that I couldn't do what he asked—but from that mo-ment on, I promised Nelson, I'd stick with his description.

Satisfied that I'd do my best, Nelson explained that before patients could get into the PNBC program, they underwent a very thorough physical screening, to eliminate medical conditions like rheumatoid arthritis or tumors, acute fracture, progressive neurological deficits, or infection. He looked for evidence of pathology: Long-standing night pain unaltered by a change in position might suggest a tumor and the need for imaging studies. A history of fever and chills, with or without a previous infection in the body would indicate the need for a bone scan, to rule out low-grade infection. But such disorders were very unusual in patients who came to PNBC.

Not everyone was a candidate. "If you had recent eye or abdominal surgery or if you're pregnant, we can't work with you," Nelson said. "If you have severe heart or lung disease, we aren't going to put you in the program, because it's vigorous exercise, and we don't want to kill you. If you are just flat-out nuts, we can't help you. We try to be compassionate, but there are certain people who aren't going to be good candidates, so they are screened out. And if they do get in, and I become convinced that they will not do well, my job is to get them out and get them help elsewhere. Holy cow, I've sent people on to surgery. To let people in who can't make it would be akin to stealing."

A patient who got the thumbs-up—and most did—was sent to the gym floor for a test of his or her spinal fitness level, to evaluate strength, flexibility, and endurance. "We believe in objective measurements," he said. "Function is a much better indicator than pain of how people are doing, because function is stable, while people with back pain tend to have good days and bad days in terms of pain. The nice thing about exercise is that it usually works, regardless of what your particular situation is—so whether you have been diagnosed with arthritis in your back, or a degenerative disc, or spondylolisthesis, exercise tends to be beneficial."

Most of the patients who came to PNBC had been doing daily exercises for years, Nelson said, "at home, or in health clubs—without benefit. The kind of exercise done in health clubs is normally of zero use, because you aren't exercising the weak link."

The first couple of weeks in the program were the hardest. "I often hear, 'You guys almost killed me,'" Nelson said. "We tell them that they will be worse before they are better, and we hand out reprints of scientific articles that describe delayed onset muscle soreness, and how it is normal if you haven't done meaningful strength training in a long time, or ever before. We want people to understand that this is what they should expect, and that we will help them get through." The typical patient, said Nelson, was significantly better in sixteen to seventeen visits.

Taking it easy didn't work for back pain, he said, because it promoted muscle atrophy, cartilage degeneration, stiffness, and depression. People with chronic spinal pain, Nelson said, quickly became experts at protecting their backs, and the longer a patient experienced chronic pain, or depended on passive care, administered in physical therapy or by a chiropractor, the more extreme the weakness, stiffness, and perceived fragility.

Often, the people who come to his clinic have been told that they have syndromes or disorders that prevent them from exercising. But, Nelson told me, "This is almost never true." For example, Heather Barnes, a star patient whom Nelson had invited to join us, had been told several years earlier that she had an autoimmune disease that would inevitably confine her to a wheelchair, in considerable pain.

"It was the spring of 2008," Barnes, an effusive blond thirty-year-old, explained, "and I'd finally decided to get into shape. Everything was going really well. I had a great job, and I'd just met the guy I knew I was going to marry." On a typical day, she spent a couple of hours at Bally Total Fitness, working to burn calories and to tone her "vanity" muscles—quadriceps, abdominals, and biceps. Because her boyfriend Troy did not like gyms, and she wanted to maximize the hours they could spend in each other's company, she began riding her bike the ten miles to and from work—about an hour in each direction. To tote her business clothes, shoes, and hair products, she stuffed everything into a backpack. Fully loaded, it weighed ten pounds.

Barnes never crashed her bike, or even bottomed out in a pothole, but two weeks after her first ride to work, her lower back began to ache. Certain the pain would abate, she continued to ride. "It didn't go away," she said. "It turned into a relentless, stabbing sensation that got in the way of everything I did."

In August, when a colleague recommended that she see a nearby "spine expert," Barnes made an appointment. The "expert" was a chiropractor whose protocol included X-rays, manual manipulation, ultrasound, ice packs, floor-based Pilates, and massage. "I paid $1,000 up front for twelve sessions," Barnes recalled, "but after a month of treatment, the pain across my low back was actually worse. Pretty much everything I did, awake and asleep, hurt me. Even taking a deep breath hurt, and so I quit, leaving quite a bit of money on the table."

After four more months of constant discomfort, her relationship with Troy was in disarray. "The pain was affecting everything, obviously," Barnes said. "I'd do the simplest thing—lean over to pick something up, and I'd scream at the top of my lungs, and I am just not that kind of person. Forget intimacy: I couldn't imagine how I could ever become a decent wife or mother."

Troy stuck it out. The couple became engaged and scheduled their wedding date for seven months later, both of them certain that there had to be an organic cause for Barnes's condition, one that could be resolved before the honeymoon. They had read the *Consumer Reports* issue that ranked spine surgery first on the list of overused treatments. And they were aware that the many spine surgeons in the Twin Cities, where they resided, were responsible for a much higher than average rate of spinal fusions.

First, they sought help at the Cleveland Clinic. Then they visited the Mayo Clinic, in Rochester, Minnesota. Barnes's MRI showed nothing remarkable. Neither institution could offer a diagnosis beyond "nonspecific back pain." One finding, established after tests at Mayo, showed that Barnes's erythrocyte sedimentation rate (ESR)—often elevated in people who are overweight, as Barnes was, and sometimes a marker of the onset of an inflammatory condition—was beyond the normal range.

"I was struggling to find hope," Barnes said, "and also to absorb the idea that maybe this would never get any better." A few months before the wedding, she saw her primary care doctor. She gave him copies of the doctors' notes from Mayo and the Cleveland Clinic. After he scanned them, he explained to her that her elevated ESR suggested that she'd developed an autoimmune condition called ankylosing spondylitis (AS), one that would eventually result in incapacitating spinal arthritis. Barnes did not know that this was a spurious correlation: Taken alone an elevated ESR level should not be considered evidence that a patient has AS.

"As I was leaving the office," Barnes said, "my primary care doctor gave me a brochure describing ankylosing spondylitis, and a prescription for strong anti-inflammatory drugs that would eventually mess up my stomach." He told Barnes to make an appointment to see a rheumatologist, who would manage her condition as it progressed. "What was in the brochure was horrible," she said. "The bones of my pelvis and spine would likely fuse. It would be very painful. I wouldn't be able to move, and I might end up so hunched over that I couldn't raise my eyes to the horizon." Instead of making an appointment with a rheumatologist, she spent the next few months on the Internet, "trying to come to terms with the fact that I was living with something that would eventually cripple me."

A little over two years after she and Troy had first met, the couple got married. A few weeks later, Barnes made her way to the rheumatologist's office. In preparation, he'd ordered a blood panel, including the test that identifies the gene HLA-B27, one that exists in 95 percent of Caucasian individuals who are diagnosed with ankylosing spondylitis. (The gene is found in 8 percent of the Caucasian population, but only 2 percent of that group will ever develop AS.) The absence of the gene did not rule out the possibility that she had the disease, the rheumatologist told her, but it made it unlikely that this was what caused her back pain.

"I remember going kind of limp," she said. "I was incredibly relieved that I did not have this crippling disease, but to be honest, I went straight from relief to 'If it's not AS, then what is it?' I realized that I was back to square one."

Over the years, her rheumatologist had sent other patients to Brian Nelson, with excellent outcomes. After twenty-eight months of relentless pain, Barnes attended her first appointment at PNBC's Eden Prairie clinic. Her first gym session was relatively gentle, but afterward she was very sore, and more than a little skeptical. "I still had the victim's mind-set," Barnes said. "I was absolutely sure that exercise was going to make me worse." For the next three months, she worked out twice a week with PNBC's physical therapy team. "When they first took me into the gym, which was full of a lot of computerized machines," she said, "I thought, 'Really? Why can't I just go back to Bally's and do this myself?'" Within a couple of weeks, she was using the lumbar extensor machine, her pelvis restrained and her thighs tightly strapped down as she struggled mightily to raise the seat back as it pressed her chest to her thighs. "It was really, really hard," she said, "but by that point, I was aware that at PNBC, you couldn't back off. The staff had expectations, and you were going to meet them, because there was a progress check at the end of each session, where you got graded. 'Plus' meant that you were working hard. 'Minus' meant that you were showing all kinds of classic pain behavior."

After a month at PNBC, Barnes felt her pain begin to abate. She stopped taking the anti-inflammatory meds. In December, as her program drew to a close, her PT designed a home exercise program for her and taught her how to use a Roman chair—as I described earlier, a platform that supports your weight at a slight angle—to work on torso rotation and spinal extension. "When they said I was done," remembered Barnes, "I said, 'Uh, no, I don't think so. I'll see you on Thursday.' But at PNBC, the premise, from the minute you start, is that this is all about learning to take care of yourself, and no longer burdening the health care system. They make sure you know exactly what you're doing, but you have to commit, from the beginning, to putting the time in to do the independent work."

"And Heather—would you say you've done that?" asked Brian Nelson, who had just returned to the conference room. Blushing just a bit, she said she felt so well that in fact she and Troy were thinking about starting a family.

I asked Barnes whether she regretted having accepted the diagnosis of ankylosing spondylitis from her primary care doctor. Had she told him he'd made a mistake? She had not wanted to embarrass him. Instead, she found a new physician. "I was always willing to let the doctors take over," she said. "I figured that they were the experts, not I. I went in trusting their knowledge, and when they talked over my head, I never questioned them. These days, however, I ask an awful lot of questions."

Brian Nelson and I saw Barnes out. When I asked to have a look at the physical therapy gym, Nelson concurred, but only if I'd promise not to interrupt anyone's workout. At one end of the facility, there was a large, mostly glass-enclosed room, home to PNBC's CORE spinal fitness program. A "No Whining" sign—the classic red circle with a diagonal line through it—hung on a bright green wall. Three PNBC clinics have CORE fitness programs, where patients who have graduated from the therapeutic program can follow their personal exercise routines, twice a week for thirty minutes, at a cost of $40 a month or $425 a year, paid out of pocket. A PNBC physical therapist is always close at hand should questions arise, but members are expected to work out on their own.

In the main gym, which is much larger than the CORE fitness glass box, I encountered Debra, a PNBC physical therapist, who on that spring day had elected to liven things up by wearing full clown makeup. Her patient was Dawn, a volunteer firefighter in her midthirties, who, despite my request that she ignore me before we both got into trouble with Nelson, stopped lifting weights to tell me that she came to PNBC after three epidural steroid injections and a microdiscectomy, none of which had resolved her pain. She started at PNBC eight weeks after the surgery. "I wish I'd come here first," she said. "I felt much better after the first week." With four or five weeks left in her program, she expected to be able to handle any recurrences on her own. "I want out of here, and I don't ever want to come back," she said. "This place is all about knowing how to help yourself, every day, so you never have to reenter the health care system."

LIKE BRIAN NELSON, Werner Kieser believed in systematic, quantitative exercise. Since 1966, when he bought the license to manufacture MedX equipment in Europe from Jones, Kieser's empire had grown from a single gym to 140 facilities, most of them established as franchises, in seven countries. In 2013, sales throughout the franchises amounted to $160 million.

For $1,050 a year, Kieser Training members are entitled to a medical evaluation and two thirty-minute workouts each week. Each gym is equipped with exactly twenty-nine exercise machines, many of them of Kieser's own invention. They are laid out in precisely the same order, no matter where in the world they stand, so that if a member from Zurich uses a gym in Belgium, there's no learning curve. The star of the show is always the computerized medical strength training machine, or MST, now running far more complicated software than it did in Arthur Jones's day.

When Werner Kieser, who is well into his seventies, picked me up at my hotel in Zurich, we walked at top speed all the way across town to Kieser Training headquarters. Back patients, Kieser explained as I trotted beside him, are patients with long-term value to the medical profession. On his fingers, he ticked off the list of practitioners in Europe, Asia, and Australia who typically profit from each spine operation: surgeons, anesthesiologists, psychologists, physiotherapists, nurses, clinic management, and occupational therapists. "Back patients guarantee repeat business, and a budgetable source of income," he said. "That's money these physicians can rely on, year after year." The medical strengthening therapy that patients used at Kieser Training, he said "is not good for business, because patients disappear from the 'back market' and they never reappear."

Today his avocation is reading the works of the great philosophers, but back in the early 1970s, when Kieser was a welter-weight boxer and running a small boxing training facility, he read the magazine *Iron Man*, and stumbled upon the work of Arthur Jones. "I realized that he was about twenty years ahead of my own thinking," Kieser said. As the first European gym owner to buy Nautilus equipment, he was also one of the first to know that Jones was about to sell Nautilus and plunge all his resources into MedX.

When Kieser arrived in Florida, anxious to see what all the fuss was about, Jones put him on the MedX lumbar extension machine. "Although I was quite strong and fit," said Kieser. "I had terrible muscle soreness the next day, in areas I had evidently never before reached in my training." He returned to Europe and read all of the research from the University of Florida Center for Exercise Science. A couple of weeks later, he and his physician wife, Gabi (who has degrees in both medicine and business administration), were back in Florida. "We bought the machines," said Werner, "and my wife opened the first European clinic for medical strengthening therapy, in the same building as our gym facility."

After a major Zurich newspaper ran an article about the Kiesers' brand of strength training, and a six-minute documentary appeared on TV, Gabi's practice was solidly booked for four months in advance. Clinicians were furious, her husband recalled. "Some doctors who worked at the clinic told us that the name 'Kieser' was forbidden to be mentioned at Schulthess Clinic in Zurich because they were getting so many requests from our MST patients to cancel operations."

Quickly, the Kiesers realized that MST did more than eliminate pain and build muscle strength. It also helped patients overcome fear-avoidant behavior. The Kiesers had planned to make MST a several-session treatment, but the patients who attributed their recovery to the lumbar extension machine insisted on continuing to use it. This was not feasible within the confines of Gabi's booked-solid schedule, so the Kiesers moved the lumbar extension machine into the main gym facility, where it became an important part of the curriculum.

AFTER WERNER KIESER took me on a brief tour of the company's unpretentious headquarters—there's a sign out front with the company motto on it: "Man grows only through resistance"—we entered the gym. It had a bright, loft-like feel, with hardwood floors and big windows, and lots of brushed aluminum and glass. The machines were lined up in rows, like so many armor-clad knights awaiting their marching orders. At eleven a.m., the place was silent—no crashing of steel plates or thumping of barbells, no clients groaning with effort, no sound except for the gentle whir of the machines' cams, gears that alter the resistance of the weight stack. A lot of things that are standard in U.S. gyms were missing: This gym had no posters encouraging you to "Just do it," no smoothie bar, no music, no flat-screen TVs, no mirrors.

This was not by accident. "It's thirty minutes of training twice a week, followed by a shower," Werner Kieser announced. "We tell people they will accomplish three things, in order of importance. First, they will get rid of pain. Second, they will become stronger. And third, they will become more attractive. The fitness industry seems to offer what is requested, but not what is actually needed. The point is to provide the correct amount and type of exercise to produce optimal results."

In the Kiesers' gyms, there would be no sauna, no steam room, no massage, and no cardio exercise equipment. When I raised my eyebrows at the prospect of a gym without a treadmill, a StairMaster, or an elliptical trainer, Kieser, who takes his hikes in the Alps, said that cardio exercise was best accomplished outside the gym, on the days between weight-training sessions, "preferably by walking in the mountains or the forest." Aerobic exercise depleted stores of glycogen, the main source of protein synthesis necessary to build muscle, Kieser explained. Jumping onto the treadmill for a half hour before perform-ing strength-training exercises was therefore counterproductive, be-cause it broke down the precious muscle you were trying to build.

JUST AS BRIAN Nelson did at PNBC, in 2002, Gabi and Werner Kieser established an internal research department that examines the data generated by three hundred thousand clients. The scientific commu-nity generally regards such in-house studies skeptically, because they lack a control group, composed of participants who do not train, or who train on different equipment.

Still, the outcomes of the Kieser Training studies have been per-suasive. "Today, many doctors send patients to our gyms," Werner Kieser said, "and most of those patients have an odyssey of useless therapies behind them." When I asked him whether—given the avail-ability of facilities and instruction—physicians would send patients for MedX or MST training in the United States, he looked skeptical. "In Europe, or in any of the countries where we have a foothold, med-ical care is the government's responsibility, so no stakeholder stands to profit greatly from treatment," he said. But in the United States, where medicine is fee-based and tests, interventions, and surgery rack up the profits, there's no incentive to order care that is effective and saves money. Times were changing, and certainly health care was becoming more cost-sensitive, but he doubted that conservative treatment and invasive procedures would be exchanged for exercise anytime soon.

IN ZURICH, PHYSICIAN Gabi Kieser is in charge of the evaluation and treatment of back pain patients, which occurs before they can start working out in the gym. (In most Kieser Training facilities, physicians perform this role, but in a few, physiotherapists handle assessments and oversee MST training.) Typically, she said, patients start to notice improvement after three or four sessions on the MST, but twelve to twenty sessions are required before the patient achieves normal strength on it. Then, he or she receives three hours of one-on-one training on the gym floor, with outcomes carefully tracked. Six solo workouts are followed by an additional one-on-one training session, to make sure that body mechanics are perfect. After every session, the patient (who is now a gym member) receives a computer printout, evaluating progress and weaknesses. Even when a gym member starts working out alone, said Werner Kieser, there are always trainers on the gym floor, checking the quality and speed of movement. They do not hesitate to interrupt and retrain a client who is moving too quickly or not concentrating.

He handed me a padlock with a key and directed me to the women's changing room. There, I found a long row of sleek, full-length, brushed aluminum lockers—nothing like the too-small-for-your-coat boxes with fussy push-button combination locks that I used at home. At the far end of the room, gleaming cylindrical shower stalls made me think of Woody Allen's infamous "orgasmatron," as featured in his 1973 feature film, *Sleeper*. I'd already let Werner Kieser know that because I was traveling with lightweight walking shoes, rather than my bulky trainers, I might not have the proper footwear for the gym. This was not a problem, he said: "In our gyms we don't run. Humans are not running animals but rather climbing monkeys."

Dressed in workout gear, I met Michael Rausch, the Zurich Kieser Training facility's manager. At forty-three, Rausch was blue-eyed, with a two-day growth of scruffy beard and an inspiring smile. When he handed me a dove-gray towel embroidered with the Kieser logo, I asked about the pocket sewn across the top. It slipped over the seat back of whatever machine the client was using, protecting it from sweat. "Mr. Kieser does not believe in doing things partway," Rausch said.

At that moment, a patient was working out on the MST, so we'd begin with the F-3, a kind of gym-floor version of the MST, with some, but not all, of its straps, buckles, rollers, cranks, and wheels. The F-3, he explained, was not quite as good at isolating the lumbar extensor musculature, but a client could use it—unlike the MST—without careful supervision.

I was to do every exercise as slowly as I could, Rausch instructed. Momentum was the enemy in strength training. "The faster you go," Rausch noted, "the less effect you have on your muscles, but you could be putting ten times as much stress on your joints."

It took me about one minute to do six very mindful reps on the F-3. I could feel my low back muscles working. For the first time, my thighs and glutes stayed out of the equation.

Over the next hour or so, we made our way around seven of the twenty-nine machines on the circuit, until finally, we reached the MST. Rausch invited me to climb into its spacious lap, explaining that the Kiesers had used the MedX as their prototype, but they'd redesigned it to make the hulking monster slightly less intimidating. After asking for my age, weight, and height, he typed the data into the software interface. He made certain that all of MST's belts and buckles were secured. Then he set the weight counterbalance, ensuring that the seat back would be just heavy enough to force my lumbar muscles into action.

Rausch was just about to hit the switch when his boss came around the corner, and asked whether I'd survived the workout thus far. I had, but like most patients who climb aboard the MST, I admitted that I was terrified that I was about to be crushed. Michael Rausch directed me to lower my torso toward my thighs, until my nose touched my knees, and then return my upper body to a seated position. In comparison with the dinosaurish MedX, the MST was a sleek Mercedes. When I finished my reps, my back and pelvis no longer felt weak and cranky. As I headed for the shower, I danced a little jig.

AS SOON AS I got home from Zurich, I started looking for a Bay Area facility equipped with a MedX lumbar extension machine. When nothing came up in Google—the nearest machine was more than an hour away, and the office assistant said she thought it was out of commission—I called practitioners who had taken part in the University of Florida's research. That's how I met physical therapist Thomas E. Dreisinger, who said that Arthur Jones had "captured" him some twenty-six years earlier, and put him to work on MedX. Ever since, Dreisinger had followed MedX's fortunes, sometimes taking a stake in a company that seemed poised to bring the machine back to life. As I had discovered, the machines were hard to find. There were a few in use in San Diego, at U.S. Spine and Sport.

But the company to watch (and one for which Dreisinger had done some consulting work) was Pure HealthyBack (PHB), owned by Scientific Exercise, Inc., in Orlando, Florida.

Pure HealthyBack's business model was based on a claim that Arthur Jones had made in the machine's heyday—that MedX, because it could rehabilitate most back pain patients and return them to work, could save American industry billions of dollars in lost workdays and insurance claims due to back injury. With the computer on board to evaluate progress, the machine could detect—as no "crying to smiling" pain scale would—who was getting better with each session, and who was just not trying. Although it is not likely that the two men ever met, Jones and Wilbert E. Fordyce, the much-maligned chair of the Task Force for Pain in the Workplace, shared the same philosophy: Individuals who didn't get better in two weeks ought to be released from employment.

There was a solid footing for Jones's claim. To determine how

MedX therapy, over the course of a year, affected the cost of low back disability claims, Vert Mooney, a prominent orthopedic surgeon from the University of California at San Diego School of Medicine and a believer in MedX, conducted a randomized, controlled investigation at the Western Energy Company Rosebud Coal Mine in Colstrip, Montana. To be taken seriously, a study must receive peer review. That meant that a group of Mooney's colleagues would have had to critique it, and find it substantial. Mooney's study was eventually published in the *Journal of Occupational Rehabilitation*, but it never received peer review, probably because the results the paper described were so good that they would have damaged the prospects of those occupational medicine practitioners who would have had to sign off on it.

Mooney described these outcomes: Prior to starting the MedX program, mine workers at Rosebud had suffered nearly three back injuries per two hundred thousand employee work hours, far in excess of what would normally occur in such a setting. On the mine site, Mooney set up a once-a-week, twenty-week MedX strength-training program for 197 workers, 90 percent of whom said they'd had ongoing back trouble. As a control, a similar group of employees were tested to determine their baseline strength on the MedX, but they were not assigned an exercise protocol. After the twenty-week training period, although the number of injuries among the MedX group declined by 82 percent, back injuries sustained among the untrained group didn't change. Still, the improvement in safety was such that Rosebud Coal Mine's average workers' compensation liability payment declined from $14,430 per month to $380 per month, for the study year.

All that was required, Arthur Jones said, to reduce the costs of workers' compensation was "one brief exercise session each week, per worker, for a period of ten or twelve weeks." If MedX could rehabilitate workers' comp patients in ten weeks, and separate the patients who wanted to get well from those who were malingering, chiropractors, physical therapists, and surgeons would certainly feel the pinch, but so would other stakeholders, including workers' comp lawyers, independent medical examiners, the administrative court system that determines such cases, and workers' comp insurers.

Pure HealthyBack had emerged from that model, said Dreisinger. And he suspected that the company could make MedX mighty again in North America. The buzzword in health care was "EBM"— evidence-based medicine—and Pure HealthyBack was all about measurement and proof. Health care providers could no longer get away with wasting money. "If you can't prove that what you are doing for a patient can be measured and actually works, then you won't be able to stay in this business in the United States," Dreisinger said.

As customers, Pure HealthyBack would pursue self-insured organizations, where claims were administered in-house. Because they decide what they will pay for, and those decisions directly affect the bottom line, such groups were especially interested in controlling costs. Pure HealthyBack would help them do that. With a proprietary computer software package that would measure patients' individual outcomes every week, it was possible to track exactly how much an organization was spending (and saving) on back pain care.

After several delays, in 2013 Pure HealthyBack opened its first facility, a thirty-five-hundred-square-foot clinic at the Ochsner Health System in Southeastern Louisiana. It would serve Ochsner's thirteen thousand employees, distributed among eight hospitals. Instead of parading through serial interventions that ran up enormous bills, Ochsner's workers would go straight to PHB's facility for treatment. Initially, only hospital employees were eligible for treatment, but as word got out about the rehab protocol, patients from all over the state asked to be included in the ten-week program.

The second Pure HealthyBack clinic to open was almost twice the size of Ochsner's. It was a joint venture between Beebe Healthcare in Sussex County, Delaware (per capita, the state fills the most high-dose painkiller prescriptions in the United States, suggesting a high prevalence of back pain), and Pure HealthyBack. Orthopedist Ronald Wisneski, previously chief of spine surgery at Ohio State University Wexner Medical Center, became the medical director. Like Brian Nelson, the Minnesota surgeon, and Vert Mooney, who before his death practiced in San Diego, he was fed up with operations that did not work.

When we spoke, Wisneski explained that prospective patients were first assessed for red flags such as cauda equina syndrome, progressive neurological degeneration, and cancer. Patients with documented severe spinal or neurological pathology were not candidates for the PHB program. But if the diagnosis was nonspecific low back pain—and it almost always was—the patient would not receive an MRI, or injections, or a referral to a spine surgeon or pain medicine clinic. Instead, he would spend ten weeks on MedX, reconditioning his back extensor muscles with Beebe HealthyBack's trainers.

Wisneski and his team were diligently collecting data on the 460 patients who by August 2014 had completed the ten-week study. The investigation's outcomes revealed an average decrease of 54 percent in pain and disability and an average 50 percent increase in strength. That kept patients on the job and made them less likely to pursue serial interventions.

"MedX by itself is not a panacea," acknowledged Wisneski. "But when it is part of a global wellness program, it's a tremendous, cost-effective resource. There's nothing else you can do in an exercise environment that gives this kind of immediate quantitative progress. It provides you with the resources to do something for yourself. It's an anti-recidivist strategy. The goal is to get patients back on track, so that they do not constantly revisit the health care system."

As I completed this book, Pure HealthyBack was expanding its operations, and had just opened four MedX-equipped clinics in Michigan. Workers' comp insurance was accepted.

WHETHER THE MEDX protocol, with its good-for-the-bottom-line focus on quantitative measurement and follow-up coaching, will flourish in clinics and hospitals throughout the country remains to be seen. If Werner Kieser can find a suitable master franchisee in the United States, one with the minimum capital investment of $5 million at the ready, North Americans could have access to his gleaming, frill-free, back pain–focused gyms, with MedX technology at their core. Brian Nelson's concept, now integral to HealthPartners, could become the go-to model for health care organizations everywhere.

But as history has proved, this could go another way. As they have in the past, stakeholders in the back pain industry could refuse to stand by and watch while MedX cannibalizes their revenue streams. All those providers with grievances could take them to Medicare, the highest court in medicine, and insist that the agency refuse to reimburse for exercise-related therapy, once again snuffing the life out of MedX.

Personally, I hope that computerized lumbar extensor strengthening, in any of its permutations, will thrive. If Kieser Training opened a gym in San Francisco, I'd be there for the ribbon-cutting, ready to push that weighty seat back into its upright position. I know many back pain patients, at the end of their rope, who would head there first, long before contemplating injections or surgery.

Periodically, I checked in with the patients who over several years had become my best sources. When I realized that I hadn't heard from Heather Barnes for more than a year, I sent a couple of e-mails to her work address, and received nothing in return. That worried me. But a quick trip to LinkedIn showed me that Barnes had moved on, and had a new job title. She was "Director of Barnes Household Operations." There was a new baby. In her profile picture, she seemed to glow with delight; and when I congratulated her, she said she owed it all to PNBC.

"I do think there's some progress being made," Brian Nelson said, when I let him know that Barnes was thriving. "With health care reform passed, and changes on the horizon, there's going to be more emphasis placed on getting the best outcomes at the least cost. It's not as if patients who aren't treated at PNBC are going to go home and do something for themselves. They will go somewhere else, and they will have diagnostic testing, injections, and narcotics. It's a matter of deciding what we want to pay for. I think we're on the right side of that argument, and I expect that this approach to spine care will prevail over the next several years."

12

The Posture Mavens

HOW TO MAKE GRAVITY YOUR FRIEND

Almost all civilized people have been brought up to think of them-
selves as ghosts in the machine . . . as souls or spirits in alien bodies,
as skin-encapsulated egos, or as psychic chauffeurs in mechanical
vehicles of flesh and bone.
—Alan Watts, British philosopher and teacher who
introduced Zen philosophy to the West

A S I HURRIED through airports and city streets, I became an ob-
sessive observer of human posture and locomotion. I yearned to
stop a group of teenage girls with curved spines, rounded shoulders,
and hips thrust forward—to tell them what kind of pain they could
expect in the future, especially if they continued to wear stiletto heels
and carry huge tote bags. Just as my parents had, I begged my own
lanky son (whose twenty-three-year-old spine, shaped like a question
mark, reminded me of mine at that age), to save himself before it was
too late.

The nagging hadn't done me a bit of good. Asking me to stand up
straight was like asking me to fly—not possible. Some of the problem
was pure self-consciousness: Having hit a gawky five foot eight when I
was barely thirteen, I developed rounded shoulders, a budding hump,
an excessive curve at the small of my back, and a chin that poked out
as if it were in a hurry to get somewhere before the rest of me.

It would not be easy to unshackle myself from my body's limited
postural vocabulary. Largely, my chains were self-imposed: I spent
eight hours a day (well, that's a conservative estimate) sitting in my

desk chair, focused on my computer monitor. Late in the day, I'd slip in forty-five minutes of strenuous exercise—and then drive home, where, after cooking dinner, I'd collapse on the sofa and sit some more.

Given the necessity of making a living in a sedentary profession, in 2007 I'd called in an ergonomics consultant who gave me a shopping list that included a lumbar support and wrist rest, a wedge for my feet, and an unwieldy document holder that might have been effective if I worked from a single document rather than from dozens of them splayed across my desk. In what was a startling recommendation at the time, she suggested that I raise my desk to standing height, by setting the legs on cinder blocks. After I stood for ten minutes, my pelvis came to rest against the edge of the desk, leaving me sway-backed and aching. Before the afternoon was out, the cinder blocks were stacked outside in the alley, where they remain today.

Since standing seemed to be out of the question, I tried to achieve the gold standard of seated postures, with hips, knees, elbows all bent at right angles, and a straight back. Sustaining this was impossible. Within seconds after I forced myself upright, my pelvis slid forward in my chair until I was sitting on the back of my tailbone rather than my buttocks. My shoulders curled forward, my chest collapsed, and, to provide a stable base for this ungainly structure, I crossed my legs at the knee.

Frankly, it didn't matter whether I was sitting in a $150 Staples task chair or one of the multitude of expensive ergonomic chairs in my personal stable. Over thirty-five years, I'd bought a basic HAG chair (circa 1980), an Aeron chair, a Freedom chair, a bespoke model from BodyBilt, an Embody chair from Herman Miller, and a very high-end Capisco chair from HAG, constituting an investment that could have paid for a decent car. I'd even spent a few uncomfortable months in a borrowed kneeling chair. In an episode that my children love to recount, but I'd prefer to forget, I rolled off my brand-new silver exercise ball when I reached for a pen that had fallen on the floor. Suffice to say that the ball joined the discarded chairs.

Although I had my doubts about ever being able to tolerate a standing desk, I thought that a walking workstation had promise. In the *New Yorker*, I read that one of my literary heroes, the author Susan Orlean, managed most of her work on a treadmill desk. She'd been a runner for years, and maybe that explained her higher-level motor skills, and her ability to mesh cognitive and motor demands. For me, simple tasks were no problem; in fact, it was a blast to chat on the phone with a friend while walking at one mile an hour and feeling virtuous about it. I could even fake-type, running my fingers nimbly over the keys. But when I set to work in earnest, the stumbling blocks were evident: My brain freaked out. Through my progressive eyeglass lenses, the words swam, making it impossible for me to read, take notes, or write a coherent sentence. I felt dizzy, and a little carsick, and, even more than usual, my back hurt. It was back to the chair—and the slouch—for me.

Research revealed that I wasn't the only one who tortured her spine while working. "The erect posture looks very nice, but it is impossible to sit this way for very long and there is no scientific basis for it," wrote A. C. Mandal, a leading Danish surgeon who dedicated most of his career to studying better options for sitting, particularly for children. "It is entirely based on wishful thinking, morals, and discipline from the days of Queen Victoria. This erect sitting posture cannot be maintained for more than one or two minutes, and usually results in fatigue, discomfort, and poor posture."

Nor is sitting "straight" the best position for office workers, school-children, or anyone else one who spends many hours in a chair. Using positional MRI, Scottish and Canadian researchers took measurements of spinal angles, spinal disc height, and movement across different positions. In the conventional 90-degree torso-to-leg angle, the pressure on the intervertebral discs was very high. Beyond that, the conventional position led to tight hips and psoas; limp glutes; poor blood circulation causing swollen ankles and varicose veins; foggy brain; and a strained neck. The better way, observed the researchers, was to sit so that the angle between torso and legs was about 135 degrees, putting much less strain on discs, ligaments, and muscles.

But opening the hip angle that way, without altering the structure of the chair, meant that the user would inevitably slide to the floor. One alternative, if you had the time, and the skill, was to design a workstation around a zero-gravity recliner, in which case you would be lying down on the job. As attractive as that sounded, it wasn't practical: In that position, there's no good place to put your paperwork, or your monitor, or, especially, a cup of coffee. The more functional option was to design a workstation that allowed the thighs to slope downward from the torso.

"No chair is perfect, because no posture is perfect," wrote sociologist Galen Cranz. The Norwegian designer of the iconic Balans kneeling chair and the adjustable child's chair, the Tripp Trapp, Peter Opsvik spent decades engineering various perches that allowed a person to rest comfortably and work at the same time. His book, *Rethinking Sitting*, is worth reading. "The best posture is always the next one," explained Opsvik, and therefore the best way to sit was to cycle through various postures during the day. He found that a high seat with a sloped seat pan and a place to rest your feet encouraged the user to perch, wiggle, and sway.

I liked that idea a lot. What if I could have the best of both worlds? What if I could move my desk up and down and fiddle and twist, but still have a place to rest my backside? With that in mind I went to see David Kahl at Fully, a design studio and shop headquartered in Portland, Oregon, with a branch in San Francisco, and another in Baltimore. A few months earlier, I'd spent a day at an office furniture expo in Las Vegas, viewing what I assumed was the last word in office furniture, including massive marshmallow-cushioned desk chairs, sized for obese Americans, and peculiarly shaped keyboards meant to fend off wrist ailments common to keyboarders whose forearms must be held at right angles to their upper arms for most of the day.

As soon as I walked into his bright San Francisco showroom, I knew that Kahl was onto something different. Nearly everything was imported from Scandinavia, where "sitting disease"—first identified in the United States around 2010—has been recognized as a problem for decades. On its website, Fully described its mission: The company was "dedicated to putting movement back into your day." You could stay very active, and still get your work done. "When you are work-ing in chairs that let you move, people feel better," said Kahl. "They're happy, and the people around them are happy." There were so many good, innovative options for sitting and standing at Fully that I knew I'd never buy another piece of office furniture without consulting Da-vid Kahl.

One particularly enticing piece of equipment was homegrown, in North Kingstown, Rhode Island. I was surprised to discover that it was the invention of Martin Keen, who also designed Keen Footwear's hiking boots and sandals. When Keen lent his acumen to office fur-niture, the result was the Locus workstation, manufactured by Focal Upright. At Fully, I tried it, and fell in love. The concept was so sim-ple: A sculptural, adjustable seat was fastened to a post, which in turn was attached to an adjustable base. The accompanying adjustable desk could be kept conventionally flat, or it could be pitched toward the user. Wisely, Keen designed accessories to accommodate the slant, preventing your MacBook and coffee from sliding to the floor.

When you are seated at the Locus workstation, the torso/thigh an-gle is the highly desirable 135 degrees. The spine stays neutral, the leg muscles and glutes are engaged, and the neck and head are positioned right where they should be. The legs, the upright pole of the seat, and the base of the desk form an isosceles triangle. There is no need for a seat back or a lumbar support, nor is there any temptation to lean backward to rest.

The comment posted to the YouTube page where Martin Keen demonstrates how to use the Locus captures the feeling: "*Daaaam-mmmn*. Someone finally got the desk thing right."

To buy the combination workstation costs a little more than $2,000, and that's before you start adding the accessories. I promised myself that if I could unload my stable of ergonomic chairs, maybe on Craigslist, I'd make the investment in maintaining my mental and physical health and my spine's well-being. It made no sense to spend the kind of time and money I was doling out for postural interven-tions and bodywork, only to ruin it all by sitting for hours in a chair that would undo all the work in minutes.

ONE DAY, WHILE thumbing through physical therapist Deane Ju-han's handbook for bodywork, I found something that rearranged my thinking. Everything in our lives, Juhan observed—"our habits, our jobs, our social situations, our general dispositions"—encouraged us to "prefer certain fixed positions over others." We developed "partic-ular fixations" and clung to them, until the possibility that "we might in fact stand up in a different way passes out of our conscious consid-eration." Those ingrained postures, he explained, create patterns of tension in our muscles, and, in time, that constant tension "alters the thickness of our fascia and the shape of our bones in order to more efficiently accommodate a limited number of positions."

We find familiar postures comforting, wrote Juhan, because they provide "sensory and psychological stability, a constant norm which we return to as to a favorite jacket or old friend." Escaping was tough: "Person, posture, and point of view become firmly welded together, unfortunately limiting all three. And what was a familiar friend can become an increasingly tormenting millstone around the neck."

To liberate myself from those millstones, I'd have to become aware of my "old friends"—postures and positions that did not help me but which I habitually assumed, such as the classic "knee-over-knee," with my body angled to the right for balance. That position, a favorite since I took it up in the classroom as a young teenager, had shortened all the muscles on the right side of my torso.

Since there were more approaches to correcting posture than I could reasonably hope to study, I stuck with six fairly accessible in-terventions. (Although not all are available in all parts of the country, in most regions you will find at least one of them.) On the list were methods that are basically European—the Feldenkrais method; Rolfing structural integration; the Alexander Technique; and Pilates and its close relative, Gyrotonic—and from the East, the practices of Iyengar yoga and the Asian martial arts Tai Chi and Qigong. Al-though several of these approaches had been properly studied in ran-domized controlled trials, others had not undergone evidence-based scrutiny. In such cases, I relied on my own experience, and on word of mouth.

Although they look and feel different, these techniques have something important in common. They rely on the brain's remarkable and sustained capacity to reorganize itself. They produce similar results, improving posture, proprioception (awareness of where your body is located in space), and movement patterns. With the exception of Tai Chi and Qigong, which are practices that cannot be attributed to any individual progenitor, these techniques were developed by unusually intuitive people who influenced one another's thinking in significant ways.

Feldenkrais

I BEGAN WITH the Feldenkrais Method of Somatic Education, usually referred to simply as Feldenkrais. There were two aspects to this form of training: Awareness Through Movement group classes and workshops, and one-on-one Functional Integration sessions. Hospital rehabilitation programs, HMOs, local gyms, and community recreation centers offered inexpensive Feldenkrais programs. Best of all, you didn't have to be fit to get started, so this practice was accessible for just about anybody.

Margaret Mead, the cultural anthropologist, was a Feldenkrais fan. Andrew Weil, the director of the University of Arizona's Center for Integrative Medicine, is also a booster, explaining that the practice allows us to "rediscover the free, effortless sense of movement we had in the first few years of life—and undo many of the aches and pains that plague us as adults who have literally become too set in our ways."

After a friend described the Feldenkrais Institute of New York, on the West Side of Manhattan, as "a kind of church . . . a temple of the human body" where she was sure I'd feel very welcome, I e-mailed the institute's cofounder and clinical director, physical therapist Marek Wyszynski.

In our initial conversation, he said that when he first saw a client, he was always curious to discover what he or she thought had brought on the pain. Both patients and physicians, as well as most physical therapists and chiropractors, dwelled on what they called the "inciting incident," but did not take into account how aberrant movement patterns, over many years, had resulted in this accumulated damage. Wyszynski said it was important to consider how the problem was related to posture, movement patterns, and behavior in general. He wanted to know what the client was doing every day that might be causing the distress.

"As you start to examine even the simplest actions," he said, "you realize that our awareness of how we do what we do is very limited." We are on automatic pilot most of the time, he added. "But when an activity starts to give us problems—like pain when getting up from a chair or difficulty climbing stairs—relying on automatic pilot leads to slower recovery or even further deterioration."

A few weeks after our initial conversation, Wyszynski invited me to attend the Feldenkrais Institute of New York's sixth birthday celebration at the organization's headquarters on West Twenty-Sixth Street. I pushed through the heavy doors of a converted loft building, where the institute occupied the immense second floor.

In preparation, I'd read several of Moshé Feldenkrais's better-known monographs, including a useful one called *Learn to Learn*. A physicist, mechanical engineer, and one of the first Western black belts in judo, Feldenkrais was born in what is now Ukraine. After immigrating to Palestine in his teens, he moved to Paris, where he received his doctoral degrees from the Sorbonne, and took a position at the Institut Curie, analyzing the prospects for nuclear fission.

At the beginning of World War II, having signed on with the British Admiralty, Feldenkrais left Paris for Great Britain, transporting precious cargo: a jar of "heavy water," in which the hydrogen in the molecules is partly or wholly replaced by the isotope deuterium, essential in the operation of nuclear reactors. After the war, he settled in the new state of Israel, to do physics research at the Weizmann Institute. In the 1940s, on board a submarine—by then he was director of the Israel Defense Forces electronics department—he slipped on the deck, reinjuring a knee that he'd damaged while playing soccer in his youth. Doctors could not promise that rehab or surgery would work; after the operation, they told him, he might spend the rest of his life in a wheelchair. Because Feldenkrais understood how the laws of gravity and motion affected the mechanics of movement, he began to develop what would become a series of short exercises that helped educate the body in easier, more efficient movement patterns.

He gave his resulting thousand "Awareness Through Movement" lessons names, like Pelvic Clock, Coordination of Flexors and Extensors, and Spine Like a Chain. From the beginning, he focused on teaching patients effective techniques for self-rehabilitation.

WHEN I STEPPED off the elevator into the Feldenkrais Institute's reception area, I walked into a crowd of extremely friendly New Yorkers, ranging in age from their early twenties to their early nineties. Moments later, there were whoops of joy from an adjacent room, as seventy newly certified Feldenkrais teachers—who had just completed their prescribed eight hundred hours of rigorous training over a three-and-a-half-year period, at a cost of about $4,500—were presented with their diplomas. Since 1999, the number of teachers worldwide has grown from three thousand to nearly six thousand, with programs in thirty-nine countries. Ready to celebrate, giddy graduates and teachers-in-training emerged from the twenty-seven-hundred-square-foot studio.

The rest of us, dressed in comfortable street clothes rather than workout gear, drifted into the enormous room and plucked wide, thick foam pads and blue blankets from a big stack. We spread them out on the wood floor, so that each of us had our own little island.

One woman of about my age walked past me with a jungle cat's confidence and grace, seemingly prepared to move in any direction, at any time, at any speed, without hesitation. Hers was what Feldenkrais would have described as a "potent posture," and it was a beautiful thing to watch.

There were no mirrors in the studio, because Feldenkrais believed that it was unproductive to imitate an external model or ideal. The impetus for movement had to come from within, and there was no right way or wrong way to do a movement.

"Do everything slowly," Feldenkrais wrote. "I do not intend to 'teach you,' but to enable you to learn at your own rate of understanding and doing. Time is the most important means of learning. . . . There should be sufficient time to perceive and organize oneself. No one can learn when hurried and hustled." As I thought about all the energetic and exhausting yoga classes I'd tried (and failed), I understood how important this was.

When the instructor joined us, he stood at the front of the room, next to a human skeleton that dangled, cranium to toe phalanges, from a metal stand. Since some of us were new that evening, he said he'd start with the basics. He'd remain at the front of the room. He would not touch or adjust anyone's posture. He would not perform the exercises himself, so there was no need to watch him. For the next forty-five minutes or so, we were to listen to his words and move as much or as little as suited us, in as much comfort as possible. The goal was to allow our bodies to discover new kinesthetic patterns—ones that might serve us better than those that were old, stiff, and stale. Then he asked us to consider something I'd never considered: exactly how our bodies were meeting the floor.

I recognized that my left foot and toes were pointed straight forward, but my right foot—in fact, my entire leg, including hip and thigh—rotated sharply to the right. The right buttock was glued to the floor, while my left cheek barely skimmed the mat. Something was seriously out of whack. As we began the Feldenkrais lesson called the Gentle Twist, the instructor issued calm, easy-to-follow directions. Quickly, I drifted into a relaxed state, alert enough to follow along but not at all anxious about keeping up. The time flew by; a knee moved up, back, sideways; the pelvis rocked, the tailbone lifted and retreated to the floor. That the practice didn't require fitness, strength, or flexibility was part of its appeal.

When the class ended, after about an hour, we were asked once again to check to see how our bodies were meeting the floor. To my surprise, my body's corkscrew twist had resolved: I lay flat. When I got to my feet, instead of moving stiffly, I felt light and energetic.

In another room, where platters of cheese, fruit, sandwiches, and salads had been set out in celebration, I met Courtney King. In her midthirties, King had soft, straight brown hair and a shy smile. "A year ago," she told me, "I was sure there were things I'd never do again, because my back was so tight and inflexible—but Feldenkrais has changed that."

She was twenty-four when the World Trade Center was attacked on September 11, 2001. That day, she felt the first twinge. Three months later, her back muscles were in such severe spasms that she couldn't stand up straight. By 2004, "there was pain I could not make go away," she remembered. She'd encountered Feldenkrais in an acting class in college, but hadn't continued. Compared with the two or three ballet classes she took every week, and her Hatha yoga practice, it had seemed unchallenging. Now, desperate for some gentle exercise, she began to visit the institute a few times a week. "I'd thought the back pain was related to the stress of yoga and dance," she said, "but as I got more involved with Feldenkrais, I realized that the pain had more to do with the way I carried myself every day."

With Feldenkrais, her back pain was gone in about two months. She resumed her yoga practice. But like many others, she stuck with her Feldenkrais lessons. "People mostly come to the institute for pain management," King said, "but they stay on because Feldenkrais makes them feel so good." There were other benefits: She was a shy person who was not often comfortable in social situations, but at the institute, she'd felt right at home. "After the lesson, when you walk down the hall," she said, "everyone you pass is wearing a big smile, and you're suffused with this sense of peace and well-being, as if you've unwound all the bad stuff—all the social constraints and habits that get in the way of making connections."

It seemed impossible that a single Feldenkrais session could reduce my pain. But the morning after, I hinged neatly at the hips when I reached for the Crest, instead of jutting out my chin and craning my neck. When it was time to go to work, without special attention from my brain, my body called upon the previous day's lesson. Instead of relying on the small muscles of the shoulder girdle to pull open a heavy door, I recruited the latissimus dorsi, the strong, broad muscles that encircled my rib cage.

Back in the Bay Area, I found physical therapist Deborah Bowes, a highly respected teacher, at the Feldenkrais Center for Movement Education in San Francisco. Bowes, who became a Feldenkrais practitioner in 1987, was one of the center's cofounders. Although Feldenkrais was very popular with younger people, many of the workshops that Bowes ran were designed for those of us who were starting to feel our age. "So many people have been injured by going to a modality that doesn't fit," Bowes said. "You have to think about what you can do that would be comfortable for you."

I signed up for a three-day, eight-hour-a-day back care workshop with Bowes. Among my classmates I found Patty, a Pilates teacher whose back pain made it hard for her to carry her own groceries. There was Lynn, a fitness instructor who had been dependent on Vicodin for about a decade. Margarita sometimes had to lie on the floor for days. Cheri, rosy-cheeked and lively in her late seventies—and who looked as if she was in the best shape of all of us—was committed to staying that way. Two younger men filled out the group— Pradip, a thirtyish engineer whose hamstrings were chronically tight and painful; and Brad, an impressively buff ice hockey player who had injured his back in training. Together, we ran through lesson after lesson with an occasional break for a lecture. It was fascinating. I could imagine coming back for more. Among the workshops Bowes offered were "Feldenkrais for Freedom from Habitual Patterns," "Walking with Ease," "Pain-Free Knees and Ankles," "Feldenkrais to Reduce Stress and Anxiety," and "Comfortable Sitting." There was a Feldenkrais workshop for people who suffered from insomnia, and one for musicians, and another called "Comfortable Feet."

In addition to the Awareness Through Movement group classes, Feldenkrais teachers offer private Functional Integration sessions. FI, as it is known, is not a replacement for ATM classes, but for many, it becomes a key adjunct to them. Many people report feeling taller, refreshed, free from pain and tension, flexible and balanced, more comfortable and confident physically, and more emotionally positive, or "lighter," after this one-on-one work. Intrigued, I decided to sign up for an FI session with Bowes.

Stretched out on the low, padded therapy table, fully dressed, I listened to her soothing voice. My body tends to tense up in the presence of an unknown massage therapist, but Bowes was so gentle that readily, I granted her admission to a very primitive part of my central nervous system. "This is about finding out where the 'noise' is," she murmured, as she ran gentle fingers over my rigid trapezius muscles. "We want to find out where the blinders are. You may have been crooked for years without noticing . . . until you do. Pain is like a garment you don't know you're wearing until you take it off." As she continued to manipulate my head and spine, I spent ninety minutes in a semiconscious state. This was not any kind of massage: It was visceral communication. It took considerable sweet-talking, but I felt the taut muscles of my low back and hip finally give up their fight.

Afterward, I bought an audio CD of Deborah Bowes's Feldenkrais lessons, all delivered in that same hypnotic way. After several weeks of individual lessons, I was moving better, with much more fluidity. My back no longer hurt, nor did my hips. It was something I knew I wanted to pursue further in the future. But for the time being, I was moving on—because who knew what I'd find down the road?

Rolfing

I CAME UPON a copy of Ida Rolf's 1978 book, *Rolfing and Physical Reality*, in the giveaway pile at the local library. The jacket was pale and tattered, but the words on the page resonated like mad: "Some individuals may perceive their losing fight with gravity as a sharp pain in their back, others as the unflattering contour of their body, others as a constant fatigue, yet others as an unrelentingly threatening environment," Rolf wrote. "Those over 40 may call it old age. And yet all these signals may be pointing to a single problem so prominent in their own structure . . . that it has been ignored: They are off-balance. They are at war with gravity."

What I thought I knew about Rolfing didn't jibe with this measured assessment. I'd spoken with people who—back in the 1970s—had undergone grueling sessions in the hands of very aggressive practitioners, who pounded them like veal cutlets in need of tenderizing.

Over the years, as Rolf Structural Integration was formalized into ten very specific sessions, that had changed. The first three were called the "sleeve sessions" because they focused on the layers of fasciae just under the skin. "Fasciae" form a translucent cocoon, slipcovering every bone, muscle, tendon, ligament, organ, and blood vessel in the body. Gossamer-thin or thick and tough, depending on their function, fasciae allow fibers to glide over one another, as if doused in olive oil. Strands of fasciae connect remote aspects of our anatomy; two strands of fasciae, for instance, anchor our thumbs and then extend up the arms and around the pectoral muscles, all the way to the rib cage. The next four sessions addressed the region between the pelvis and the top of the head. The final three sessions integrated all parts of the structure—thus, the name.

Until I found Rolf's book, I'd never heard of fasciae—but I was intrigued. "If there is constant excess muscle tension," wrote researcher and physical therapist Tom Myers, who has devoted his career to investigating a part of the anatomy that most physicians fail to acknowledge, "the *fasciae* over time must compensate by making more 'fabric,' ultimately forcing the body into a straitjacket of limitation and distortion." I suspected the constriction of my own fasciae might explain why I could not hold my torso erect for more than a few minutes, before returning to my original question mark shape.

On the jacket of the book I found at the library, there was an image of Ida P. Rolf, white-haired, with kind eyes and a large flower pinned in her hair. I thought I'd learn that she was a 1960s flower child, but I couldn't have been further off. Born in 1896, she received her PhD in biological chemistry, and accepted a job at the Rockefeller Institute of Medical Research, where she investigated the role of collagen in wound healing. Because fasciae are collagen-based tissue, she also considered their physiological function, discovering a passion that would engage her for the rest of her life.

Rolf took a leave of absence from Rockefeller in 1927, moving from New York to Zurich, where she studied mathematics and atomic physics. But when she fell in with a less academic crowd, she began to explore Tantric yoga, mysticism, and the Alexander Technique, and developed the technique she called "structural integration." In the mid-1960s, having achieved some influence in Europe, she brought structural integration to California's Esalen Institute, on the cliffs of Big Sur. At a time when medical science wholeheartedly embraced the Cartesian mind-body split, Rolf insisted that there was no such bifurcation, and started teaching.

WHEN I CALLED the Rolfing Structural Integration headquarters in Boulder, Colorado, for a referral in the Bay Area, the woman who helped me told me that I should definitely look up Michael Salveson, but that it would be almost impossible to get in to see him. He treated only eighteen to twenty people per week, and he was booked up six months in advance. Four decades earlier, he'd been one of Ida Rolf's star students at Esalen. The two had remained close friends until Rolf died, at the age of eighty-three.

Rolf structural integration is never cheap, but when I learned that Salveson charged $300 per ninety-minute session, about double the standard fee, I was taken aback. Later, the expense would make sense: The basic training involved in becoming a Rolf practitioner costs about $18,000 and requires more than seven hundred in-person, on-site hours, over a span of twelve to eighteen months. Becoming an advanced certified Rolfer (and those are the ones you want to see) takes years, and much more coursework. Still, I was in luck. Because the winter holidays were upon us, many of his clients were away. Michael Salveson would not be able to complete my Ten Series, but he could find me a spot for a couple of sessions, and would refer me to someone who could finish what he'd started.

Still worrying that what lay ahead might be exceptionally painful, I drove to Salveson's house in the Berkeley Hills. When he collected me from his book-and-art-filled living room, with floor-to-ceiling windows with a view of San Francisco Bay and the city beyond, I followed him through the kitchen and down a narrow flight of stairs to his studio. On the way, I turned a tight corner and knocked two framed charcoal drawings off the wall. Neither broke, and Salveson said nothing as he set them back on their hooks. But later, he'd explain that "the rehabilitation of internal subjective awareness" was at the heart of what he did. His job was to slip in "under the radar of conscious cognitive processes, to make contact with the parasympathetic nervous system and to help the body make whatever internal corrections were necessary." I could only hope that making those internal corrections would eliminate the kind of clumsiness that caused me to walk into things and take artwork off walls.

Once again, it would be necessary to conduct research attired only in my underwear. Salveson asked me to take a walk around his big motorized treatment table, broader and lower than an ordinary massage table, while he took a good look at what time and fasciae had wrought. As directed, I stretched out on my belly. Within two minutes, as his enormous hands traveled over me, I'd handed over my parasympathetic nervous system. I understood what he'd meant by "slipping in under the radar of conscious cognitive processes." As he deftly pried apart fasciae that had been tightly bound over a lifetime, there was physical discomfort but no sense of suffering.

Halfway through the session, Salveson asked me to climb off the table, and to take another walk around the room. My legs felt like tree trunks, heavy, numb, and unyielding. But when I finally got to my feet, I was acutely conscious of the sensation of the carpet under my soles.

He put me back on the table for another forty-five minutes. When the session ended, I was standing much taller. The angle of my chin to my chest had opened. My clavicle, usually pointed toward the ground, was high and proud. My neck was long, my lungs took in more air, and my shoulders had broadened. But I was also slightly disoriented: With my head properly situated, and my chin raised, I was staring through the bottom section of my progressive eyeglass lenses, meant for reading the small print, instead of looking through the upper region, intended for distance.

I should take the rest of the day off to let this new pattern settle in, Michael Salveson said. There would be no working out, and no sitting at my desk slumped over my laptop. As soon as he could find a slot, I would come back for my second session in the Ten Series.

A month later, I was less nervous. As Salveson probed the taut piano wires at the base of my neck, some kind of emotional dam crumbled. Sniffling and apologizing for the waterworks, I reached for the tissues. I was not to worry about it, he said. Rolfing almost always provoked emotional arousal. If it didn't, something was wrong. If I'd been looking for a way to debunk Cartesian theory, I'd found it.

Because the holidays were over, Salveson's appointment book was full—for the next year. So that I might complete the remaining eight sessions, he referred me to an advanced certified Rolfer, who worked closer to home.

His referral, James Schwartz, was tall and thin, and very well read. While I was on the table, he was inclined to produce on-target metaphors that I couldn't write down and had to try to remember. In one of the eight sessions, he compared the situation in my right hip and low back to a brawl: "It's a lot like trying to calm down a mob," he said, pensively. "It's tempting to intervene with riot police and mace and clubs, but it's usually more efficient to look for the ringleaders—the ones that are spearheading all this trouble—and to try to negotiate with them."

Often, I was relaxed enough to fall asleep on the table. However, during Rolfing session number seven, during which the therapist inserts his latex-gloved fingers into the client's mouth and works (painfully) to release the jaw, you'd better believe that I was wide awake.

Ida Rolf made no bones about it: When the Ten Series was a fait accompli, you were on your own; your Rolfer did not want to see you again, unless you had a baby or a traumatic injury. It was the client's job to develop a personal practice—yoga, Feldenkrais, Tai Chi—that would sustain the improvements.

Although he was trained in the practice, James Schwartz no longer worked within the boundaries of classical Rolfing. His clients rarely wanted to leave after ten sessions. I understood that: I'd made a lot of progress, and I wanted to keep going. That's when Schwartz went to work on the twenty-three inches of fasciae known as the "mesentery," attached to my small intestine. I'd always wondered why constipation, even for a short time, exacerbated back pain, and he could explain it. When the small intestine became packed with stool, it tugged unceasingly on the lumbar spine, compressing the nerves and causing discomfort. Plunging his fingers into the muscles around my navel, he went after the mesentery with gusto. Just as he predicted, a trip to the loo followed. Until bowel constriction set in once again, my back felt great. It made me wonder how many people who think they're suffering from back pain (especially those who take constipation-inducing opioids) are actually struggling with a lackadaisical bowel.

I would love to have seen James Schwartz every week, but I knew how risky it could be to depend on someone else to fix you. It was up to me to find a practice I liked and could pursue on my own, thereby fulfilling Ida Rolf's decree.

Alexander Technique

FROM AT LEAST a dozen people, including actors, writers, and musicians, I'd heard that the Alexander Technique had made a big difference in their lives. Among the well-known adherents were Kenneth Branagh, William Hurt, Kevin Kline, Jeremy Irons, James Earl Jones, Kelly McGillis, Paul Newman, Lynn Redgrave, Maggie Smith, Robin Williams, Paul McCartney, Sting, Julian Bream (the classical guitarist), James Galway (the classical flutist), and Yehudi Menuhin (violinist and conductor). The attraction was long-standing: In the 1930s, such luminaries as George Bernard Shaw, Aldous Huxley, Lewis Mumford, and Leonard and Virginia Woolf had taken AT lessons.

But the Alexander Technique also worked for people who were not celebrities. David Homan, the executive director of the America-Israel Cultural Foundation, said that in his early thirties, he'd started Alexander lessons, which made him aware of the habits that brought on his pain. He learned to recognize how he puffed out his chest and thrust his hips forward in an effort to disguise the size of his abdomen. But that position accentuated the curve in his low back, sending his stress straight to his spine.

Before he "found Alexander," he had tried yoga, Pilates, and Feldenkrais. None of these had prevented his back from going into such severe spasms that on multiple occasions, he spent part of the workday stretched out on the long table in the foundation's conference room. But after six months of AT lessons, he was standing taller. People knew that he had changed in some way, but they couldn't say what it was. They asked if he'd gotten a haircut or was wearing new glasses. "I was suddenly in control of something I'd thought was uncontrollable," he said.

"Now, when I'm heading for trouble, I can recognize it. I feel sort of awkward and haphazard and uncoordinated, and everything hurts from the neck down," he said, "and I can take some time to intervene on that. Before AT, I had no idea of how to stop my back from hurting except to lie down. Now I can activate the parts that are underworking and deactivate the parts that are overworking."

The origins of the Alexander Technique lie with F. M. Alexander, a Tasmanian actor and orator who, in the late 1800s, was trying to make a living by declaiming Shakespeare in stentorian tones. But his terrible stage fright, shortness of breath, and fear-induced laryngitis threatened to derail his career.

In an effort to overcome these problems, Alexander recited his lines before a mirror. As he spoke, he saw that in preparation, he sucked in his breath, as if before a long underwater swim. He stiffened his neck, pulled his head back, and depressed his larynx. When he relaxed, allowing his neck to move naturally and his spine to lengthen, as if a string pulled the top of his head toward the sky, the laryngitis, breathlessness, and anxiety disappeared.

Alexander performed for another decade, but he also helped other actors and musicians leave behind the habitual motor patterns he called "debauched kinesthesia." In 1904, a prominent British surgeon who learned about Alexander's technique helped finance a move to London. Each night, before the curtain rose, Alexander was on call at West End theaters, helping actors warm up before they performed. A decade later, when he took the practice to Broadway, he attracted the attention of Columbia University professor James Harvey Robinson, who described his encounter with F. M. Alexander in the *Atlantic Monthly*.

Robinson was a self-acknowledged slouch, and he hoped that Alexander could help him do something about it. "Those of us who are conspicuously slovenly in our carriage are urged by parents, teachers and friends to 'brace up,'" he wrote in the *Atlantic*. "I have given myself this order and received it from others since childhood, but have found that my best efforts failed. Now I see the reason. No one explained to me what it was to 'brace up'; and I assumed that an effort to elevate my chest, buckle in my back, and bring my shoulder-blades as nearly together as possible was the desired end. This is what most people do when they endeavor to straighten themselves. While there might be worse positions, this one involves a great deal of strain; it tends to throw out the abdomen and does not really increase the freedom of the lungs."

Robinson wrote of a "bodily dogmatism . . . which shows itself in a strong reluctance to grant that our habitual posture and movements are wrong." That insistence on doing things the way you'd always done them had to be banished, Robinson realized, while working with Alexander. Slumping was a habit, and it was one that could be broken—but it would not disappear in a vacuum. It was essential to provide the body with an alternative.

CLINICAL TRIALS OF expensive drugs and devices are common, while investigations of protocols or products that won't make hundreds of millions of dollars are rare. Still, there are exceptions, and the Alexander Technique, which has received considerable attention in peer-reviewed medical journals, is among them. Thirty-three years after F. M. Alexander left Tasmania for the West End of London, a group of nineteen doctors composed and signed a letter to the *British Medical Journal*, endorsing his approach. Noting that they had seen "beneficial changes in use and function with the technique in their patients and themselves," they urged that such training should be incorporated into medical school curricula, to be taught by F. M. Alexander himself. Poor "use" of the body, they wrote, predisposed a patient to disorder and disease, including back pain, and they thought that the Alexander Technique might be the antidote.

From what I could see, that advice was ignored. But seventy-one years later, the *BMJ* published the outcomes of a large randomized controlled trial, funded by the United Kingdom's Medical Research Council, which is in turn funded by the government. University researchers had recruited about five hundred patients from sixty-four general medicine practices. Prior to starting the trial, the patients, all of whom had experienced at least five years of back pain, made lists of tasks they could no longer perform. When the study ended, the plan was to evaluate whether anything had changed. One group of participants received "normal" care, that is, physiotherapy (as physical therapy is referred to in Britain) or an educational booklet. Another got massage therapy. The third group engaged in six lessons in the Alexander Technique, and the fourth group had twenty-four AT lessons, in combination with a walking program.

Those who were massaged were the first to experience relief, but when the massages ran out, so did the benefits. The physiotherapy patients and those who had six AT sessions saw less improvement than those who took twenty-four Alexander lessons and joined the walking program. In that group, the number of "things I can no longer do" decreased by more than 40 percent.

Instead of inspiring admiration, the study upset both allopathic physicians (who practice conventional Western medicine) and holistic practitioners, who feared that the British National Health Service (NHS) would bail on standard conservative treatments for back pain, ruining their practices. Normally, after a paper appears in an eminent scientific journal, a few comments, phrased with great deference to the authors, are published or posted online. But after the paper describing the Alexander Technique study appeared in *BMJ*, it generated sixty-seven such comments within days, mostly from physicians. Few of them were even marginally polite.

Just as UK physicians had anticipated, or feared, the NHS embraced the Alexander Technique as part of its revised guidelines, and declined to allow epidural steroid "jabs" for most common low back pain conditions. From there, it got ugly. In July 2009, Paul Watson, at the time the head of the British Pain Society, who had been involved in developing the new NHS guidelines, and thus put the kibosh on injections, was ousted from his leadership post, in what members described as an "extraordinary row."

AS THE BATTLE over the usefulness of the Alexander Technique raged in the United Kingdom, I prepared for a session with Judith Stern, a teacher who had been helpful to David Homan, who no longer had to seek relief from his back pain upon his organization's conference room table. As I watched some lessons on YouTube, I was puzzled. The AT teacher followed a student around a small room, minutely adjusting the position of his head and neck. The changes were so minor that it was hard to imagine how they could be effective.

Judith Stern had taught the Alexander Technique to clients for more than twenty-five years, lecturing widely to medical school students and other physician groups. Working mostly from her office in Rye, just north of New York City, Stern also saw some clients in Manhattan. A forty-five-minute session cost $95, which was about average for an AT lesson. Within moments of meeting at her Manhattan office, she explained that she would try to undo my unconscious habits and help me develop "'conscious control', which would permit my system to come back into balance." This idea, I recognized, was also intrinsic to Feldenkrais and Rolfing.

Most AT work occurs while the student is upright and walking.

But in my initial session with Stern, I found myself on the table, her hands cradling my head, while she gently shifted it by millimeters. If I could locate a position of ease while lying down, she explained, I'd be able to find it again, while standing, sitting, and walking. Her work, she explained, was not so much about "fixing" bad habits as it was about inhibiting them, so that innately good habits could take over. "When you've been in chronic pain for years," she said, "you've spent a long time detaching yourself from your body's sensations, out of self-preservation. It can take a while to tune in to what your body is doing."

After about a quarter hour, Stern asked if I could feel a difference between my right and left legs, while lying on my back on the table. "My left leg is alive," I said without hesitation. "My right leg feels dead." "That's a great kinesthetic distinction to make," she said. "You're constantly holding and guarding your right hip. It's such an entrenched habit that you won't even let go when you're well supported and lying down. You do it when you walk and sit, but you also do it when you're sleeping." The tightness in those muscles, Stern observed, was the physiological equivalent of a knot tied in a garden hose. It impaired my circulation and sent other muscles into spasm, cutting down on my resilience and making me more vulnerable to new injury.

She asked me to allow my torso to release away from my limbs, to let it widen and soften. My intellect said "Huh?" but my body was on board: I could feel the tension lessen in my hip as my shoulders and rib cage spread like pudding across the table.

"Your brain is convinced that hanging on like this is the way to help you survive, the only way to keep you safe," she said, "and that it would be unwise to let go. My job is to serve as a guide, to show you that it is safe to give up this holding. It's to show you how to do less and still be yourself. I want to introduce you to the two-year-old Cathryn, who knew perfectly well how to be easeful and upright and how to play. You don't need to be this wired to be effective."

Although in real life I almost never cry, once again I dissolved into tears. Stern handed me a box of tissues, asking me what it might be like if I could ratchet down the intensity with which I did everything in my life. "We don't know how much unnecessary work we're doing," she said, "until someone shows us how to do something different. You're storing a lot of fear and pain and anxiety in those muscles, and it's my job to give you a sense of what it's like to let your head and neck rest, to take all those muscles off duty."

I would have been pleased to allow Judith Stern to whisper to my arms, legs, torso, and head for the rest of the day. But after a half hour, she asked me to let myself go as floppy as a marionette, while she guided me into a seated position. "Dangle from my hand," she said. "Don't worry about your spine: I'll hold it for you. Now, let's take a little walk, like you're a dangling skeleton with your head and neck free, and the pelvis hanging down." Following her instructions, I could sense that I had made peace with the forces of gravity, at least briefly.

"That looks good on you," Stern observed. Finding my balance would take time, she added. "If, as you have been, someone has been dramatically separated from her body in order to survive," she said, appraisingly, "it tends to be a longer journey."

Back on the sidewalk, a chilly wind blowing straight off the Hudson hit me. But instead of hunching my shoulders against it, or screwing up my face in useless, icy misery, I thought about allowing my head to move forward and up, released my legs from my torso, and made my way toward the subway at Columbus Circle, for the moment feeling very free.

Yoga

HAVING MADE MY way through these predominantly Western techniques, I moved on to studying traditionally Eastern approaches that held promise for back pain patients. Among them were yoga and, later, Tai Chi and Qigong.

In 2015, nearly twenty million people in the United States were practicing yoga, contributing to an industry that was worth $10 billion a year, according to a study conducted on behalf of *Yoga Journal*. Many devotees had started going to class because they thought it would be good for their backs. But the outcomes of a Columbia College of Physicians and Surgeons survey, polling thirty-three thousand yoga teachers, therapists, and other clinicians around the world, showed that this wasn't necessarily true. In fact, low back trauma was the most common type of yoga injury.

Because chronic back pain patients were often weak and deconditioned, they overworked the lumbar and cervical regions of the spine. Improperly executed forward bends—even simple forward bends—presented a great risk; so did headstands, performed before the shoulder girdle and thoracic spine were strong enough to provide the necessary support. Gentle, restorative yoga, which many back pain-inhibited people pursue as a good place to start, was great for relaxation, but it wouldn't make a back patient any stronger, build bone, or improve balance.

Few people consider checking a yoga teacher's credentials before unrolling a mat, but how an instructor has been trained is a very important consideration. Phenomenal yoga teachers are out there, of course, but the world is rife with frighteningly inexperienced ones, often certified in one hundred hours of training by "yoga teacher mills." Some have done their coursework online, without ever setting foot in a classroom. Even teachers who claim to be "yoga therapists" may be unseasoned.

I learned that two styles of yoga, Viniyoga and Iyengar, were the most suitable options for people with orthopedic and musculoskeletal problems. (Some people refer to Iyengar yoga as "furniture yoga," because the class incorporates blocks, belts, blankets, and sandbags, as well as folding chairs, stools, wall ropes, benches, and "tresslers" of various sizes, all of which are used to facilitate various poses.) In the past, these practices were studied in clinical trials that focused on posture, pelvic and spinal alignment, and training muscle groups to work properly together. The outcomes, published in the *Archives of Internal Medicine* and the journal *Pain*, showed that a well-designed yoga program not only decreased the perceived intensity of back pain, but also improved people's ability to accomplish their daily tasks, and reduced their reliance on pain medication, the last by a very impressive

88 percent. More studies were needed, but those were not statistics you could ignore.

It was probably no coincidence that to become a Viniyoga or an Iyengar instructor required enrollment in lengthy teacher-training programs. It took five hundred hours to become a Viniyoga therapist, and about five years before aspiring Iyengar teachers were allowed to call themselves instructors. In Iyengar yoga, reaching junior instructor level could take a decade of work and testing. In the United States, only two Iyengar instructors, Patricia Walden and Manouso Manos, had achieved the level of advanced senior teachers. Both traveled and taught other instructors for most of the year. I didn't think I had a prayer of getting to know either of them. But then, I met a teacher at the local high school. It was her misfortune that would get me an audience with Manouso Manos.

I THOUGHT I knew a little about yoga. Way back in 1982, I'd joined a Manhattan studio and spent a couple of evenings a week attempting to mimic poses that were far beyond me. Too often, I wound up rigid with muscle spasms. Finally, the instructor grew tired of waiting for me to recover and get off the floor so she could lock up, and suggested that I might take up something less taxing.

In 2010, ready to try again, I bought a monthly pass at a Northern California studio with a yard-long list of offerings, from which I'd selected a Level One class. Among sleekly muscled women dressed in the kind of yoga outfits that can readily go out for dinner, I could barely find a place to put my mat. After three of about thirty Sun Salutations, I collapsed, out of breath, wondering who in hell could survive Level Two. The instructor suggested that I stick to restorative classes, which were better "for people like me."

When I met Lisa Miller, she'd been attending the same yoga class twice a week for six years. But half a dozen years before that, she'd struggled with back pain. There were several inciting incidents, none of them serious enough to explain the kind of pain she was in. Over the years, she'd seen twelve chiropractors, and failed multiple sessions of PT. The physiatrist at the local spine practice recommended IDET (intradiscal electrothermal treatment), without mentioning that studies had recently shown that it was no more effective than a placebo, or that, as a result, insurance providers had stopped paying for it. When Miller demurred, the physiatrist sent her over to the hospital for discography (another procedure that would soon have its comeuppance). The technician at the radiology suite warned her that it was going to hurt. "But when that needle went into the disc at L5-S1, I screamed," she said. "And I'm not a screamer."

Based on the results of the discography, Miller was scheduled for a lumbar spinal fusion with a titanium cage. "The surgeon told me I could expect a 90 percent pain reduction," she said, "and when I looked skeptical, he said that he wouldn't do it if it shouldn't be done." She had six weeks of summer break to get her back on her feet, before she would return to teaching auto shop in the fall, she told him. That meant, she added, that she'd be "pushing up and down off a cold concrete floor, while dealing with twenty-five kids and five to ten cars each day."

In August, after the surgery, she was very impaired. Although she could barely walk or carry anything, she tried to go back to work. But eventually, prepared to make it her full-time job to heal, she took a leave of absence in the middle of the school year, and moved in with a friend in Los Angeles. There, she went to see an eminent neurosurgeon, who told her that she should fax him her application for Social Security Disability because she was never going back to work. The damage from the surgery was such that her life was going to be about pharmaceutical pain management.

Miller kept searching. "I was willing to try anything," she said, "no matter how 'out there.'" After a bout of crystal therapy—she'd lie on the table with crystals placed all around her, and on her abdomen—she saw a psychotherapist. That didn't help either. "Frankly, I was ready to die," she said.

Although Miller was so disabled that she had to crawl to the bathroom, she decided to try a few private Iyengar yoga lessons with instructor Karin O'Bannon. But fixing what was wrong with her was beyond O'Bannon, who arranged to take Miller to a Manouso Manos workshop. In preparation, Miller read up on B. K. S. Iyengar.

"When we got there," Miller remembered, "there was this long line—about eighty people—who were waiting to see him." He sent Miller and O'Bannon to an area in the back of the studio, where he could provide some individual attention during class. After Miller collected her "props," and before class started, Manos spoke to her again. He directed her to stop trying to ignore the pain. Obviously, that wasn't working. She was to go and find it; to confront it head-on. Once again, Miller was skeptical. Every practitioner she'd seen before told her to try everything possible to distract herself from thinking about how much she hurt.

"When Manouso said that, it dawned on me," said Miller, "that I was going to have to push through the pain, that this was the only way out." With Manos at her side, staring into her eyes, she went ahead. "I was crying, and pouring sweat, a flood of it," she recalled. Finally, Manos said that she'd done enough and told her to sit down. "It was the first pain relief I'd had in so many years," she said. "And I recognized that I'd found a man who could help me get out of this horrible mess."

WHEN LISA MILLER suggested that I might like to come with her to class, I quickly agreed. A couple of weeks later, after a hour-long drive in heavy commuter traffic, Miller and I were standing outside the Abode of Iyengar Yoga, in Glen Park, a residential neighborhood in the southern part of San Francisco.

We walked through a very ordinary front door and found ourselves in a gorgeous yoga studio, illuminated by a skylight. The place was jammed; later Manouso Manos would tell me he usually had about sixty students. "Some people call it 'hope for the hopeless,'" Miller said softly, steering me toward a line that had formed in front of Manos, who sat on the floor at the front of the room. "There are countless numbers of us," she added, "with surgeries gone wrong, and really significant pain issues—and somehow, he manages to address all our needs while running the class."

Manos wore an old T-shirt and a pair of bloomer-like yoga shorts. When I finally reached the front of the line, I squatted down next to him, prepared to give a full account of my condition. He asked me to point to the problem, so I did. My right hip ached as usual. "What about the other one?" he asked. That was fine, I said. "Okay," he said. "We can fix it." Just as he had with Lisa Miller, he sent me to the back of the room.

After dragging clanking yoga chairs—these are folding metal chairs, minus their standard backrests—out of the closet, everyone in the class took the first pose. When we began a series of spinal twists, Manos arrived at my side, directing two assistants to position my body so it was squeezed between the wooden tressler—which looks something like a gymnastic balance beam—and the wall. Trapped between the two, I had no alternative but to keep my spine straight, while I turned from the hips.

As the assistants helped me move on to other poses, Manos came back to rearrange me. Just when I thought the pain could get no worse—I believe I was in Half Moon pose, with one leg elevated on the tressler, with sweat pouring into my ears and expletives tumbling from my mouth—the pain simply expired. Like Miller, I had let it do its worst; it had no more to give.

Limply draped over the tressler, I looked at Manos, astonished. "There is a hardening that has taken place on one side of your back," he said. "The first step to getting the thing to go free is to unlock it. I work it to allow it some elasticity, and then I work to make it so that all the parts can find their way back to where they belong. Human nature will tell you if you injure something, you should leave it alone and let it rest. That works in many cases, but there are injuries that aren't going to be helped that way. You are going to have to grit your teeth, bite down a bit, and go through some pain."

Nor should I think I was out of the woods (yet), he said. "You know when you chase a mouse how it doesn't head straight for the door?" he said. "First, it runs wildly all over the room. I guarantee that it will be that way with your pain. It will try every trick in the book and be all over your body before we get rid of it."

Later, I'd ask Manos how he was able to identify my shortcomings so quickly. "This thing I do is an amazing kind of dance between two people, and it takes a leap of faith," he said. "When you do what I do for years, you make a lot of mistakes along the way. But you gain adeptness, and hopefully you remember that the condition of the person in front of you is like another person's condition, so that you're not reinventing the wheel every single time."

I wanted more Iyengar, and I wanted it right away. But I would not be permitted to return to Manos's class at the Abode until I had studied the form for at least six months. When I asked him to refer me to another great teacher, he suggested Claire Colvin, who had been his student for years. A full-time accountant, she taught her own class two late afternoons each week, in a bare-bones single-room studio, in a town very near mine.

If I'd known that the class included ten regulars who had been coming for about a decade, and that no one just walked in, I would never have summoned the nerve to attend. But when I showed up—a time-sucking newbie with a tendency to groan, tip over, or even fall sound asleep in Savasana (Corpse Pose)—both Colvin and her students assured me that I was welcome. They'd been at it forever, and most had daily practices, but it had taken them just as long as it took me to learn to fold and stack the supportive blankets properly, and to figure out how to loop and buckle themselves into the woven cotton belt that was required for many poses. My progress was slow. I still staggered like a drunk every time I came out of Warrior pose. But no intervention helped me more. For a while, I forgot what it was like to hurt. And when my husband and I headed back east to care for our aging parents, Colvin's class was what I missed most. She e-mailed me regularly, to find out how things were going and to tell me that everybody missed me.

Pilates

ALTHOUGH TWENTY-FIVE MILLION people pursue Pilates in the United States, with a million more adherents in the United Kingdom, I'd never caught the bug. In New York, Pilates was all the rage, however. When I began to look for workout options in the neighborhood, I discovered that there were several second-floor Pilates studios located nearby. It was a form of training that preternaturally skinny New York women loved because, in theory, it stretched, strengthened, and balanced the body, without building the bulky thigh, glute, and arm muscles you get from doing three reps of fifteen squats with free weights in both hands. Other advertised benefits included improved posture, better blood circulation, and increased lung capacity.

Joseph Pilates, who created the practice, was a German circus performer and boxer. In 1912 he left for London, where he served as a physiotherapist to Scotland Yard personnel. Despite his status at the police department, when World War I broke out, as a German national, he was sent to a string of internment camps, where he taught floor exercises to weak and ill prisoners. Because many were bedridden, he developed an early version of his bed-like Reformer, using springs he yanked from the camps' discarded mattresses.

Back pain patients who swear by Pilates training believe that it helps them develop a strong "core," thereby ending their discomfort. For some people it worked: My friend Jennifer, decked with low back pain after years of carrying twin infants and their older sibling, felt that Pilates twice a week was all she needed to stay strong. Others told me that Pilates had not worked for them at all: In the end, there had only been more pain.

The well-known Pilates routines exercise the body in two planes. The spine bends forward and arches backward, but the bends, twists, and turns that are part of regular life are rarely practiced, leaving students unprepared for the rotating motion required to pluck a toddler from a car seat or to lift a roll-aboard into the overhead compartment.

Almost as soon as I joined Jennifer in a Pilates mat class, I remembered why I didn't like it. The "Rolling Like a Ball" exercise involved rocking back and forth on my bony, flexed spine, bruising it. The next exercise, the Pilates "One Hundred"—in which you stretched out on your back with your shoulders and trunk slightly raised and your legs elevated and bent at ninety degrees, your low back in "neutral," and your navel "scooped in"—strained my lumbar extensors, although it was intended to strengthen my core. I wasn't the only one in the room who was using the back muscles instead of the hard-to-recruit transversus abdominis muscles in the lower abdomen, but I was probably the only one who knew I was doing it wrong. In the front of the room, the instructor, flapping her arms, breathing rhythmically, and counting, could not see us, or correct our misguided efforts.

Stuart McGill, the human biomechanics expert we met earlier, would have been horrified. No fan of Pilates, he said that there was no known benefit to "drawing your navel to your spine," to get into a position called "neutral," and that "hollowing (or scooping) in," that is, pressing the low back to the floor, could exacerbate a back pain patient's condition, by reducing the stability of the spine.

MANY STUDIES HAVE examined the role of Pilates in treating low back pain, but the outcomes aren't impressive—and uneven teacher training may be to blame. Joseph Pilates trained his teachers for two or three years before he allowed them to work with their own clients, but today, certification requirements are minimal. The person who opens a tiny single-Reformer studio on Main Street may have taken teacher training for months or even years. But it is equally possible that after she took a few classes herself, her formal training lasted only for several weekends.

If you intend to sign up for twice-a-week classes, in the hope of resolving your back pain, you should find a a doctorate-level physical therapist with OCS, PMA-CPT after his or her name, standing for orthopedic clinical specialty, Pilates Method Alliance-Certified Personal Trainer. Such practitioners are difficult to locate, and I'd almost given up hope when I met Dan Santi, a seventy-three-year-old biotech entrepreneur, with an MD, a PhD, five start-ups under his belt—and a very bad neck and back. He invited me to come watch what he did with his trainer, the legendary movement expert Elizabeth Larkam.

At the crack of dawn, on a soggy and cold San Francisco morning in March, I climbed a steep flight of stairs to the second floor of a town house in the Lower Pacific Heights neighborhood, where Santi and Larkam were already at work. Things were looking up for Santi now, but when I met him six months earlier, he was sick of working with certified personal trainers who treated him as if he were thirty-five, until he got hurt. Larkam was different, he told me: She respected who he was and what he could do, and she pushed him just enough.

When I arrived, Santi was standing on the Reformer, while Larkam, her blond hair pinned up, dressed in a gray tweed jacket, a red turtleneck, and a pair of bright socks made with individual compartments for the toes, put him through a series of lunges. Then he stretched out on his back, with his knees crooked in frog position. Before he could go any further, Larkam repositioned his pelvis so that it was two millimeters to the left—because she knew it would make a difference.

As a dance medicine specialist at the Center for Sports Medicine at Saint Francis Memorial Hospital in San Francisco, Larkam had developed Pilates protocols for orthopedic, spine, and chronic pain diagnoses, building a program that drew physical therapists from all over the United States for training. She had expanded awareness of Pilates in the United States, spreading the word about its therapeutic potential.

But after many years of promoting Pilates as a stand-alone treatment for back pain rehabilitation, Larkam had second thoughts. The practice reinforces spinal flexion—the shrimplike C curve—and in a world oriented toward devices and laptops, she did not believe this was what people needed. Among back pain patients, she'd found, the C curve was endemic, and it was her job to fight it. All types of training had benefits and kinesthetic blind spots, Larkam said, so in addition to using Pilates, she also drew the best from yoga, Feldenkrais, and a type of exercise you may not have heard of: the Gyrotonic Expansion System.

Increasingly, Larkam used Gyrotonic with her clients. "Unlike most trainers," she said, "I don't think about muscle strengthening. I think about the components of movements, and the optimal sequence of movements, to reflect what you actually have to do to get from one part of your life to another." The Gyrotonic protocol, developed by Juliu Horvath (that unusual spelling of his first name is correct), incorporates the principles of yoga, dance, Tai Chi, and swimming. It consists of about 150 exercises, performed on four different machines equipped with springs and pulleys. They are all relatives of the Pilates Reformer, with one important difference: In three dimensions, they allow for spiraling, circular, arching movements, which flow together seamlessly in rhythmic repetitions, with corresponding breathing. The joints move through a natural range of motion without jarring or compression. These carefully crafted sequences create balance, efficiency, strength, and flexibility. Gyrotonic is beautiful to watch. With its emphasis on spinal extension (many exercises involve slight back bends), it was an excellent antidote to the *C* curve and the relentless constriction of my desk chair.

Although there was a well-equipped studio very close to my house, Gyrotonic is nowhere near as easy to find as Pilates. That's because it takes two years of study to become a fully accredited trainer, and the pulley-equipped machines, which run as smoothly as skate blades over fresh ice, are costly to acquire. Many of the 10,500 trainers (in fifty-two countries) teach at studios that primarily focus on Pilates; often there's one Gyrotonic bench in a room full of Reformers. Before you sign up for a Gyrotonic class—the cost is approximately the same as a Pilates session—take some time to assess the qualifications of the instructor, seeking one who has a Gyrotonic Expansion System Level 2 Master Trainer certification.

Tai Chi and Qigong

THERE WAS ONE other practice I wanted to explore—but what I thought was one in fact turned out to be two. There are Tai Chi ("tie chee") and Qigong ("chee-gung") classes in most U.S. cities and towns. Classes are priced at about $125 for ten sessions, which makes Tai Chi and Qigong the most economical interventions described in this book. Fit, younger clients often participate, but because of their gentle, joint-sparing nature, Tai Chi and Qigong classes are especially suitable for older back pain patients. Anyone who can walk can do Tai Chi, and even those who are wheelchair-bound can take on Qigong. Beyond improving back pain, the exercises have been shown to enhance cognitive abilities; help prevent osteoporosis and arthritis; and improve balance, gait, and posture. A 2015 study showed further benefits in terms of reducing insomnia and systemic inflammation. Classes are conducted in welcoming groups, both indoors and outdoors. For recovering from back pain, the exercise is helpful, but so is getting together regularly with people who share your interests.

Dwight Etheridge, a fifty-three-year-old IT (information technology) consultant from Anacortes, Washington, spent thirty years running marathon races. "I also worked a lot, and drank a lot of coffee to keep going," he said. "And in 2008, I got to the point where I was still running, five to ten miles a day, but I wasn't doing enough cross-training. My back started to tense up, and I felt really weird in the hips." His primary care doctor told him that sitting at his desk for twelve hours was his problem. An MRI showed no anomaly that could be considered a target for surgery. Physical therapy helped, but only briefly. "I didn't change my lifestyle," Etheridge said. "I couldn't sleep at night. Sometimes it would take me an hour to get out of bed, because my back was just frozen in spasms. Finally, I reached a point where everything just collapsed."

In 2013, he gave up work and stopped running. Overcome with anxiety, he watched his muscle tone disappear. That's when he found his way to Embrace the Moon, a Chinese fitness and martial arts school in Seattle, and into a class that taught an athletic Qigong form called the Hands of the Eighteen Luohan. (A Luohan is a person who has achieved a high level of spiritual cultivation.) Exercises included the poetically named Lifting the Sky, Shooting Arrows, Plucking the Stars, and Carrying the Moon.

After four months of group practice, several times a week, Ether-

idge could run again, and his energy had returned. After three decades of constant employment, he decided not to return to his IT job.
"I kind of retired," he said. "I sold my house and moved up to a resort community." Etheridge gave Tai Chi a try but preferred the slow
and repetitive approach of Qigong. He developed a home practice,
which starts with fifteen to twenty minutes of meditation. "I go to
class about once a week," he said, "but I practice every day, usually
outdoors and barefoot." He's running again, without pain, but he's
not running races; it's just for fun.

Many of the people who attend his Qigong class, he said, are much
older than he is, which he finds encouraging, because it means that
this practice will serve him well for years to come.

Talking to Etheridge made me want to sign up immediately for
Qigong. I'd always found it fascinating. On a reporting trip in my
mid-twenties I woke up in Shanghai and peered out of my hotel room
window as the sun rose over the Bund. I watched as a hundred or so
older people dressed in Mao suit trousers, their jackets buttoned to
their chins, performed Qigong, as synchronized in their movements
as a flock of sandhill cranes. Such spontaneous gatherings would soon
come under close government scrutiny in China, as possible meeting
places for what the government perceived as cults and gangs.

Today, Qigong in China remains strictly regulated: It is part of the
Chinese National Health Plan and is practiced in schools, universities,
and hospitals. In the United States, both Qigong and Tai Chi have
flourished: According to the National Institutes of Health, more than
2.3 million Americans practice either Qigong or Tai Chi.

THE CHINESE PHILOSOPHY of Taoism emphasizes the natural balance, fluidity, and change of all things and the importance of living
in spiritual and physical accord with the patterns of nature. Although
both Tai Chi and Qigong can be classified as "moving meditations,"
there are differences between them.

Tai Chi originated as a martial art in the 1600s, and there are five
popular family styles of the art: Chen (the original), Yang, Wu, Hao,

and Sun. Each has its particular flavor but all are based on correct rules of body mechanics, "qi" or energy flow, steady breathing, and calm mental attitude. Tai Chi emphasizes the relationship between correct posture and relaxation. With practice, the body becomes pliant, elastic, and fluid. Every exercise set emphasizes the whole body and mind working together to move continuously, and over time this increases range of motion, strength, coordination, and balance. The movements are circular and never forced, the muscles are balanced, the joints are never fully extended, and connective tissues are not overly stretched. Tai Chi is practiced with relaxed hips, as though one is sitting back slightly, with great emphasis on the big muscle groups of the legs and glutes. The knees are always kept soft and in correct biomechanical alignment. A Tai Chi routine can be as short as five minutes or can take as long as forty minutes to perform.

Whereas Tai Chi and Qigong share the country, culture, philosophy, and medical framework of China, in practice they are different. Qigong, the study of "qi" or bio-energy, predates Tai Chi by several thousand years. Generally speaking, its choreography is simpler and most people find it easier to learn. There are ten thousand different types of Qigong practiced today, focused on health, strength, and spiritual development. The forms can range from very active to quite still.

To learn how Tai Chi and Qigong worked to alleviate back pain, I spoke with Nicholas Griepentrog, who grew up doing physical labor on a farm, where hauling bales of hay or wielding a pitchfork didn't bother him. He never had back pain until he left the farm and started college, where he attended classes as a full-time student and also held down a forty-hour-a-week job. He thought the back pain would end with graduation, but when he moved to Southern California and took an office job, it got worse.

About three years after he graduated, Griepentrog started taking Tai Chi at the local community college. "It took a while for the aches and pains of getting active again to wear off," he said, but he could tell that it was working. After several years of practice, he started to teach at a local studio. Then a move for a new job increased the length of his commute, making it impossible for him to teach or attend class.

The back pain returned—and stayed with him through a move to Seattle. "I got married, and there was a new job, and increased stress, and another long commute," said Griepentrog, "and all that meant that my back was worse than ever." In January 2014, his wife signed up for a Tai Chi class that was around the corner from her office—and Griepentrog joined her. "There was fairly quick improvement," he said. "As I began to practice more often and go to more classes, my body started to change. I didn't really notice it, but one day I realized that things didn't hurt the way they used to." He felt his low back expanding; it was as if the muscles could relax, giving the discs more room to breathe. His hips opened up.

Today, he doesn't have pain, aside from a dull ache if he sits for too long. He devotes more than six hours a week to practicing and spends about $1,500 a year on workshops with Tai Chi luminaries, but his Tai Chi goes far beyond the *kwoon*, or training hall. "This is a constant thing," he said. "Even when I'm standing in line at the grocery store, I practice. I'm shifting my weight, and I'm doing other little things that make a huge difference."

When he meets people with back pain, he tells them to start Tai Chi. "I say, 'This will fix it,' but most don't want that level of involvement. They want to go to the doctor and have it go away. But that is not how Tai Chi works. You have to do it, from this moment forward. The physiological changes take years. The longer you have been messed up, the longer it takes to unwind it."

Both Tai Chi and Qigong have been studied extensively in clinical trials. The research that really piqued my interest came from the Australian George Institute for Global Health, where, in 2009, investigators addressed the effect of Tai Chi on arthritis and chronic back pain. Their first study, a placebo-controlled trial, demonstrated that Tai Chi improved pain and disability among arthritis sufferers and also showed its potential to improve overall health. The follow-up randomized controlled trial, which incorporated eighteen sessions over ten weeks, focused on the therapeutic effect of Tai Chi on chronic low back pain, addressing postural and body awareness, arm and leg strengthening, balance, and gentle upper back stretching. Participants in the Tai Chi group were encouraged to find ongoing practice in their neighborhoods, while those in the control group pursued their usual health care routine. When investigators examined the outcomes, they found that those in the Tai Chi group reported a 23 percent improvement in back pain and a 32 percent reduction of disability. The control group showed no such improvement.

The George Institute investigators have continued to study Tai Chi, in an effort to discover precisely what factors are in play. Does the improvement stem from the relief of psychological stress? Is it the result of being part of a group? Are the benefits from meditative, regular, diaphragmatic breathing, or perhaps from the movement itself? There is a great deal more research in the hopper, and it will be exciting to see what emerges. In the meantime, because my motor memory is probably not good enough to allow me to acquire a long series of Tai Chi movements, I'm joining the friendly Qigong group that practices nearby and often goes out for refreshments when class is over.

NOT EVERYONE CAN get out to a class. Primary care physician Paul Lam took up Tai Chi when he was still an undergraduate, to counter his painful arthritic condition. He's taught the practice for three decades at the Tai Chi for Health Institute in Sydney, Australia. For $30, Lam sells an eight-hour DVD called *Tai Chi for Arthritis* that breaks down the Sun Tai Chi form into individual movements and teaches them slowly, in a sequential manner.

In April 2013, the U.S. Centers for Disease Control and Prevention recommended Lam's DVD as a way to improve balance and reduce falls in elderly individuals. The Arthritis Foundation seconded that appraisal, endorsing the Sun style as a low-impact exercise that can reduce joint pain. The Arthritis Foundation of Australia and Arthritis Care in the United Kingdom followed suit.

If you can get to a class to learn Tai Chi and Qigong, it's certainly preferable to learning from a DVD. Although it's hard to hurt yourself in either practice, finding the right instructor for this approach is even more of a problem than it is in other disciplines. There are no state or federal licensing requirements, nor is there a standard training protocol. In Chinese martial arts, a student works with a master teacher until the master teacher invites him or her to lead a group.

Part of the beauty of Tai Chi is just how non-Western it is, says Stanwood Chang, an instructor at the Benson-Henry Institute for Mind Body Medicine, part of the Harvard-affiliated Massachusetts General Hospital. "The philosophy is 'relax and be comfortable,'" said Chang in the *Harvard Health Letter.* That made me think of what Moshé Feldenkrais said about his own practice: "Do everything slowly. . . . There should be sufficient time to perceive and organize oneself. No one can learn when hurried and hustled." I remembered how Judith Stern, the Alexander teacher, asked me to allow my "neck to be free so that the head can go forward and up," a directive reminiscent of the Tai Chi instruction "to suspend the spine like a string of pearls from heaven." In fact, the more I studied these postural interventions, the more relationships and cross-pollination I noticed. Each had its disciples, and a million fine distinctions could be drawn among them. But in the end, their goals were the same.

Slowly, over the months and years that I worked with and interviewed experts, my posture and gait changed. Finally, I could "stand up nice and straight," as my late father had so often requested, although at six foot four, he couldn't do it himself. The slump returned only when I was very tired. The changes were obvious, and also expensive: I could no longer squeeze my shoulders into my wardrobe of jackets; larger sizes were required. As I'd first noticed at Michael Salveson's studio, once I lifted my chin, my progressive lenses went wonky. These, too, needed to be replaced. As the curve in my upper back flattened, and my shoulders, rib cage, and back broadened with muscle, my reptilian spine went under cover. The changes were so significant that my own reflection in a shop window surprised me.

As I gained control over my own body, I felt different about myself, as if I had added a new room to my personal architecture. For the first time in my life, I had a strong and confident physical presence. I was no longer a brain on a stick. I still had some distance to go—and I suspected the next stage might take a lifetime—but I was not shackled to a crumpled posture.

I knew things had changed when, at a school event, I found myself talking to an extremely tall and impressively upright gentleman, about ten years my senior. As we chatted, he stood perfectly straight, like a fire tower in a forest of teenagers. Just as I was about to comment on his carriage, he offered me a compliment. "You have lovely posture, you know," he said. "And that's very unusual in a woman of your height."

Conclusion

SIX YEARS LATER

IN NOVEMBER 2009, IN the first year of my research, I attended the North American Spine Society's annual meeting in San Francisco. Roughly four thousand spine medicine professionals filled the vast Moscone Center. In the auditorium, we sat cheek by jowl in rows as long as city blocks, as researchers took the podium to describe new developments, devices, and techniques.

The atmosphere was electric with prospects. In the exhibition hall, easily as large as two football fields, there were richly carpeted kiosks, the broadloom embossed with device manufacturers' logos. Tables overflowed with the usual swag; tote bags, pens, mugs, also branded. Young, attractive sales reps pulled espressos from steaming machines and handed out chocolate truffles, while others hawked jewel-colored titanium hardware displayed on velvet in glittering chrome and glass cases. Here and there, a raw turkey breast, a bloody T-bone, or a nice thick cut of London broil rested on a cutting board, thus prepped to allow surgeons to test the new instruments. In 2009, the spine business was still Wall Street's darling, experiencing predictable double-digit growth annually. Manufacturers continued to make lucrative deals with key opinion leaders. Few had an inkling of the explosive and drastic changes that lay just ahead.

Six years later, in 2015, I headed back to NASS, this time to Mc-Cormick Place in Chicago for the society's thirtieth annual meeting. I anticipated the same mob scene, but when I finally found the west entrance, marked by a few lonely NASS banners flapping in the wind, the meeting lobby was so silent and deserted that I thought for a moment that I'd flown to Chicago on the wrong weekend. I had to ask two guys who were pushing mops for directions.

The atmosphere in the auditorium felt more melancholic than enthusiastic. The go-go years were over. Many seats were vacant. Surgeons were no longer in charge. The 2015 NASS president, physiatrist Heidi Prather (who you met in chapter 2), now vice-chair of the Department of Orthopaedic Surgery at the Washington University School of Medicine, is a doctor of osteopathy, rather than an MD. Outspoken, female, and barely in her fifties, Prather's comments revealed a great deal about the future of the back pain industry.

"We need to look from the outside in and look at how we, as specialists, contribute to the crazy road trip patients are placed on, in hopes of eventually finding what they need," she told the audience. "I refer to it as 'the specialty fishing pond.' The patient is fished out of the pond [by] one specialty. If they don't fit . . . they are thrown back into the pond, only to be fished out again. This costs a lot of time and money and promotes the evolution of a chronic problem. Chronic problems . . . are costly; lost time from home and work activities, increased anxiety and depression [and] increased health-care spending."

Prather advocated a change in the way that back pain patients were treated. Physicians and health care plans had to give up their allegiance to fee-for-service billing, she said, or "we are going to lose the ball game." They had to start sending patients to interdisciplinary rehab programs. "We don't get reimbursed for educating and communicating," she said. "Being paid only by what we do limits us to being mere technicians."

It was essential to remember, Prather said, that "people are complex organisms . . . they don't always fit in a box." While she spoke— her expressive face looming huge on a couple of video screens—I checked out the reactions of the people sitting around me. Younger people—many of them might have been physical therapists or physiatrists, engaged in rehab—nodded in agreement; Prather was their hero. But all around me, spine surgeons sat there slack-jawed, pale, and probably feeling a little ill.

Ken Robinson, the British author, educator, and motivational speaker whose subject is creativity and whose TED talks have been viewed by around three hundred thousand people in 150 countries, followed Prather on the podium.

This was a tough and possibly very depressed audience, but Robinson tried his best to liven things up. The last time he'd spoken at a medical conference, he said brightly, he delivered the keynote to an audience of pathologists and, in return, left with an offer of a free autopsy when the time came. This time, he said naively, clearly unaware of the issues that plagued such operations, he hoped to leave NASS with a coupon good for one spine surgery. The joke landed with a deafening thud.

Medical meetings have complex agendas, published well in advance, so that attendees can allocate their time to their preferred tracks. In 2009, talks focused on surgery and interventional pain management, with sessions on new methods of spinal fusion—BMP-2 was still riding high—disc replacement, vertebroplasty, and kyphoplasty. There were free lunches, cocktail events, and gala dinners. For every twenty events scheduled, there was maybe one that focused on rehabilitation.

In 2015, the "interdisciplinary spine forum" track, barely in existence six years earlier, was much more prominent. Rehab experts had been imported from Europe and Australia for the occasion; the speakers were physical therapists, physiatrists, psychologists, and social workers rather than surgeons, interventional pain physicians, and pain management docs. There was a seminar on central sensitization, another on the role of fear-avoidant behavior, one on how to care for the opioid-addicted patient, both pre- and post-surgery, and another that taught participants how to identify—while patients were still in the acute phase—those who were at risk of developing chronic back pain.

When Robinson completed his talk, a few people wandered out to find coffee, which was not being served. Hardly anyone headed for the exhibition hall, where all the deal-making had taken place in previous years. I walked over, to find a room that was oddly quiet and mostly empty. The extravagant kiosks that I remembered from 2009 were largely absent, as was the massive swag. The sales reps looked bored and they were not as young or as sexy; the huge commissions were largely a thing of the past.

Medtronic's opulent circus tent had always occupied the center ring at NASS. But in 2013, in the wake of the BMP-2 scandal, the device manufacturer had abandoned the dog-and-pony show. That year, Medtronic staffed some desks with employees from its medical affairs group. In 2014 and 2015, even that small presence was gone: Medtronic was completely absent from the meeting. For NASS, this was a body blow. It was as if Ford Motor Company had declined to bring cars to the world's biggest auto show.

Just across the corridor from the exhibition hall, there was a dedicated exercise booth, with inspiring photographs of people on gym balls, performing core-enhancing planks. That seemed promising: Maybe spine surgeons could pick up some tips. But when I stepped inside to see what was going on, I found two massage tables—and not much else. There were no gym balls, free weights, or TRX cables on hand, not even a foam roller. Two young McKenzie practitioners who were standing around said that several surgeons had stopped by, to ask for help managing their own back pain. But in an oversight, the exercise committee had failed to equip the booth with gym equipment or an exercise specialist.

Later that morning, I was paying close attention to the words of several important rehab experts from Australia when a massive hand fell upon my shoulder. I looked up to find Brian Nelson, the Minnesota surgeon who built Physicians Neck and Back Clinic. After walking a half mile or so through McCormick Place's deserted corridors, we finally found a place to get a cup of coffee.

He was retiring, he told me—now that he was in his late sixties, he and his wife wanted to leave ice-cold Minneapolis for the comparatively warmer climes of southern Colorado. He knew that PNBC was in good hands with HealthPartners; he believed that the model he had built would be implemented by health care organizations everywhere. He was not nearly as certain that spine surgeons, working in single-discipline practices, would do what was right, prescribing aggressive exercise regimens before they put their patients on the surgical schedule. They were just not familiar with exercise as a treatment—and he couldn't see how that would change. "That's too bad," Nelson said, "because you can get wonderful outcomes with exercise, and you need to give people that chance—because surgery is where the enormous costs are coming from."

He doubted that health care plans would continue to pay for interventions for which there was little scientific evidence, and where iatrogenic outcomes were common, Nelson said. Lumbar fusion for degenerative disc disease, injections, opioids—these treatments were on their way out, but as long as the insurers' fee-for-service arrangement remained, and reimbursement was forthcoming, spine surgeons would help develop devices, and interventional pain physicians would invent new technologies. Until insurers began paying for intensive exercise and rehab, and refused to pay for other approaches, said Nelson, patients would suffer, costs would soar, and nothing much would change.

TO MY CONSIDERABLE frustration, as I wrote this book, every time I thought I'd put a chapter to bed, the story evolved, in ways that were too significant to ignore. At times, the task seemed Sisyphean: I'd thought I'd never find the perfect moment to stop researching, rewriting, and updating. But if I refused to let the manuscript go, I'd never accomplish my goal of helping readers understand what they were being offered and what it was worth to them. The best approach was to continue my exploration, well into the future, on my website at cathrynjakobsonramin.com. Now that you've come this far, I hope that you'll visit it regularly. It will serve as a valuable adjunct to what you've just read, and also as a way for me to continue to offer my thoughts as they evolve. Please help me by contributing your own thoughts and comments. It's easy to do, and your personal experience—triumphant or bleak—will benefit all of us.

As for my back—well, let's say that most of the time, the truce prevails. I'll have turned sixty by the time you read these pages, and

I can honestly say that I'm stronger and physically much tougher than I was at fifty. And yet, I'm not bulletproof; like all of us, I have some really bad days. The difference is that I know how to embrace exercise and push through the pain, without allowing it to overwhelm me. I know that I can't take to the couch, or the hot tub, or the heating pad, however attractive those options seem. Check with me on the day after a six-hour flight, or a long drive, and I'll be on the floor, struggling to do Stu McGill's Big Three.

By the way, you might like to know that I did get the chance to join my friend Stacey on that long-awaited hiking trip in the Peruvian Andes. We climbed to thirteen thousand feet on the Salkantay Trail, taking the back (hard, slow, highly vertical) way into Machu Picchu. There were times when the air was so thin that I thought I'd never catch my breath or lift my foot to take another step. When we reached Machu Picchu, I was worn out, and ready to inhale deeply at the relatively gentle altitude of eight thousand feet. But my back wasn't a problem—not once. It was no longer holding me hostage.

Acknowledgments

IF I COULD, I would thank each of the six hundred people I interviewed for this book. But just listing them would fill another very long chapter. Suffice it to say that if your name appears anywhere in these pages—as an expert or as a patient—you have made an essential contribution. Still, I can't close without recognizing some of the many individuals who guided me on this long journey.

At the top of that list is the longtime editor of the *Back Letter*, Mark L. Schoene, smart, incredibly well informed, and always patient. There was no question he couldn't answer. Charles Rosen, the Orange County surgeon who fought for transparency in revealing physicians' financial conflicts of interest, made a huge difference in my understanding. Brian Nelson, the Minnesota orthopedic surgeon who built Physicians Neck and Back Clinic, was always ready to talk, often as he drove from one of his clinics to the next. Stuart McGill, the human biomechanist, cleared up many mysteries—and I think of him every day, as I tackle the Big Three. Andrew Kolodny, the founder of Physicians for Responsible Opioid Prescribing, responded to e-mails both day and night, as he walked me through the intricacies of opioid marketing and the neurobiology of addiction. Diana Williams, Vinnie LaSpina, Brian Beaudoin, and James Schwartz have my lifelong allegiance for making me truly strong and training me in the best ways to tackle my physical shortcomings.

When I finish reading any book, I study the acknowledgments for insight into how the author handled what is always a daunting process. Mom and Dad are usually mentioned, as well as the author's friends, the agent, and the editor. But too frequently, the names of the real heroes are absent. In my case, these would be the investigative journalists, often working for news organizations, who laid the groundwork, probing, prying, crunching reams of data, and providing me with the clues I needed to proceed. That's why I want to thank John Fauber, Kristina Fiore, Ellen Gabler, David Armstrong, Barry Meier, Duff Wilson, Reed Abelson, Simon Singh, Maggie Mahar, Gina Kolata, Denise Grady, Jane Brody, Sabrina Tavernise, Mina Kimes, Peter Loftus, Peter Waldman, Peter Whoriskey, Dan Keating, Pia Christensen, Shannon Brownlee, Robin Young, Biloine Young, John Carreyrou, Tom McGinty, Linda Greenhouse, Walter Eisner, Doug J. Swanson, Lou Grieco, Barbara Hansen, Catherine Larkin and David Olmos, Linda Greenhouse, Jim Spencer, Jodie Tillman, Ben Eisler, Greg Noble, Susan Taylor Martin, Rhonda L. Rundle and Scott Hensley, Melissa Davis, Ford Vox, Michael J. Berens, Ken Armstrong, Celine Gounder, Elisabeth Rosenthal, Charles Ornstein, Tracey Weber, Katherine Eban, Lisa Giron and Karen Kaplan, Kirsten Stewart, Yvonne Abraham, Stephanie Smith, Susan Heavey, Milton J. Valencia, Roni Caryn Rabin, John Tozzi, Stephen S. Hall, Peter Eisler, Aaron Glantz, Jason Cherkis, Joshua Davis, Lee Fang, Pippa Wysong, Edward Siedle, Tony Schwartz, the staff of ProPublica, the staff of the Center for Investigative Reporting, Gretchen Reynolds, Shayla Harris, Patti Neighmond, Jerome Groopman, Chris Newmarker, Patricia Sullivan, Steven Koepp, Charles Duhigg, William Broad, Jennifer Wolff Perrine, Pamela Paul, Courtney Rubin, Ellen Barry, Michael Richards, Paul Thatcher, and Liz Szabo. I'd also like to thank Vauhini Vara, the newyorker.com editor who encouraged me to break the story on Zohydro, a powerful opioid that—in the midst of a public health crisis—nonetheless slipped through the FDA's approval process and into the market.

Completing a work of this scope demands a stellar and dedicated team of editorial assistants, researchers, fact-checkers, copy editors, bean counters, and hand-holders. My assistant, Elizabeth Savage, worked meticulously and untiringly, managing to keep up with not only my requests, but also with the needs of her two young children, both of whom were born during the years we spent on this book. My thanks to my untiring and exacting fact-checkers, Rob Liguori at Verificationist and Melissa Chianta, as well as copy editors Lily Casura, Molly Bradley, Gretchen Schrafft, Mandy Erickson, and Natalie Jones, and researchers Deanne Carter, Marissa Barkey, Tracy McIntosh, and Katherine Takeshita. All worked ceaselessly to keep the facts accurate, the files organized, and the project moving forward. Thanks to Holly Alexander at TopSpin and Jonathan Manierre at Turkois Design for digital services, to Sonja Holmberg for her painstakingly detailed anatomical renderings for the title page, and to Jessica Jones for producing the videos on my website, in which I get myself in and out of spine-hostile situations.

I want to thank my remarkable agent and dear friend, Inkwell Management's Michael Carlisle, whose encouragement, warmth, and passion for this project never faltered over eight years, and also his assistant Mike Mungiello, who graciously handled a million details. And I have the utmost affection and respect for my editor, HarperCollins's Gail Winston, whose talent, kinship, and unerring judgment have truly spoiled me for all others. Her assistant editor, Sofia Groopman, is also a rare treasure, on top of her game and bound for a great future in publishing.

Thanks to my professional colleagues for their continual support and kindness: Katy Butler, Jason Roberts, Jane Isay, Michelle Slatalla, Josh Quittner, Elizabeth Sanger, Jeffrey Trachtenberg, and Jillian Keenan. Then there are the friends, relatives, and associates who held my hand as I inched my way through this project: my siblings, of course, Tom and Amy Jakobson, Peter and Lisa Jakobson, and Holly and Neil Alexander; my aunt Helen Mintz and all the Mintz and Greenwald cousins, Joel and Marikay Raphaelson, Nancy and David Lowenherz, Michele and Michael Lash, Janet Sher and Jim Wilson, Michele Berdy, Robin Sherman, Alice and Ira Steinman, Nicki and Alon Adani, Ted Dreisinger, Catherine Joei, Anthony Alofsin, Jennifer Fearon, Daniela Castillo, Bonnie Sudler, Hans Li and Jennifer

Kouvant, Nancy Abraham, Sid and Gloria Ramin, Margaret Klaw, Meg and Sam Flax, Alan Metcalfe, Stacey Spector, Ira Brind, Deborah Aal Stoff, and Mei-Ling Fong. Thanks, especially, to Howard Schatz and Beverly Ornstein.

And finally, my everlasting appreciation and love to Ron Ramin, my husband of nearly three decades; and to our two sons, Avery and Oliver, who managed to grow up to be fabulous men, in spite of having a mother who was always on a tight deadline. And my heartiest thanks to our dog, Dasch, who went to work with me, but never sat for long. Every two hours, like clockwork, he insisted that I get up and take us for a walk, thereby saving my back.

A final note: I have made every effort to provide accurate and timely information. If, as the reader, you find that you have something to add, please e-mail me at crookedthebackbook@gmail.com. I will carefully assess your recommendations and make appropriate changes in subsequent editions.

Notes

Here, you'll find intriguing material that adds context and depth to the information in the book.

More detailed source endnotes are posted on my website, at www .cathrynjakobsonramin.com, to give researchers and other interested individuals the opportunity to examine specific topics and studies in much greater depth. Nearly all are hyperlinked, for easy access.

Introduction: A Terrible Affliction

2 **lumbar spinal fusion:** Spinal fusion is surgery to permanently join two or more vertebrae, eliminating any movement between them by creating a single, solid bone.

Chapter 1: Back Pain Nation

7 **my primary care doctor:** Primary care doctors are either general practitioners or internists; some refer to themselves as family practitioners, which means that they also see children.

8 **dose of radiation:** In terms of radiation, one spine or neck X-ray equals seventeen lung X-rays.

8 **worth their weight in gold:** A good source for a PM&R (physical medicine and rehabilitation) doctor is the American Academy of Physical Medicine and Rehabilitation: https://members.aapmr.org/AAPMR/AAPMR_FINDER .aspx.

9 **"shared decision-making":** One reason that shared decision-making often backfires is that the medical literature is itself biased. Notes Fiona Godlee,

editor in chief of the *British Medical Journal*, studies with positive outcomes are much more likely to be published, while studies showing negative results often are missing from the medical literature. Those that aren't missing often have flawed methodology, observes Godlee. So when patients use decision aids and engage in shared decision-making with their physicians, they are often exposed to a biased view of the evidence. See Fiona Godlee, "Optimism and Consent to Treatment," *British Medical Journal* 349 (2014): g6118, http://dx.doi.org/10.1136/bmj.g6118; and "Overconfidence Continues to Plague Spine Care—Are There Any Innovative Ways of Countering This Risky Bias?" *Back Letter* 31, no. 4 (2016): 37–43, doi: 10.1097/01.BACK.0000482344.95364.61.

9 **two cervical and two lumbar X-rays:** The human spinal column is made up of thirty-three bones—seven vertebrae in the neck, or cervical region; twelve in the upper back, or thoracic region; five in the low back, or lumbar region; five in the sacrum; and four in the coccyx. The vertebral bodies are built like little barrels, with round walls made of relatively stiff cortical bone. The tops and bottoms of the barrels are made of a more deformable cartilage—the end plates—which are porous, to allow the transport of oxygen and glucose. The insides of the barrels are filled with springy, cancellous bone. This unique architecture allows the vertebrae to bear high compressive loads.

9 **a disc herniation**—defined as a bulging or extrusion of the nucleus pulposus inside the disc—is not typically a sudden event. It is the result of repeated cycles of flexion that allow the thick collagen layers of the annulus to slowly delaminate, while the material of the nucleus pulposus gathers slowly between those layers.

11 **the 90/10 hypothesis:** The source of the 90/10 hypothesis was not a scientific investigation; rather, it was drawn from the rheumatologist Allan St. J. Dixon's anecdote-filled 1973 talk at the annual meeting of the British Association for Rheumatology and Rehabilitation. Dixon observed that in his clinical experience, 44 percent of patients who sought advice about their back pain from family doctors were better in one week, and 86 percent were better in a month. No one asked to see his records. But two years later, in 1975, an eminent Swedish spine specialist, Alf Nachemson, mentioned the hypothesis in a speech, instantly converting Dixon's unsubstantiated experience into fact. See Allan St. J. Dixon, "Progress and Problems in Back Pain Research," *Rheumatology and Rehabilitation* 12, no. 4 (1973): 165–75; and Alf Nachemson, "The Lumbar Spine: An Orthopaedic Challenge," *Spine* 1, no. 1 (1976): 59–71.

11 **Primary Care Musculoskeletal Research Centre:** The center, now called the Arthritis Research UK Primary Care Centre, is located within the Research Institute of Primary Care and Health Sciences at Keele University. Peter Croft stepped down as director of both the center and the institute in 2011 but continues to work there as a professor of primary care epidemiology.

14 **workers' compensation underwriters:** Ever-escalating costs, coupled with the prospect of long-term payouts to workers for years to come, mean that workers' compensation underwriters can raise a company's premiums

every year, while accumulating a large reserve of cash that the insurer may invest. In what is referred to as a "perverse incentive," the more workers' compensation underwriters spend on patient treatment, the greater their potential profits.

15 a world that is increasingly virtual and screen-based: Such rampant deconditioning isn't anything new. In the mid-1950s, back pain expert and physiatrist Hans Kraus launched a study that showed, most controversially, that American children were much less fit than European children. Dwight Eisenhower acknowledged this political hot potato when he was in office but took no consequential action. Subsequently, he lobbed the fitness issue to president-elect John F. Kennedy, who was astounded to learn that one out of every two young Americans drafted by the military he relied on to keep Americans safe in the shadow of the Cold War had been "rejected by Selective Service as mentally, morally or physically unfit."

With that as his inspiration, JFK (who, as we will see later, suffered from chronic back pain, but not because he was injured on a PT boat, as most people think) wrote an article for *Sports Illustrated* called "The Soft American." In that forum, he took the nation to task. "Our struggles against aggressors throughout our history have been won on the playgrounds and corner lots and fields of America," he wrote. "Thus, in a very real and immediate sense, our growing softness, our increasing lack of physical fitness, is a menace to our security." In acknowledgment, the *New York Times* ran an article headlined, "President-Elect in Magazine Article Says 'Flabbiness' Menaces U.S. Security."

As president, JFK established a White House Committee on Health and Fitness and an annual Youth Fitness Conference. Physical fitness became a major theme in education. Meredith Wilson, creator of the Broadway musical *The Music Man*, composed a song officially called "The Youth Fitness Song," but most people renamed it the "Chicken Fat Song." The refrain, as those of us of a certain age will recall, was "Go, you chicken fat, go." Robert Preston, the star of *The Music Man*, recorded a six-minute version to be played while schoolchildren performed the accompanying workout. But the movement toward childhood fitness was not sustained.

See John F. Kennedy, "The Soft American," *Sports Illustrated,* December 26, 1960, http://armymedicine.mil/Documents/Panel%20C%20-%201960 -Kennedy-Soft-American.pdf; "Kennedy to Push Fitness Program," *New York Times,* December 21, 1960, 21; Al Baker, "Despite Obesity Concerns, Gym Classes Are Cut," *New York Times,* July 10, 2012, http://www.nytimes .com/2012/07/11/education/even-as-schools-battle-obesity-physical-educa tion-is-sidelined.html?pagewanted=all&_r=0; and Centers for Disease Control and Prevention, "Youth Risk Behavior Surveillance—United States, 2011," *Morbidity and Mortality Weekly Report* 61, no. 4 (2012): 37, http://www.cdc.gov/ mmwr/pdf/ss/ss6104.pdf.

17 persistent pain: Researcher Daniel Clauw observes that pain can fall into three different "buckets": (1) nociceptive pain, where pain stems from damage or injury to local tissues in the periphery (i.e., the spine, knee, hip, ankle, elbow, wrist, etc.); (2) peripheral neuropathic pain, where pain originates from injury or damage to nerves in the periphery of the body; and (3) centralized pain, where some type of disturbance in the central nervous system leads to the amplification or augmentation of that pain. See Daniel Clauw, "Are Opioids Preferentially Effective in Treating Different Underlying Mechanisms of Chronic Pain?" NIH Pathways to Prevention Workshop: The Role of Opioids in the Treatment of Chronic Pain, Bethesda, Maryland, September 29–30, 2014.

Chapter 2: A Tale of Two Tables

19 "vertebral subluxations": Chiropractors define subluxation as a health concern that manifests itself in the skeletal joints and through complex physiological relations. It affects the nervous system and may lead to reduced function, disability, or illness.

21 psychiatrist Stephen Barrett: There are some groups whose members think that Barrett, and the organization he runs, Quackbusters, is part of a scam—"an organized assault by a well-funded group, against companies, and practitioners, offering alternatives to the drugs/surgery paradigm." Barrett was the cofounder of the National Council Against Health Fraud, which some say was created to deflect attention from health scares associated with toxic chemicals, redirecting federal scrutiny to quackery in alternative medicine, including homeopathy, chiropractic, and naturopathy. See Tim Bolen, "Who Are These So-Called 'Quackbusters'?" accessed September 9, 2015, http://www.health-report.co.uk/quack_busters_scam_revealed.htm.

24 the group's website: www.chiropracticstroke.com is a website with useful information on this topic.

26 In response, Chicago chiropractor Chester Wilk: Wilk's lawsuit referenced (among many other offenses) the organization's effort to sully chiropractic's reputation by co-opting television and screenwriters to include negative portrayals in their work, and influencing the advice doled out by syndicated newspaper columnist Ann Landers.

29 "practice-building": That's the subject of a textbook by James W. Parker, who emphasized that the chiropractor's main task was not to cure the patient but to sign him up for as many sessions as his pocketbook will tolerate. "One adjustment for each year of age," Parker recommends, "is a rough thumbnail guide of what people will willingly accept and pay for." In the tellingly titled 1995 book, *Chiropractic: The Victim's Perspective*, George Magner mentions that mid-twentieth-century "practice-building consultants" promised to teach chiropractors to build million-dollar practices. They focused on how to achieve what they called "the optimum gettable" with every patient. See James W. Parker, *Textbook of Office Procedure and Practice Building for the Chiropractic Profession*, 4th edition (Fort Worth, TX: Parker Chiropractic Research Foundation,

1975); Stephen Barrett, "Some Notes on James W. Parker, D.C.," *Chirobase*, January 16, 2012, http://www.chirobase.org/12Hx/parker.html; and George Magner, *Chiropractic: The Victim's Perspective* (Amherst, NY: Prometheus Books, 1995).

30 **no shortage of chiropractors:** Preston Long, a chiropractor who regularly provides legal testimony about chiropractic fraud in personal injury cases, and who wrote *Chiropractic Abuse: An Insider's Lament*, said that the market is effectively glutted with chiropractors who have hundreds of thousands of dollars in school loans to pay off and cannot make a living. Long, who resides in Arizona, cited a recent chiropractic newsletter that reported that insurance company denials in his state have resulted in "hundreds of Arizona chiropractors closing their doors and filing for bankruptcy." Some practitioners, he indicated, were selling their equipment from the trunks of their cars. See Stephen Barrett, "Chiropractic Income Has Been Dropping Steadily," *Chirobase*, March 20, 2014, http://www.chirobase.org/02Research/income.html; and Preston H. Long, *Chiropractic Abuse: An Insider's Lament* (New York: American Council on Science and Health, 2013).

31 **International Society of Clinical Rehab Specialists:** To find a rehabilitation specialist through the International Society of Clinical Rehab Specialists, go to http://www.rehab2performance.com/find-a-provider/.

31 **author of two insightful books and two DVDs:** See http://www.amazon.com/Craig-Liebenson/e/B005711JLQ.

31 **"E-meter":** The Church of Scientology, taking a page from chiropractic treatment, used E-meters extensively until the U.S. FDA seized more than a hundred of them in 1963. The device is still used today in the "auditing" process, to "locate areas of spiritual distress or travail," but FDA regulations preclude Scientologists from suggesting that E-meters can treat physical or mental illness. See Simon Singh and Edzard Ernst, *Trick or Treatment: The Undeniable Facts About Alternative Medicine* (New York: W. W. Norton, 2008), 163–64; Hugh B. Urban, *The Church of Scientology: A History of a New Religion* (Princeton, NJ: Princeton University Press, 2013), 49; and "What Is the E-Meter and How Does It Work?" Scientology website, accessed September 9, 2015, http://www.scientology.org/faq/scientology-and-dianetics-auditing/what-is-the-emeter-and-how-does-it-work.html.

31 **Hippocratic bench:** The Hippocratic bench employed traction and cranks to stretch the spaces between the vertebrae. The disc decompression machine works in much the same way.

32 **CPT code:** Current Procedural Technology code

35 **he started the McKenzie Institute:** Robin McKenzie's legacy lives on—and a person who is suddenly besieged with leg pain resulting from a herniated disc would do well to find a certified MDT (medical diagnosis and therapy) practitioner in the clinic directory: http://www.mckenziemdt.org/clinics.cfm?section=int#ClinicDirectory.

35 **locate a doctorate-level PT (DPT):** The American Physical Therapy

Association's website, Move Forward (http://www.moveforwardpt.com), has a search function that can help locate board-certified PTs in various specialties. After selecting your location, check the box labeled "musculoskeletal." Then look for therapists in private practice who have the abbreviation OCS (orthopedic clinical specialist) or SCS (Sports Certified Specialist) after their names—or preferably both. Also, the American Academy of Orthopaedic and Manual Physical Therapists has a "find a fellow" search function that will provide you with contact information throughout the United States and Canada for active exercise-focused, hands-on physical therapists—the opposite of the shake 'n' bake, bells-and-blinkers breed. Finally, you can check out the "faculty" tab on the Evidence in Motion website (http://www.evidenceinmotion .com/who-we-are/faculty/), where you will find the résumés of practitioners who are some of the best in the business.

36 **eighteen states allow unlimited direct access:** Unlimited direct access is available in Alaska, Arizona, Colorado, Hawaii, Idaho, Iowa, Kentucky, Maryland, Massachusetts, Montana, Nebraska, Nevada, North Dakota, Oregon, South Dakota, Utah, Vermont, and West Virginia. See "Levels of Patient Access to Physical Therapist Services in the States," American Physical Therapy Association, March 2016, http://www.apta.org/uploadedFiles/APTAorg/ Advocacy/State/Issues/Direct_Access/DirectAccessbyState.pdf.

36 **seven states insist:** Alabama, Illinois, Louisiana, Mississippi, Missouri, Texas, and Wyoming have the most restrictive rules.

36 **barely made inroads into the rest of the world:** There are very few chiropractors in Europe, but they do exist in South Africa and Australia.

36 **a Scandinavian and central European export:** What we know today as "physical therapy" is based on the work of Per Henrik Ling, who in the early 1800s founded the Royal Central Institute of Gymnastics, which focused on active therapeutic exercise for those who were ill or injured. Later, in Czechoslovakia, the Prague School of Rehabilitation became the main center of physiotherapy, and the training grounds of internationally important practitioners such as Václav Vojta, Vladimir Janda, and Karel Lewit. The Prague School's approach, which emphasizes the neurological aspects of motor control, spread far beyond its center at Motol University Hospital, on the outskirts of the city, to influence how physical therapy is performed around the world.

38 **an episode of television's *The Dr. Oz Show*:** Presented prior to Mehmet Oz's 2014 grilling by the congressional Subcommittee on Consumer Protection, Product Safety, Insurance, and Data Security. See Jen Christensen and Jacque Wilson, "Congressional Hearing Investigates Dr. Oz 'Miracle' Weight Loss Claims," *CNN*, June 19, 2014, http://www.cnn.com/2014/06/17/health/ senate-grills-dr-oz/.

38 **"the benefits of active care":** In 2014, as part of the American Board of Internal Medicine Foundation's Choosing Wisely campaign, the American Physical Therapy Association (APTA) published a "what not to do" list. Heat therapy, electrical stimulation, ultrasound, and other "passive physical agents"

almost never help, according to the list. Instead, the primary goal of physical therapy is to get a patient to adopt an exercise program that will increase strength and mobility. See "Physical Therapy: Five Treatments You Probably Don't Need," Choosing Wisely, http://www.choosingwisely.org/patient-resources/physical-therapy/.

40 **proprioception:** Proprioception is the sense of where your body is in space, determined by a feedback cycle between the brain and receptors in muscles, joints, and ligaments.

41 **my real problem was self-inflicted:** In early 2009, a team of researchers at UC San Diego published the results of a study that showed that most spine procedures disrupt the multifidi, destabilizing the spine, resulting in discomfort that may be more extreme than the pain that initially led to the procedure. See Samuel R. Ward et al., "Architectural Analysis and Intraoperative Measurements Demonstrate the Unique Design of the Multifidus Muscle for Lumbar Spine Stability," *Journal of Bone and Joint Surgery* 91, no. 1 (2009): 176–85, http://dx.doi.org/10.2106/JBJS.G.01311.

Chapter 3: Hazardous Images

45 **bone spurs:** Osteophytes are tiny bone spurs that form on the facet joints and in the foramina, the small hole through which nerve roots exit the spine. When a bone spur is impinging on a nerve in the lumbar spine, it can cause symptoms: radiating pain, weakness, tingling, or numbness in the legs and feet. See "Lumbar Osteophytes (Bone Spurs) Video," *Spine-Health*, http://www.spine-health.com/video/lumbar-osteophytes-bone-spurs-video.

46 **evidence of spinal stenosis:** In a younger spine, the ligaments exert a contracting force on the vertebral arches, keeping them together and aligned. Normal pressure inside the disc is required to maintain that ligament tension. When the discs begin to flatten, the ligaments become lax and the spine sacrifices stability. The skeleton constantly seeks to create as much stability as possible. Its response to increased pressure on facet joints and vertebral end plates is to create more bone. Osteophytes develop on all bony structures, disrupting the fit of the facet joints and forming obstructions that impede nerves, both inside the spinal canal and in the neural foramina, through which the nerves exit. In addition, one of the most critical ligaments, the yellow ligamentum flavum, begins to droop into the spinal canal, impinging on spinal nerves. Spinal stenosis typically involves leg pain, referred to as neurogenic claudication, characterized by a weak, tired feeling across the buttocks and down the thighs with pain, numbness, and cramping in the legs. The pain in the legs is far more intense when the patient is walking or standing, and usually stops when he or she sits down or bends forward.

47 **evil humor:** The four humors of Hippocratic medicine are black bile, yellow bile, phlegm, and blood. Phlegm—with a different meaning than it has today—was thought to cause rheumatism, as well as tumors and anemia.

47 in Shakespeare's plays: The Bard's protagonists and their enemies suffered alike: "Thou cold sciatica," he wrote in *Timon of Athens*, "cripple our senators, that their limbs may halt as lamely as their manners." In *Measure for Measure*, his characters greet one another with inquiries about the state of their suffering: "How now! Which of your hips has the most profound sciatica?" and proceed to discuss the diseases they have "purchased" from their favorite prostitute, the gloriously named Mistress Overdone.

48 Unlike CT (computerized tomography) scans and X-rays: The average radiation exposure from lumbar radiography—X-rays of the low back—is seventy-five times higher than it is for chest X-rays. Before you rush out to get one, you should know that the amount of gonadal radiation (radiation of the pelvic organs) from obtaining a single plain X-ray of the lumbar spine—which provides two views—is equivalent to being exposed to a daily chest X-ray for several years. See Erin Futrell, "Do I Need an MRI/X-Ray/CT Scan?" *Joint Ventures' Blog*, July 2, 2012, http://www.jointventurespt.com/blog/Do_I_Need_an_MRIX-RayCT_Scan/.

Meanwhile, a CT scanner can emit one hundred to five hundred times as much ionizing radiation as a single X-ray. According to the National Cancer Institute, over the next three decades, the seventy-two million CT scans performed in 2007 in the United States alone will translate into twenty-nine thousand cases of cancer, some twelve hundred of which will be attributable to CT scans of the lumbar spine. It is very rare for a patient to be told of this risk, or to learn that there is a huge variation in radiation doses from CT scans, depending on the age and quality of the machine. See Jane E. Brody, "Medical Radiation Soars, with Risks Often Overlooked," *New York Times*, August 20, 2012, http://well.blogs.nytimes.com/2012/08/20/medical-radiation-soars-with-risks-often-overlooked/; and "CT Scanning = 15,000 Deaths?" *Back Letter* 25, no. 2 (2010): 19, doi: 10.1097/01.BACK.0000368163.33395.7d.

48 Physicians Neck and Back Center: At the time of my interview with Brian Nelson, the center was called "Physicians Neck and Back Clinic."

49 the Agency for Health Care Policy and Research: The name has since been changed to Agency for Healthcare Research and Quality, and the agency is now one of the branches of the U.S. Department of Health and Human Services.

50 Thousands of new diagnostic radiologists: In his 2007 book, *How Doctors Think*, Jerome Groopman describes the findings of Ehsan Samei of the Advanced Imaging Laboratories at Duke University Medical Center, who noted, "The average diagnostic error in interpreting medical images is in the 20 percent to 30 percent range. These errors, being of either the false-negative or false-positive type, have significant impact on patient care." There is no question that some radiologists are far more competent than others at reading scans. Groopman cites Dr. E. James Potchen at Michigan State University, who looked at more than one hundred radiologists' performances in reading chest X-rays. "Remarkably," writes Groopman, "60 percent of the radiologists failed to identify the missing clavicle." They disagreed among themselves more than 20 percent of the time about whether the film was normal, and sometimes had different opinions when shown the same film twice at different times of day. What was surprising was the level of confidence that the radiologists expressed—they were very confident that they were right, even when they were wrong. See Jerome Groopman, *How Doctors Think* (New York: Houghton Mifflin, 2007), 179, 181.

52 **"Black" discs:** Black discs are not truly black in situ but look that way on scans because they lack sufficient hydrogen protons to generate a signal.

Chapter 4: Needle Jockeys

56 **In the United States more than ten million:** Between 1994 and 2001, the number of epidural steroid injections administered each year increased by 270 percent, and fees collected for those injections rose by 629 percent. Needle-based procedures, despite their shortcomings, became part of the clinical armamentarium. See Janna Friedly, Leighton Chan, and Richard Deyo, "Increases in Lumbosacral Injections in the Medicare Population: 1994 to 2001," *Spine* 32, no. 16 (2007): 1754–60, doi: 10.1097/BRS.0b013e3180b9f96e.

58 **There are two dominant techniques:** In an interlaminar injection, the steroid is delivered over a wide area. Similarly, the caudal approach uses the sacral hiatus (a small bony opening just above the tailbone) to allow for needle placement into the very bottom of the epidural space, and thus for the steroid to spread over several spinal segments and cover both sides of the spinal canal.

With a transforaminal ESI (epidural steroid injection), the needle is positioned along the nerve at the point where it exits the spine, and medication is injected into the "nerve sleeve." From there, the medication moves up the sleeve to the epidural space. This method gives a more concentrated delivery of steroid to a single nerve.

59 **In "blind" injections:** Blind injections are administered mostly in rural or disadvantaged regions where guidance under fluoroscopy is not available.

59 **fluoroscopic guidance:** When the procedure is done with fluoroscopic guidance, the physician employs an X-ray imaging technique, known as fluoroscopy, to guide the placement of the needle.

59 **"blood patch":** A blood patch is a surgical procedure that uses autologous blood in order to close a puncture in the dura mater of the spinal cord. The clotting factors in the blood close the hole.

59 **when the needle actually punctures the dura mater:** Other outcomes include paraplegia, quadriplegia, spinal cord infarction, and stroke. Potential causes of these adverse events include technique-related problems such as intrathecal injection, epidural hematoma, direct spinal cord injury, and embolic infarction after inadvertent intra-arterial injection. See "FDA on Epidural Injections," *BackLetter* 30, no. 12 (2015): 133–42, doi: 10.1097/01.BACK.0000475388.37495.3e.

60 vials were contaminated with a deadly fungal mold: When the FDA sent its inspectors to NECC's premises, they found black fungus floating in vials of methylprednisolone acetate, "thick residue" on areas used to prepare sterile products, and insect infestation within just a few feet of areas where sterile drugs were produced, not to mention a bird flying around inside the building. In the putatively sterile prep room, counters were stained, pools of standing water led to a leaky boiler, and the entrance mat was brown and soiled. According to *Newsweek*, Glenn A. Chin, who supervised production at NECC, had elected to shortcut proper sterilization procedures. As *Newsweek* described it, instead of heating the drugs with 121-degree high-pressure saturated steam in an autoclave for a minimum of twenty minutes, he may have told his subordinates to worry less about sterilization and more about raising production to meet demand. He may have also ordered them to falsify paperwork documenting the facility's sanitation procedures. See Form FDA 483, inspection reports of New England Compounding Center and Ameridose, LLC, http://www.fda.gov/downloads/AboutFDA/CentersOffices/%20Officeof GlobalRegulatoryOperationsandPolicy/ORA/ORAElectronicReadingRoom/ UCM325980.pdf and http://www.fda.gov/downloads/AboutFDA/CentersOf fices/OfficeofGlobalRegulatoryOperationsandPolicy/ORA/ORAElectronic ReadingRoom/UCM327729.pdf; and Kurt Eichenwald, "Killer Pharmacy: Inside a Medical Mass Murder Case," *Newsweek*, April 16, 2015, http://www .newsweek.com/2015/04/24/inside-one-most-murderous-corporate-crimes-us -history-322665.html.

61 In December 2012, NECC filed for bankruptcy: By the summer of 2015, thirty-four hundred claims had been filed in the compounder's bankruptcy proceedings. The *Boston Globe* reported that roughly one thousand of those claims were those of patients who were seriously injured, or made by relatives of those who died. In an effort to establish a victim compensation fund of $210 million, plaintiffs' lawyers subpoenaed eighty health care providers who could be held liable for having given the injections, as well as some NECC vendors. Other sterile bulk drug compounders came under increased FDA scrutiny. See Kay Lazar and Jack Newsham, "Tainted Drugs Settlement Fund Grows to $210 Million," *Boston Globe*, March 6, 2015, http://www.bostonglobe.com/ business/2015/03/06/tainted-drugs-settlement-fund-grows-million/9YyHqgi Aq6jw09bl3pbkcK/story.html.

61 The wheels of justice turned slowly: Daily, there were reports of other large sterile compounders found to be operating under profoundly unsterile conditions. But as multiple bills entered the legislature and foundered there, it became clear that Congress did not intend to alter the way that compounding pharmacies are regulated, or legislate the FDA's increased surveillance. Playing catch-up, in November 2013 President Obama signed the Drug Quality and Security Act, legislation that offers bulk compounding manufacturers the opportunity to register voluntarily with the FDA as "outsourcing facilities," making them subject to the same requirements that are imposed on conventional manufacturers, including reporting of adverse events. For compounders, such registration is costly: It means paying user fees for regular FDA inspections, just as pharmaceutical companies do. The expectation is that market pressures will force bulk compounders to register if they wish to do business with hospitals, which are their major clients, but it is by no means certain that this will occur. See Sabrina Tavernise, "Bill on Drug Compounding Clears Congress a Year After a Meningitis Outbreak," *New York Times*, November 18, 2013, http://www.nytimes.com/2013/11/19/us/bill-on-regulating-drug-compounding-clears-senate.html.

65 **glucocorticoids could make her bones fragile:** Even with doses equivalent to 2.5 to 7.5 milligrams a day, there is an increased risk of vertebral and hip fractures. See T. P. Van Staa et al., "Use of Oral Corticosteroids and Risk of Fractures," *Journal of Bone and Mineral Research* 15, no. 6 (2000): 993–1000, doi: 10.1359/jbmr.2000.15.6.993.

67 **Synthes's chief executive officer, Hansjörg Wyss:** Wyss was also the company's major shareholder and chairman of the board.

68 **four of Synthes's top executives:** Michael D. Huggins, who was chief operating officer; Thomas B. Higgins, president of the Synthes spine division; Richard E. Bohner, who was vice president of operations; and John J. Walsh, who had been director of regulatory clinical affairs.

69 **offered significant benefits:** In 2014, Jensen cowrote a position paper stating that vertebroplasty was safe, and that it could prevent patients who would otherwise be confined for several weeks to bedrest from losing significant bone density and muscle strength, as well as from developing cardiovascular problems, http://www.jvir.org/article/S1051–0443(13)01487–5/pdf.

71 **False Claims Act:** When a company that develops medical products markets a product off-label, that company is making a "false claim" for its efficacy. Since most medical products companies are government contractors—their products are used in procedures involving Medicare and Medicaid patients—off-label marketing defrauds the federal government, which subsidizes those entities. See "Looming Legal Challenges," *Back Letter* 29, no. 8 (2014): 85–95, doi: 10.1097/01.BACK.0000453375.66539.ad.

Chapter 5: The Gold Standard

73 **recommending lumbar spinal fusion surgery:** Lumbar fusion surgeries can be performed in a number of different ways. A procedure in which the surgeon accesses the spine through an incision in the back is called a posterior fusion, as opposed to accessing the spine through an abdominal incision, which is called an anterior fusion. When the spine is accessed through an incision in the psoas muscle—which is located at the side of the lumbar region and extends into the pelvis—it is called an XLIF, or extreme lateral interbody fusion. When a surgeon approaches through both the abdomen and the back, in two separate incisions, it's called a 360-degree fusion.

76 **most European and UK surgeons:** In the European Union, Germany leads the way in spinal fusion surgery, with about 6 percent of the global market. See GlobalData MediPoint, *Spinal Fusion: Global Analysis and Market Forecast*, June 2014, http://www.marketresearch.com/product/sample-8230547 .pdf.

77 **Ghanayem's surgical fellow:** The term "fellow" refers to a physician who, after residency, receives additional training in a specialized field such as spine surgery.

79 **Because in heavy smokers:** The rate of nonunion among smokers is about 40 percent; among nonsmokers, it's about 8 percent. See C. W. Brown, T. J. Orme, and H. D. Richardson, "The Rate of Pseudarthrosis (Surgical Nonunion) in Patients Who Are Smokers and Patients Who Are Nonsmokers: A Comparison Study," *Spine* 11, no. 9 (1986): 942–43.

Nicotine interferes with the flow of nutrients and oxygen-rich blood to the discs; it also triples or quadruples the speed of disc degeneration while reducing calcium absorption, which helps build the new bone essential to forming a solid fusion. In smokers, incisions heal more slowly and are more prone to infection because nicotine reduces the oxygen available to the healing wound, impairing collagen production. In one investigation, 90 percent of the postoperative infections observed in the study group had occurred in patients who smoked. See "Does Your Back Hurt? Then Put Down That Butt!" North American Spine Society, accessed October 2, 2015, http://www.knowyourback.org/Pages/SpineInTheNews/FeatureArticles/BackHurtPutDownthatButt.aspx.

A Northwestern University study published in October 2014 in the journal *Human Brain Mapping* found that smokers are three times more likely than nonsmokers to develop chronic back pain. "Smoking affects the brain," said Bogdan Petre, lead author of the study and a technical scientist at Northwestern University Feinberg School of Medicine. "We found that it affects the way the brain responds to back pain and seems to make individuals less resilient to an episode of pain." Over the course of a year, 160 adults with new cases of back pain were given five different MRI brain scans and were asked to rate the intensity of their back pain and complete a questionnaire on their smoking status and other health issues. Thirty-five healthy control participants and thirty-two participants with chronic back pain were also followed in the study. Scientists looked at activity in the nucleus accumbens and medial prefrontal cortex to see how smoking increased or decreased communication between these areas. This circuit, said Petre, was "very strong and active in smokers," but there was a dramatic decline in activity when the patients quit smoking during the study. Their experience of chronic pain lessened. See Bogdan Petre et al., "Smoking Increases Risk of Pain Chronification Through Shared Corticostriatal Circuitry," *Human Brain Mapping* 36, no. 2 (2015): 683–94, doi: 10.1002/hbm.22656; and Erin Spain, Northwestern University, "Smoking Is a Pain in the Back," news release, November 3, 2014, http://www.northwestern .edu/newscenter/stories/2014/11/smoking-is-a-pain-in-the-back.html.

79 **he was also obese:** Although the presumption is that after spine surgery an obese patient will be more active, exercise vigorously, and therefore
lose weight, this is not generally how it works. In a study from orthopedic
surgeon Ryan M. Garcia, patients in the study—despite post-surgical improvement in spinal stenosis symptoms and walking ability—had gained
weight, on average, two to four years after surgery. See "Does Spine Surgery Promote Weight Loss?" *Back Letter* 23, no.7 (2008): 75, doi: 10.1097/01
.BACK.0000327744.08065.11.

79 **dependent on painkillers:** A study published in the *Journal of Bone and
Joint Surgery* in 2014 directly linked opioid use prior to spine surgery to less
improvement and higher levels of dissatisfaction following spine surgery. The
median preoperative dose was a conservative 8.75 milligrams of morphine,
which is equal to 6 milligrams of oxycodone or approximately 2 milligrams
of methadone. Patients taking double that amount had significantly worse
mental and physical health and disability scores. "We have demonstrated that
increasing amounts of preoperative opioid consumption may have a harmful
effect on patient reported outcomes in those undergoing spinal surgery," said
lead study author Clinton J. Devin, an orthopedic surgeon at the Vanderbilt
Spine Center. See Dennis Lee et al., "Preoperative Opioid Use as a Predictor
of Adverse Postoperative Self-Reported Outcomes in Patients Undergoing
Spine Surgery," *Journal of Bone and Joint Surgery* 96, no. 11 (2014): e89, http://dx
.doi.org/10.2106/JBJS.M.00865; Opioid Dose Calculator, version 1.91, Agency
Medical Directors' Group, http://www.agencymeddirectors.wa.gov/Calcula
tor/DoseCalculator.htm; and American Academy of Orthopaedic Surgeons,
"Opioid Use Prior to Spine Surgery Linked to Diminished Patient-Reported
Outcomes," news release, June 12, 2014, http://newsroom.aaos.org/media
-resources/Press-releases/opioid-use-prior-to-spine-surgery-linked-to-dimin
ished-patient-reported-outcomes.htm.

80 **The bands of collagen:** On the subject of the biology of the intervertebral
disc, I had a long and fascinating conversation with Jill Urban, a now-retired
professor in the Department of Physiology, Anatomy, and Genetics at Oxford
University. Urban devoted most of her career to studying cartilage metabolism
in the intervertebral discs. The discs, which serve as the joints of the spine, she
explained, made up about one-third of the length of the spinal column. She described the behavior of macromolecules, which produce collagens and proteo-
glycans, the building blocks of disc tissue. In the human fetus, the disc tissue
was composed of notochordal cells—the same cells that populate the spines
of fish. Later—around the age of four—those notochordal cells evolved into
mesenchymal cells. In adults, the discs were mostly water, with cells making
up about 1 percent of the volume in the nucleus pulposus. Throughout the life
span, the discs struggled to get enough oxygen and glucose, essential for cellular metabolism and hydration. Deprived, the disc discolors, and cracks and fis-
sures form. See J. P. G. Urban, S. Roberts, and J. R. Ralphs, "The Nucleus of the
Intervertebral Disc from Development to Degeneration," *American Zoologist*

40, no. 1 (2000): 53–61, http://www.jstor.org/stable/3884378; and Jill Urban, in discussion with the author, October 29, 2009.

82 the FDA's newly established and still amorphous device approval process: The Medical Device Amendments, a 1976 federal statute, sought to prevent dangerous devices from entering the market. Devices that were in use before 1976 were mostly "grandfathered in," meaning that no additional testing was required. For new devices, there were two routes: The first, referred to as "510(k)," required only that a product be "substantially equivalent," perhaps the most confusing concept you'll encounter in this book. Substantially equivalent meant it had to be as safe and effective as an existing product—even if the older product, introduced years earlier and "grandfathered in," was untested and considered unsafe. The ease with which 510(k) devices entered the market would have unforeseen consequences. The second route, called "post-market approval" (PMA), required a manufacturer to jump through the many hoops involved in conducting clinical trials, making the process longer and much more costly.

Long bone screws, the kind that surgeons use to set broken limbs, were among the products that were grandfathered in under the Medical Device Amendments. Although the details are lost to history, AcroMed's 510(k) application may have suggested that the Steffee plates were meant to be used in long bone surgery, fulfilling the same purpose as screws, and thus satisfying 510(k) requirements.

See "Medical Devices and the Public's Health: The FDA 510(k) Clearance Process at 35 Years," Institute of Medicine, report brief, July 29, 2011, http://www.nationalacademies.org/hmd/Reports/2011/Medical-Devices-and-the-Publics-Health-The-FDA-510k-Clearance-Process-at-35-Years.aspx.

82 The green light allowed Steffee: Although physicians can use any FDA-approved drug or device in any manner they see fit, manufacturers are prohibited from wooing physicians to use products in "off-label" applications, meaning for purposes beyond what is specifically noted in the FDA approval.

82 closed its doors: The company would be sold to DePuy Spine.

83 Larry Kessler: Dr. Kessler is now a University of Washington professor of health services.

84 Because the federal antikickback statute: According to a special fraud alert issued by the Office of the Inspector General in March 2013, "When remuneration is paid purposefully to induce or reward referrals of items or services payable by a federal health care program, the anti-kickback statute is violated." Under this statute, hospitals and ambulatory surgical centers that buy from PODs can also be held criminally liable for participating in a "kickback transaction." See "Special Fraud Alert: Physician-Owned Entities," Office of Inspector General, Department of Health and Human Services, March 26, 2013, http://oig.hhs.gov/fraud/docs/alertsandbulletins/2013/POD_Special_Fraud_Alert.pdf.

85 orthopedic surgeon Scott Boden: As a young researcher, Boden had disputed the usefulness of imaging in back pain treatment. By the time he began to study BMP-2, he had become the director of Emory University School of Medicine's spine center.

87 **big payday could sway the judgment of a group of eminent surgeons:** It has long been established that industry-supported trial results are unreliable: Such trials report positive results for products under study 85 percent of the time, while government-supported studies, conducted through the National Institutes of Health, find positive results about half the time. In 2008, Marcia Angell, former editor in chief of the *New England Journal of Medicine*, had observed in *Journal of the American Medical Association* that "it would be naïve to conclude that bias is only a matter of a few isolated instances. It permeates the entire system. Physicians can no longer rely on the medical literature for valid and reliable information." Financial conflicts of interest permeated professional journal publications. Many felt that it would be impossible for a clinical researcher, dealing with human subjects in a trial, to be financially engaged and dispassionate at the same time. See Marcia Angell, "Industry-Sponsored Clinical Research: A Broken System," *JAMA* 300, no. 9 (2008): 1069–71, doi: 10.1001/jama.300.9.1069.

87 **Within months, surgeons who might have performed:** In 2010 in the *Journal of the American Medical Association*, Rick Deyo, the Oregon Health and Science University researcher, set out to investigate the usefulness of such multilevel spinal fusions, especially when performed to correct spinal stenosis. Deyo revealed no benefit to multilevel fusion over a simple and relatively safe (and cheaper) decompression surgery, where bits of bone and ligament were removed to make more room for the spinal nerves. The mean cost of a surgical decompression was $23,727, while the mean cost of a complex spinal fusion was over $80,000. Fusion surgery was associated with three times as many life-threatening complications, including heart attacks, strokes, blood clots, rehospitalizations, and deaths. And hospitals were able to bill out the cost of spinal implants and associated products to insurers at up to ten times their cost. See Richard A. Deyo et al. "Trends, Major Medical Complications, and Charges Associated with Surgery for Lumbar Spinal Stenosis in Older Adults," *JAMA* 303, no. 13 (2010): 1259–65, doi: 10.1001/jama.2010.338.

However, more recent research, published in 2015, shows that there may not even be an advantage to the often-recommended decompression surgery—a "decompression laminectomy"—for spinal stenosis. Especially in an older population (the group most commonly afflicted by stenosis), surgery may provoke complications, including (but not limited to) spinous process fracture, coronary ischemia, respiratory distress, hematoma, stroke, risk of reoperation, and death due to pulmonary edema. A recent Cochrane Collaboration review looked at patients who underwent decompression procedures and/or spinal fusion, and those who had nonoperative care—and found no difference in pain levels at six months. Another study from Finland showed that patients who underwent surgery felt briefly better than subjects who received nonoperative care—but the advantage was not sustained; eight years out, the surgical group had lost its advantage. The jury is still out on this one, and the decision must be weighed carefully—but in an older person who is willing to go to rehab after surgery, even half a year of restored mobility may be worth the risk. See Fabio Zaina et al., "Surgical Versus Non-Surgical Treatment for Lumbar Spinal Stenosis," *Cochrane Database Systematic Review* 2016; doi: 10.1002/14651858. CD010264.pub2; and Antti Malmivaara et al., "Surgical or Nonoperative Treatment for Lumbar Spinal Stenosis? A Randomized Controlled Trial," *Spine* 32, no. 1 (2007): 1–8, doi: 10.1097/01.brs.0000251014.81875.6d.

91 Medtronic's marketing department, the *Wall Street Journal* **contended:** A Medtronic employee had recommended excising a list of side effects from one article about Infuse. Another member of the marketing team, well aware that studies demonstrated no such benefit, wrote in a 2001 e-mail to a surgeon author that "a bigger deal should be made of elimination of donor site pain with Infuse. I would put that front and center in results, discussion and conclusion, so that 'equivalent' results aren't perceived to be a letdown." See John Carreyrou, "Medtronic Documents Spur New Questions," *Wall Street Journal*, October 25, 2012, http://www.wsj.com/articles/SB1000142405297020453050457 8076993827301944.

91 In August 2011, Medtronic commissioned: Medtronic did all it could to spin the story in its favor. During an investment conference that occurred shortly after the Yale University Open Data Access Project (YODA) began working with the data, Christopher J. O'Connell, then vice president of Medtronic's Restorative Therapies Group, said, "We've been very patient with BMP as these external reviews conducted by Yale have been underway to try to clear the air on some questions that have been raised a few summers ago by a particular author of a journal. And it's an example of Medtronic taking the high road and being extremely transparent with all the patient data and letting a third party really evaluate that rather than getting into a debate with that author." See "Marginalizing the BMP-2 Controversy," *Back Letter* 28, no. 5 (2013): 58, doi: 10.1097/01.BACK.0000430548.39301.59.

91 "Science has the power to be self-correcting": Today, fewer than 30 percent of clinical trials publish all their results within four years of completion. Data that are negative or inconclusive rarely see the light of day, and this can skew regulatory opinion, allowing an inferior product to reach the market. Within the next few years, the United States government will require that all data from key clinical trials are published and freely shared. Companies that do not comply with this requirement may receive fines of up to $10,000 a day. The mandate applies to any product that seeks FDA approval, including drugs, devices, and biologics like Infuse. See "National Institutes of Health to Mandate That Important Data from Clinical Trials Be Published and Shared," *Back Letter* 30, no. 1 (2015): 5, doi: 10.1097/01.BACK.0000459760.35630.26.

91 In June 2013, YODA released independent reports: At the 2013 meeting of the International Society for the Study of the Lumbar Spine, one session was devised as a town hall–style debate, with two surgeons taking opposing sides before 175 attendees. While one physician argued the proposition that using Infuse Bone Graft in an LT-Cage should continue to be considered the gold standard in spinal fusion, the other contended that Infuse was too risky for general use. When the audience voted, only three members were in favor of Infuse. Of those, two had been involved in BMP-2 research from the start.

That year, in the Medtronic pavilion at the annual conference of the North American Spine Society, there were no chatty sales reps or frothy cappuccinos. Instead, an austere canopy hovered over drab furniture. Medtronic's medical affairs personnel, trained and authorized to answer questions related to scientific and clinical evidence for Infuse, sat at desks, usually quite alone. See "BMP-2: The Bloom Is Off the Rose," *Back Letter* 28, no. 7 (2013): 84, doi: 10.1097/01.BACK.0000432159.51547.c6.

92 **implanted in a million patients' spines:** After analyzing FDA data, reporters at the *Milwaukee Journal Sentinel* found that more than sixty-five hundred reports of Infuse-related issues had been registered with the agency's medical device reporting system over eleven years. Half of those reports were filed in 2013 alone. See John Fauber, "Trials of Spinal Surgery Option Infuse Were Too Little, Too Late," *Milwaukee Journal Sentinel*, May 17, 2014, http://www.jsonline.com/watchdog/watchdogreports/trials-of-spinal-surgery-option-infuse-were-too-little-too-late-b99244456z1-259690251.html.

92 **"vigorously defend the product and company actions in the remaining cases":** Those "remaining cases" piled up quickly. By February 2014, there were at least four hundred cases on file. By late spring, Humana, the large managed care organization, had sued Medtronic for falsely representing Infuse as safe and effective in spinal surgery, and by making "sophisticated and deeply deceptive" statements that probably led Humana to pay for the product in many thousands of surgeries. Humana alleged that Medtronic violated the federal RICO (Racketeer Influenced and Corrupt Organizations) statute by paying prominent spine surgeons and other key opinion leaders millions of dollars to promote off-label uses of BMP-2, observed the *Back Letter*. Humana hoped to recover the money it had paid for those surgeries involving BMP-2, including revision surgeries, when less costly procedures could have been performed with superior outcomes. See Susan Kelly, "Humana Sues Medtronic over InFuse Bone Growth Product," Reuters, June 2, 2014, http://www.reuters.com/article/2014/06/02/medtronic-humana-lawsuit-idUSL 1N0OJ1OE20140602; and "Racketeering Allegations Involving Controversial Bone Grafting Drug BMP-2," *Back Letter* 29, no. 8 (2014): 86, doi: 10.1097/01 .BACK.0000453376.43668.13.

92 **on the hook for $22 million:** Even before the *Annals of Internal Medicine* published its findings, personal injury lawyers were salivating at the prospect of handsome settlements.

92 **"immunity by federal preemption":** In Minnesota, home not only to Medtronic but also to several high-volume spine surgery clinics, Medtronic's lawyers summoned the principle of federal preemption immunity, by which

federal law supersedes a conflicting state law, preempting any state claims. Medtronic argued that the FDA, a federal agency, had approved Infuse—therefore, it fitted the rubric of federal preemption immunity, and any liability claims brought in state court should be barred. But in August 2013, Arizona judge G. Murray Snow ruled that Medtronic had "changed the calculus of preemption by promoting off-label use of Infuse," and that the case could go to trial. "While permitting health care providers to use devices in ways other than those anticipated by the FDA, the FDA prohibits device manufacturers from promoting the off-label use of their product. By engaging in off-label promotion, the manufacturer may misbrand a device," Judge Snow wrote in his August 2013 ruling. "When Medtronic allegedly violated federal law by engaging in off-label promotion that damaged the Plaintiff and thereby misbranded the Infuse device, it departed the realm of federal regulation and returned to the area of traditional state law remedies." Therefore, the court ruled, the claims against Medtronic were not preempted. See Jim Spencer, "Judge Says Federal Law Blocks Medtronic InFuse Suits," *Minneapolis Star Tribune*, August 7, 2013, http://www.startribune.com/business/218743511.html; Ramirez v. Medtronic, Inc., 961 F.Supp.2d 977 (D. Arizona 2013); and Jane Mundy, "Medtronic Infuse Bone Graft Lawsuits Filed by Injured and Investors," LawyersandSettlements.com, December 30, 2013, http://www.lawyersandsettlements.com/articles/medtronic-infuse-bone-graft/medtronic-lawsuit-bone-graft-13-19390.html.

93 **the Physician Payments Sunshine Act (PPSA):** In September 2014, as the Physician Payments Sunshine Act had mandated, the Centers for Medicare and Medicaid Services published a searchable website of corporate payments to physicians. (This list can be viewed at cms.gov/openpayments.) As journalists and diligent patients dug into the bottomless pit of data, the American Medical Association sent out an urgent message to doctors, warning them, in the wake of newly public information, to "be prepared for inquiries from the media, your patients and your friends." See "Physician Financial Transparency Reports (Sunshine Act)," American Medical Association website, http://www.ama-assn.org/ama/pub/advocacy/topics/sunshine-act-and-physician-financial-transparency-reports.page?.

94 **Increasingly, before health care plans would agree to pay:** In 2014, at a major orthopedic meeting, David Mino, the medical director for orthopedic surgery and spinal disorders at Cigna Insurance, presented findings from an analysis that tracked spine care after fusion surgery for 1,422 patients with "degenerative disc disease." Mino found that, of Cigna policyholders who had lumbar fusion (at an average cost of $100,000), nearly 90 percent were still in so much pain two years later that they required ongoing treatment. There were repeat and revision surgeries, either from complications or because pain did not resolve. Of patients who had been reliant on opioid medications before surgery, 95 percent remained dependent on the drugs, a habit that cost Cigna $2,600 per patient each year. Post-surgery claims for the group totaled a whopping $11 million, raising rates for everyone. See Jodie Tillman, "Spinal Fusion

Costs Spur Insurance Changes, but Can Medicare Follow," *Tampa Bay Times*, June 20, 2014, http://www.tampabay.com/news/health/spinal-fusion-costs -spur-insurance-changes-but-can-medicare-follow/2185334.

95 **To gain access to Chinese doctors and patients:** The *Wall Street Journal* quoted Medtronic CEO Omar Ishrak: "'We're completely bullish on China,' Mr. Ishrak said. Despite challenges including sudden regulatory shifts and a health care system rife with corruption, the executive said he sees China's rewards outweighing its risks. 'It's a numbers game,' he said. 'This will be the largest market and it's not a debate. It's a matter of when.'" See Laurie Burkitt and Jeanne Whalen, "Medtronic on Hunt for Deals in China," *Wall Street Journal*, May 26, 2015, http://www.wsj.com/articles/medtronic-on-hunt-for-deals -in-china-1432642292.

96 **physician-owned medical device distributorships:** Most of these PODs operated under the financial umbrella of larger holding companies that arranged for monthly profit distribution.

101 **According to** *Orthopedics:* In June 2015, after Atiq Durrani turned up at a clinic in Lahore, *Orthopedics This Week* did a great job of unearthing the details. https://ryortho.com/2015/06/spine-fugitive-durrani-found-in-pakistan/

102 **no board actions against him:** There are other egregious cases. When the *Wall Street Journal* identified Portland, Oregon, neurosurgeon and MBA Vishal James Makker as performing the nation's highest rate of multiple-level spinal fusions on Medicare patients of any surgeon in the country, he lost his operating privileges at Providence Portland Medical Center. Eventually he surrendered his Oregon medical license. Makker operated at more than ten times the national average; records show that in some cases, he operated more than seven times on the same patient. For every hundred spinal fusions he performed, reported the *Wall Street Journal*, Makker returned to the OR to do thirty-nine revision procedures; this was the highest revision rate in the nation. He lost his surgery privileges at local hospitals and more than thirty medical negligence lawsuits were filed against him. Just before he surrendered his medical license in 2012, Makker, whose LinkedIn profile notes that he did his neurosurgery training at Brown Medical School, posted on Facebook that he intended to volunteer as a surgeon in developing countries for an organization called the Foundation for International Education in Neurological Surgery. "I will likely be doing this until I can find a position that suits me as a practicing Neurosurgeon," he wrote on Quora, a website that declares that its mission is to "share and grow the world's knowledge." Makker describes himself online as being "Board Certified by the American Board of Neurological Surgery," but the search function of the American Board of Medical Specialties brings up no record of his membership. See John Carreyrou and Tom McGinty, "Doctor in Repeat-Surgery Probe Gives Up License," *Wall Street Journal*, October 11, 2012, http://online.wsj.com/articles/SB100008723963904432949045780508608 16091972; John Carreyrou and Tom McGinty, "Medicare Records Reveal Troubling Trail of Surgeries," *Wall Street Journal*, March 29, 2011, http://www.wsj

.com/articles/SB10001424052748703858404576214642193925996; Oregon Medical Board, Stipulated Order—Vishal James Makker, MD, https://techmedweb
.omb.state.or.us/Clients/ORMB/OrderDocuments/5eadfcda-33df-4648-be1c
-aaf168ed97f3.pdf; and James Makker MD's page on Quora, accessed October
1, 2015, https://www.quora.com/James-Makker-MD.

Chapter 6: Google Your Spine Surgery

104 why in the past I'd avoided spinal injections: When my first son was
born, in preparation for a C-section, the pre-op nurse had curled my body like
a shrimp while the anesthesiologist inserted a long needle. I experienced a
sensation very much as if I'd put both my hands on an electric fence.

104 discography: At that time, Eugene Carragee had not yet publicly disputed diagnostic discography.

104 electromyography (EMG): Which would reveal nerve dysfunction, muscle dysfunction, or problems with nerve-to-muscle signal transmission.

105 fellowship-trained in this superspecialty: Minimally invasive spine surgery fellowship-trained surgeons go through medical school, then residency
in orthopedics or neurosurgery, and then commit one to two years to specialized training in minimally invasive approaches. Such surgeons practice at
NYU's Langone Medical Center, Chicago's Rush University Medical Center,
Northwestern's Feinberg School of Medicine, L.A.'s Cedars-Sinai, and the University of California San Diego's Health System.

106 "endoscopic": Which, not quite accurately, are sometimes referred to as
"laparoscopic" or "arthroscopic."

113 another procedure at L5-S1: Later, I'd learn that subcutaneous lidocaine,
used as a local anesthetic, can rapidly reach a neurotoxic dose. That's a serious
limitation because it meant that Laser Spine Institute doctors could operate on
only a single vertebral level. When I asked why LSI didn't use general anesthesia, I learned that it was necessary to have patients minimally conscious so that
they could identify the location of the pain, and that "twilight" anesthesia was
considered to be safer in an ambulatory surgery center.

113 if I'd been a fly on the wall: Later, in February 2010, I'd return to Tampa
to watch founder and chief surgeon James St. Louis perform a series of procedures.

117 Laser Spine Institute's CEO, Bill Horne: I found Bill Horne to be an exceptionally kind and thoughtful man—one who suffered from neck pain that
the doctors at LSI had not been able to completely resolve. Horne and I would
stay in touch for several years, engaged in frank conversation, until one day
he told me that he would have to put me in touch with LSI's chief marketing
officer, who would handle my requests for information from that point on.

121 a conventional steerable catheter: The FDA had approved this catheter
in 1996 for diagnostic purposes and drug delivery.

122 In April 2013, the State Medical Board of Ohio: So how could Lawrence

Rothstein and Alfred Bonati's high jinks have continued for so long? To better understand this, you need to grasp how state medical boards function—or, more accurately, why they so often fail to do so. State medical boards are overseen by the Federation of State Medical Boards, a national nonprofit organization that represents the seventy state medical and osteopathic boards in the United States and its territories. Individual state medical boards license physicians, investigate complaints, discipline physicians who break the law, administer physician evaluations, and see to the rehabilitation of physicians where appropriate. But often, state governors appoint their friends and colleagues (who are often not doctors) to seats on state medical boards. That means that if a physician in trouble makes a well-timed donation to an upcoming campaign, or otherwise supports a candidate, the state medical board's appointees may be inclined to forgive and forget. In many states, it can take five or more years to move a pending case through the system, during which time the physician may continue to work unfettered. See *U.S. Medical Regulatory Trends and Actions* (Federation of State Medical Boards, May 2014), available at https://www.fsmb.org/Media/Default/PDF/FSMB/Publications/us_medical_regulatory_trends_actions.pdf.

122 **North American Spine would be folded into a larger company:** North American Spine came under the umbrella of Athas Health, a private company focusing on spine and migraine care.

124 **or the Joint Commission, for short:** Which accredits and certifies more than 20,500 health care organizations and programs in the United States.

125 **the FDA had not approved any kind of stem cell protocol:** The dichotomy regarding stem cells is this: Because they are extracted from and transplanted into the same person, one side of the argument goes, endogenous adult stem cells do not qualify as drugs any more than saliva does. The other side of the argument says that the implanted stem cells are significantly different from those that are originally extracted, that this makes them pharmaceutical in nature, and, therefore, that FDA regulations do apply.

126 **A new lawsuit had been filed by Alfred Bonati:** It was not clear that Bonati was a reliable witness: In 2011, customs officials at the Fort Lauderdale–Hollywood International Airport accosted him after he stepped from a private plane accompanied by a gun-toting companion. Bonati was carrying a Degas painting, which, loosely wrapped in cloth, he had tucked under his arm. Bonati told attorneys and authenticators (whose fees he apparently declined to pay) that the Degas was just one in a collection of twenty-six paintings obtained by his grandfather years earlier: a collection that was now worth about a billion dollars. See Susan Taylor Martin, "Doctor's Legal Battle Reveals Potential Art Trove," *Tampa Bay Times*, March 5, 2011, http://www.tampabay.com/news/courts/civil/doctors-legal-battle-reveals-potential-art-trove/1155579.

127 **By that time, LSI had expanded:** Laser Spine Institute has locations in Tampa, Scottsdale, Philadelphia, Oklahoma City, Cleveland, St. Louis, and Cincinnati.

127 **five thousand spine operations annually:** Given the high volume of spine surgeries performed at LSI, mishaps were inevitable and not surprising. Any large and prestigious hospital would also have its share of post-op problems, but it would have the inpatient beds necessary to handle them. LSI had no true hospital facility, and in October 2014, the *Tampa Bay Times* reported on a particularly dramatic medical malpractice lawsuit brought by Ronald R. Davis, a patient from Ohio who had sued LSI after a seven-hour spinal procedure failed, leaving him disabled. Reasonably enough, Davis, who had viewed LSI's commercials on daytime CNN, believed he was flying to Tampa for what to him sounded like a minor operation. According to his lawyer, Steve Yerrid, he didn't learn until the middle of his pre-op evaluation that in fact he was scheduled for "minimally invasive stabilization" at two levels in the thoracic spine, a very delicate spinal fusion operation that is the exclusive métier of highly specialized surgeons. According to the complaint, after the operation Davis could not stand and he had no sensation in his thighs. LSI sent him to a nearby hospital, Largo Medical Center, where he remained for eleven days.

His attorney, who has himself undergone two spine surgeries at major university hospitals, described Davis as "a hardworking, forty-four-year-old equipment operator, who is now chronically and permanently injured. He can't care for his family or himself," Yerrid said. "This was far from the Band-Aid surgery he envisioned. He didn't know what was going to happen until he had already traveled to Tampa." The Davises had lost their car, Yerrid said. Their home was in foreclosure, and Ron Davis lived in excruciating pain. "Instead of realizing the hope he was promised, he is now living a nightmare." See Jodie Tillman, "Laser Spine Institute Sued over Spinal Fusion Surgery," *Tampa Bay Times*, October 22, 2014, http://www.tampabay.com/news/courts/civil/laser-spine-institute-sued-over-spinal-fusion-surgery/2203277; and Steve Yerrid, in discussion with the author, December 8, 2014.

127 **The website still bristled with testimonials:** The website continued to add glowing testimonials. But on Facebook, where the company posted yoga poses that might be therapeutic for back pain patients, effusive comments were few and far between. Even a website that charged companies a fee to be included, consumeraffairs.com, gave LSI just three and a quarter stars out of a possible five and, among a few glowing reviews, posted many more that were startlingly bad. See https://www.consumeraffairs.com/doctors/dr_fl_laser_spine.html.

130 **philanthropic work at an African clinic:** In 2008, Kaul established the Spine Africa Project. When he could no longer practice in the United States, he made plans to devote himself to the charity, with plans to set up a surgical facility at Panzi Hospital, in the Democratic Republic of Congo. In a YouTube video about the Spine Africa Project, Kaul performs a surgery on a boy under exceedingly primitive conditions. With water dripping in a dirty sink, he made the incision with a discolored electrosurgical scalpel. During the procedure, the power went down, making it necessary for the anesthesiologist to

manually ventilate the boy. Although Kaul hoped to raise the necessary funds to bring in a CT scanner, he felt that a minimally invasive approach would be well suited to a hospital with limited equipment. See Alex Hannaford, "Trust Me, I'm a Doctor: The Case of the Rogue Spinal Surgeon," *Guardian*, November 1, 2014, http://www.theguardian.com/society/2014/nov/01/uk-an aesthetist-practised-as-us-spinal-surgeon; and "The Spine Africa Project Full Documentary," YouTube video, 23:03, posted by Richard Kaul, November 13, 2011, https://www.youtube.com/watch?v=Zu50ik2l2Sc.

Chapter 7: Replacement Parts

132 **sitting for more than ten minutes was still very difficult:** Whenever I could, I worked in a reclining position, on a set of three vaguely pyramidal cushions that formed the Contour Backmax Support System.

132 **President John F. Kennedy:** Despite JFK's cultivated image of athletic vigor and sexual prowess, he had undergone several failed spinal surgeries and spent most of his life in miserable back pain. Steadfastly avoiding all activities that might tax his lumbar spine, he hobbled on crutches in private, always wearing a restrictive brace that encircled his torso and thighs. He steamed himself in hot baths and traveled with a special mattress. To get through his days, he relied on injections of anesthetics, corticosteroids, and amphetamines. This story is told exceptionally well in Susan E. B. Schwartz, *JFK's Secret Doctor* (New York: Skyhorse Publishing, 2012).

136 **in its clinical trial, the Charité disc was compared:** To get a new device through the FDA, it is not necessary to show that it is superior to existing devices. Often, the standard is "non-inferiority"; the device must not be less effective than an already-approved device.

136 **Later, Cunningham would become CEO:** Gemma Cunningham's company is http://truthmd.com.

137 **the ProDisc-L Total Disc Replacement:** The "L" stands for lumbar; there is also a ProDisc cervical implant.

137 **choosing a 360-degree spinal fusion:** Several years later, in *the Journal of the American Medical Association*, epidemiologist Rick Deyo would denounce the 360-degree fusion as ineffective, risky, and costly—and therefore not a good way to evaluate the safety and effectiveness of a new device. See Richard A. Deyo et al., "Trends, Major Medical Complications, and Charges Associated with Surgery for Lumbar Spinal Stenosis in Older Adults," *JAMA* 303, no 13 (2010): 1259–65; doi: 10.1001/jama.2010.338.

139 **Brian Bohn:** Bohn described his experience on YouTube: https://www.youtube.com/watch?v=25NZ47SKWqw.

140 **he started Global Patient Network:** The site is still on the Web at http://www.globalpatientnetwork.com/.

141 **I sent a request:** By 2015, Stenum Hospital was no longer affiliated with Malte Petersen. In fact, the web page describing his exit warned patients that he had set up shop elsewhere, and that they should be cautious about doing business with him.

141 **the Spinal Kinetics M6:** In fact, the M6 would never make it through the FDA.

143 **a forty-five-year-old disabled Medicaid patient:** We don't know the nature of this patient's disability, but it may be that he was not capable of understanding the risks involved in participating in the clinical trial.

144 **acupuncture:** Each year more than three million Americans undergo acupuncture for musculoskeletal complaints, primarily involving back pain. But acupuncture for back pain is a very controversial treatment. The best controlled studies show that the outcomes of acupuncture do not depend on where needles are inserted—or even on actual needle insertion. Several investigations have shown that sham acupuncture—in which toothpicks are pressed on the back, without actually puncturing the skin, or needles are inserted randomly and superficially—is just as effective as traditional Chinese medicine (TCM) acupuncture.

Puzzled researchers are still trying to figure out how this works. Some believe that both "real" acupuncture and "sham" acupuncture offer what is called a "super placebo effect," stimulating the central nervous system to release endorphins. A German study showed that acupuncture activated key areas of the cortex and limbic regions that sense and process pain, as well as regions that govern the expectation of pain. See Michael Haake et al., "German Acupuncture Trials (Gerac) for Chronic Low Back Pain: Randomized, Multicenter, Blinded, Parallel-Group Trial with 3 Groups," *Archives of Internal Medicine* 167, no. 17 (2007): 1892–98, doi: 10.1001/Archinte.167.17.1892. Other researchers hypothesize that there are hundreds of additional acupuncture points (beyond the recognized ones) on the body, and therefore there may be no such thing as an inactive sham. Either way, the placebo effect is impressive: The German study showed that patients who received two thirty-minute treatments per week for six months, of either "sham" or "real" acupuncture, required significantly lower doses of opioids to treat their back pain than patients in standard care.

While scientists and practitioners try to figure out how TCM acupuncture works, orthopedic and sports medicine acupuncturists have adopted a technique called "dry needling." The theory behind dry needling (which can be painful, although very slender Japanese acupuncture needles are used) is that muscles become metabolically overloaded and habitually contracted. They "forget" how to relax. Dry needling interrupts that process by increasing electrical activity and blood flow in the muscle.

Hawaii-based acupuncturist Whitfield Reaves, with a clinic on the island of Maui, is one of the pioneers of dry needling to treat back pain and sciatica. After twenty years of treating back pain patients with acupuncture and achieving little success, he decided that traditional Chinese medicine was irrelevant in the treatment of back pain. "It's not about the gallbladder meridian or the kidney meridian," he said. "And it's not about qi, or the flow of anything. This makes no sense to me, and it never did."

To be effective in treating back pain, Reaves recognized, you first needed a Western diagnosis of the problem. Two key muscle groups—the quadratus lumborum and the gluteus medius—were inaccessible on the standard acupuncture meridians. "When those muscles are out of whack, they are capable of wreaking havoc on every aspect of pelvic and spinal anatomy, especially the sacroiliac joint," he said. His approach—which I observed at his clinic in Boulder, Colorado, before he moved his practice to Maui—is to use a dozen or so needles to break up nodules in the muscles, getting the blood flowing, relaxing the muscles that don't need to contract, and waking up the muscles that are not doing their jobs. When muscles are turned off and weak—or tight and overprotective, said Reaves, "postural problems develop. The sacroiliac joints are either lax and clicking and popping, or tight and locked up."

Acupuncture for back problems has been around since 1072 BCE, said Reaves, but our backs are not the same as Chinese backs of that period. "They had no chairs," he says. "They didn't sit for seventy or eighty hours a week. Our problems are different.

"If you are a back pain patient and you want to see an acupuncturist," said Reaves, "look for someone with a background in anatomy, trigger point training, and experience in orthopedic and sports medicine acupuncture, versus pure TCM." (Whitfield Reaves, in discussion with the author, October 29 and 30, 2012.)

Sports medicine acupuncture is becoming more common in the United States. Check out Matt Callison at the University of California–San Diego Sports Medicine RIMAC (Recreation, IntraMural, Athletic Complex) (https://www.sportsmedicineacupuncture.com/certification-program/faculty/matt-callison-m-s-l-ac/), Whitfield Reaves in Maui (http://whitfieldreaves.com), Chad Bong (who has a master's degree in exercise science) in Philadelphia (www.phillysportsacupuncture.com), and physiatrist and acupuncturist Alex Moroz, who directs the musculoskeletal rehabilitation program at New York University (https://doctormoroz.com).

145 **Republican senator Charles Grassley:** At that time, Grassley was chairman of the Senate Finance Committee, the body that oversees the U.S. Department of Health and Human Services.

146 **In response to Milgram's salvo:** Whether she departed of her own volition is unclear, but six months after she wrote her letter, Milgram, who had served under New Jersey governor Jon Corzine, stepped down as the attorney general, declining to serve under governor-elect Chris Christie, who was known for currying favor with New Jersey's medical manufacturers. (In 2012, the pharmaceutical industry contributed an estimated $33.5 billion to GDP in New Jersey, according to a study from Rutgers released in 2014.) See Joseph J. Seneca, Michael L. Lahr, and Will Irving, "Contribution of the Life Sciences Industry to the New Jersey Economy," June 2014, http://bloustein.rutgers

.edu/wp-content/uploads/2015/03/Economic-Contributions-of-Life-Sciences
-EJBPPP.pdf.

146 **Rick Delamarter:** Rick Delamarter would become codirector of Cedars-Sinai
Spine Center in 2009.

Chapter 8: The Opioid Wars

154 **a crystallizable isolate of opium:** Opiates are substances such as morphine and heroin, derived directly from the opium poppy, while opioids, like
hydrocodone and oxymorphone, are synthesized products.

155 **capsicum plasters:** Even today, such plasters are available over the
counter, under brand names such as Salonpas, Icy Hot, and Bengay. Most
contain methyl salicylate, a nonsteroidal anti-inflammatory that is absorbed
through the skin, but some capsicum patches are still on the market.

156 **Arthur Sackler died:** His memorial was held at New York's Metropoli-
tan Museum, where the Sackler family had financed the transportation from
Egypt and the on-site reconstruction of the Temple of Dendur.

159 **COX-2 inhibitors:** Although two COX-2 inhibitors, Bextra and Vioxx,
were removed from the market in the mid-2000s, the FDA allowed another—
Pfizer's blockbuster drug Celebrex—to remain, with a black box warning
about possible heart attack and stroke risks, pending further research. Later,
the FDA expanded the black box requirement to all prescription NSAIDs,
which included diclofenac, commonly prescribed by the brand-name Voltaren.

In response, Pfizer launched (and paid for) a massive international clinical
trial called PRECISION, intended to evaluate the relative safety of COX-2
drugs versus standard NSAIDS. In November 2016, after roughly a decade,
the study's researchers reported that Celebrex was no riskier than ibuprofen
(Advil) or naproxen (Aleve).

What we won't learn from the PRECISION trial—because it would not be
to the advantage of opioid manufacturers for us to have that information—is
whether, even with the cardiovascular risks, the relative risks of COX-2 drugs
are lower than the risks of opioid prescription for patients with chronic musculoskeletal conditions.

160 **But the company sent out a specially trained team:** In 2001 and 2002,
Purdue funded a series of nine programs throughout the United States to
educate hospitals, physicians, and staff about JCAHO's pain standards for
hospitals. See United States General Accounting Office, *Prescription Drugs:
OxyContin Abuse and Diversion and Efforts to Address the Problem*, GAO-04-110
(Washington, DC: US General Accounting Office, 2003), 23.

164 **"piriformis syndrome":** The piriformis is a small cone-shaped muscle,
located deep beneath the gluteus muscles in the buttocks. When it's in spasm,
there's a dull ache in the middle of the buttock, tenderness in that area when
pressure is applied, and pain in the hamstrings. When the piriformis is in
spasm, it may strangle the sciatic nerve as it passes through the pelvic girdle.

Certain activities such as prolonged sitting, twisting, and rotating the torso can exacerbate it, and there can be difficulty walking up stairs and hills, as well as trouble rotating the hip outward. See Jane E. Brody, "Personal Health," *New York Times*, January 12, 1994, http://www.nytimes.com/1994/01/12/us/personal-health-848026.html.

164 **Laude decided to go cold turkey:** The term "cold turkey" refers to the gooseflesh that covers the body of a person who tries to withdraw too rapidly from opioids.

165 **the source of many of his other symptoms:** When taken long-term, opioids alter activity in several regions of the brain, including those that regulate reward, memory and learning, motivation, stress response, and hormonal response. Other disturbing symptoms include weight gain, osteoporosis, muscle wasting, fatigue, mood swings, depression, anxiety, sexual dysfunction, testicular shrinkage, dry mouth, and immune system suppression, as well as impaired respiration, disordered sleep, impaired cortisol production, and constipation. See Stephen Colameco and Joshua S. Coren, "Opioid-Induced Endocrinopathy," *Journal of the American Osteopathic Association* 109, no. 1 (2009): 20–25, http://jaoa.org/article.aspx?articleid=2093682; Nathaniel Katz and Norman A. Mazer, "The Impact of Opioids on the Endocrine System," *Clinical Journal of Pain* 25, no. 2 (2009): 170–75, http://www.mascc.org/assets/doc uments/pain_Impact_Opioids_Endocrine_Katz.pdf; Joseph Pergolizzi et al., "Current Knowledge of Buprenorphine and Its Unique Pharmacological Profile," *Pain Practice* 10, no. 5 (2010): 428–50, doi: 10.1111/j.1533-2500.2010.00378.x; and Y. Xia et al., "Sexual Dysfunction During Methadone Maintenance Treatment and Its Influence on Patient's Life and Treatment: A Qualitative Study in South China," *Psychology, Health and Medicine* 18, no. 3 (2013): 321–29, doi: 10.1080/13548506.2012.729845.

167 **"breakthrough pain":** The concept of "breakthrough pain" was first introduced by Russell Portenoy in 1990. See Russell K. Portenoy and Neil A. Hagen, "Breakthrough Pain: Definition, Prevalence and Characteristics," *Pain* 41, no. 3 (1990): 273–81, doi: 10.1016/0304-3959(90)90004-W.

168 **Institute of Medicine (IOM):** As of March 15, 2016, renamed the Health and Medicine Division (HMD).

173 **To date, it remains unclear whether buprenorphine offers the best solution:** But it is certainly making a king's ransom for those who manufacture and dispense it. Already, buprenorphine accounts for sales of about $1.5 billion a year, exceeding those of other top-selling drugs such as Viagra and Adderall. As we have seen, whenever a drug is worth that much money to stakeholders, it's likely that somebody will behave in an undisciplined manner. (In a 2013 *New York Times* article called "Addiction Treatment with a Dark Side," the authors observed that physicians in West Virginia whose names appear on the federal buprenorphine locator were five times more likely to have been disciplined than doctors in general. "Nationally, at least 1,350 of 12,780 buprenorphine doctors have been sanctioned for offenses that

include excessive narcotics prescribing, insurance fraud, sexual misconduct and practicing medicine while impaired," the reporters noted.)

As I finished writing this book in April 2016, there were still stringent controls on bupe prescription, exceeding those that exist for standard opioid painkillers. The maximum caseload was restricted to one hundred patients, and before a doctor could prescribe, he had to complete an eight-hour class and obtain federal certification from the DEA. At that point, his name would be added to the federal buprenorphine treatment locator. According to one report, with one hundred patients, a doctor could expect to earn a half a million dollars a year.

But given the size of the epidemic of addiction at hand, under thirteen thousand certified buprenorphine doctors are not nearly enough. Some clinics have a waiting list of over a thousand patients, and in the time those patients wait—often for weeks or months—they are especially likely to overdose. Under a new bill called TREAT, The Recovery Enhancement for Addiction Treatment (at the time of writing, it had made it through committee, and awaited a full Senate vote), many more doctors would be certified, and the individual cap on a doctor's buprenorphine caseload would be lifted to five hundred patients, which means that about a million more patients would receive medically assisted treatment.

For a very detailed and excellent explanation of the bupe controversy, see Jason Cherkis, "Dying to Be Free," *Huffington Post*, January 28, 2015, http://projects.huffingtonpost.com/dying-to-be-free-heroin-treatment. See also Deborah Sontag, "Addiction Treatment with a Dark Side," *New York Times*, November 16, 2013, http://www.nytimes.com/2013/11/17/health/in-demand-in-clinics-and-on-the-street-bupe-can-be-savior-or-menace.html?_r=0; Drug Enforcement Administration Office of Diversion Control, "Buprenorphine," July 2013, http://www.deadiversion.usdoj.gov/drug_chem_info/buprenorphine.pdf; and ASAM Staff, "TREAT Act Legislation Proposes Increasing Buprenorphine Prescribing Cap," *American Society of Addiction Medicine Magazine*, August 12, 2014, http://www.asam.org/magazine/read/article/2014/08/12/treat-act-legislation-proposes-increasing-buprenorphine-prescribing-cap.

Chapter 9: Head Case

192 **Ken Malloy developed patient training videos:** Today, Malloy sells these DVDs on the Internet for $49.95 at http://www.healingbackpain.com/products.html.

195 **Although several important and widely published studies:** Several groups of investigators have compared lumbar spinal fusion and chronic pain programs in randomized controlled trials, and found in favor of chronic pain programs. Jens Brox explored the question in 2003 and 2006, and Jeremy Fairbank in 2005. In another study, in 2001, Peter Fritzell showed spinal fusion to be slightly more effective. Subsequently, researcher Anne Mannion reviewed the four studies and wrote an excellent analysis that presented the rehabili-

tation approach as the winner. Her paper was selected for one of the world's major spine research awards. As Mannion prepared to fly to Scottsdale, Arizona, to accept her prize in 2013, Fritzell's 2001 team of investigators suddenly withdrew their data—twelve years after the fact. Mannion could not receive an award for a paper based in part on scientific data that had been withdrawn. Later, some critics said that Fritzell's researchers withdrew the data because, in their design of the trial, they had intentionally crippled the rehabilitation arm of the study so that it would show spinal fusion to be superior. See Jens I. Brox et al., "Lumbar Instrumented Fusion Compared with Cognitive Intervention and Exercises in Patients with Chronic Back Pain After Previous Surgery for Disc Herniation: A Prospective Randomized Controlled Study," *Pain* 122, nos. 1–2 (2006): 145–55, doi: 10.1016/j.pain.2006.01.027; Jens I. Brox et al., "Randomized Clinical Trial of Lumbar Instrumented Fusion and Cognitive Intervention and Exercises in Patients with Chronic Low Back Pain and Disc Degeneration," *Spine* 28, no. 17 (2003): 1913–21, doi: 10.1097/01 .BRS.0000083234.62751.7A; Jeremy Fairbank et al., "Randomised Controlled Trial to Compare Surgical Stabilisation of the Lumbar Spine with an Intensive Rehabilitation Programme for Patients with Chronic Low Back Pain: The MRC Spine Stabilisation Trial," *British Medical Journal* 330, no. 7502 (2005): 1233, doi: 10.1136/bmj.38441.620417.8F; Peter Fritzell et al., "Lumbar Fusion Versus Nonsurgical Treatment for Chronic Low Back Pain (A Multicenter Randomized Controlled Trial from the Swedish Lumbar Spine Study Group)," *Spine* 26, no. 23 (2001): 2521–34; and "Landmark Study Comparing Fusion Surgery to Nonoperative Care—And an Ethical Dilemma," *Back Letter* 28, no. 9 (2013): 97–105, doi: 10.1097/01.BACK.0000434493.56718.5a.

195 **nonspecific back pain of long duration:** At the Mayo Clinic, patients who enter the program have, on average, been in pain for about eight years.

195 **the widely prescribed barbiturate Miltown:** In 1956, a year after Miltown was introduced, roughly one in twenty Americans had tried it. Two decades later, when minor tranquilizer use peaked, Americans were filling more than one hundred million prescriptions for them each year—about 15 percent of the population said they had used one in the previous year. See Allan V. Horwitz, "Book Review Happy Pills in America: From Miltown to Prozac; The Age of Anxiety: A History of America's Turbulent Affair with Tranquilizers; Before Prozac: The Troubled History of Mood Disorders in Psychiatry," *New England Journal of Medicine* 360 (2009): 841–44, doi: 10.1056/NEJMbkrev0809177.

197 **the number of disabled worker beneficiaries increased:** By 2013, almost 20 percent of those who were disabled would claim back disorders as their primary impairment. Fewer than 1 percent of those who were approved for Social Security Disability Insurance at the beginning of 2011 would manage to return to the workforce by 2014, and disability-related claims would account for the majority of the costs of treating back pain in the United States. See Chana Joffe-Walt, "Unfit for Work: The Startling Rise of Disability in America," *NPR*, http://apps.npr.org/unfit-for-work.

198 **The Cleveland Clinic:** The Cleveland Clinic's interdisciplinary rehab program is more than thirty-five years old. It uses a model that integrates cognitive behavioral therapy, group psychodynamic psychotherapy, and physical rehabilitation. The staff includes five psychologists and four physicians, in addition to physical and occupational therapists—an enormous staff for a program that manages the rehabilitation of only forty patients each month. In a video posted on the clinic's website, psychiatrist Edward Covington, the program's director, tells visitors that the most important psychotherapy patients receive occurs in the gymnasium, when they learn to recapture the power of their own bodies, re-create the endurance that they lost, and learn to see themselves not as helpless and powerless to deal with their situations but as having the ability to cope physically. At Cleveland Clinic, patients are universally weaned off opioids and other drugs, legal or not, such as cocaine, heroin, marijuana, and benzodiazepines. Regardless of their status, nearly all patients leave clean—although a few remain on maintenance doses of buprenorphine—and very few relapse. "Just about all of us have special training in pain, as well as in treating substance abuse. People come in cognitively soggy and leave much clearer," said Judith Scheman. "A lot come in with unhealed trauma. And while they are here, they heal from the trauma." Every day, every patient gets ninety minutes of psychotherapy, in a group of about ten people. "It's like watching a light come on in a room," said Scheman. "There are a lot of Kleenex around, because these people are dealing with a huge amount of destruction and devastation. There are a lot of reasons to cry. These people have been hearing, 'we can't help you' for a long time. They are anxious and fearful. They are miseducated about what is causing their pain." The Cleveland Clinic's program makes a point of scrutinizing family dynamics. This makes a huge difference in how well a patient does after he or she graduates. "It's essential to help a patient find a new identity," said Scheman, "beyond sufferer." Retraining family members is key: They are often even more depressed than the person in pain. It's critical to examine what the role of the "sick" person is in the family, and how that role is enabled by other family members. There are patients who leave CPRPs very well, and almost immediately return to the role of invalid, because this is what the family structure requires. See Cleveland Clinic Chronic Pain Rehabilitation Program, http://my.clevelandclinic .org/services/neurological_institute/center-for-neurological-restoration-pain/ treatments-services/chronic-pain-rehab-program; and Judith Scheman, PhD, in discussion with the author, February 5, 2014.

198 **Mayo Clinic:** The Mayo Clinic pain rehabilitation program, one of the oldest and largest in the country, was created in 1974, and since then has treated more than five thousand patients at its Rochester, Minnesota, facility. In October 2011, the program expanded to Mayo Clinic's Jacksonville, Florida, campus, where four hundred patients are treated each year. The program runs Monday to Friday from 8:00 a.m. to 4:30 p.m. over a three-week period. The daily schedule includes physical therapy focused on gradual physical strength-

ening, proper body mechanics, and cardiovascular conditioning; three one-hour group therapy sessions per day where participants discuss stress management, sleep strategies, and cognitive-behavior therapy; and one hour of occupational therapy per day. They also have weekly biofeedback sessions. See Christopher D. Sletten et al., "Economic Analysis of a Comprehensive Pain Rehabilitation Program: A Collaboration Between Florida Blue and Mayo Clinic Florida," *Pain Medicine* 16, no. 5 (2015): 898–904, doi: 10.1111/pme.12679.

199 **Steven Stanos:** Steven Stanos left RIC in the autumn of 2014 for a new job at Swedish Hospital and Medical Center in Seattle, Washington, where he would have the opportunity to create a rehabilitation-based pain management program in a large hospital system. See "Steven Stanos, DO," Swedish Medical Center, accessed April 1, 2015, http://www.swedish.org/physicians/steven-stanos; and Steven Stanos, DO, in correspondence with the author, March 19, 2015.

199 **Feldenkrais class:** We'll explore this practice in detail in chapter 12, "The Posture Mavens."

200 **benefits of meditation in the treatment of chronic pain:** In 1979, MIT biologist Jon Kabat-Zinn began teaching a ten-week program at the University of Massachusetts medical school to help chronic pain patients develop better coping skills. His original study produced surprisingly good results—out of fifty-one patients, two-thirds showed pain reduction of at least 33 percent, and half showed reduction of at least 50 percent. In 1990, he published his book *Full Catastrophe Living*, describing his technique, which he called "mindfulness-based stress reduction," and MBSR took root around the world. Other researchers have duplicated his outcomes in patients of all ages. Caryn Feldman has accumulated many resources for patients interested in meditation, and they can be found in my website resource section at http://cathrynjakobsonramin.com/re source-subjects/meditation/.

A number of mindfulness-based practices—including meditation, yoga, Tai Chi, and the Feldenkrais method, all of which we examine in later chapters— have been reported to decrease both chronic and acute pain sensations, according to David J. Linden, a neuroscientist at Johns Hopkins, whose book, *Touch: The Science of Hand, Heart, and Mind*, is worth reading. Different forms of meditation and exercise practices address a variety of pain mechanisms and pain pathways that sustain chronic pain. Not all forms of meditation have similar effects, observes Linden: For chronic pain, mindfulness-based stress meditation seems to work best. Another book worth studying, because of its focus on meditation and chronic pain, is Ronald Siegel's *The Mindfulness Solution*. Mindfulness practice, says Siegel, can help a patient separate the pain from the suffering. There is good evidence that mindfulness meditation has a significant impact on pain and anxiety levels, because it allows the patient to observe and acknowledge thoughts, sensations, emotions, and perceptions as they arise, moment by moment, without judging them as good or bad, painful or pleasant. "You can stop thinking about 'how should I sit, what surgical intervention should I try next?' And move on to 'okay, what's scaring me now?'"

See Jon Kabat-Zinn, *Full Catastrophe Living: Using the Wisdom of Your Body and Mind to Face Stress, Pain, and Illness* (New York: Bantam Books, 1990); "Is Medicine Ignoring Key Influences on Chronic Pain? And Important Therapeutic Solutions?" *Back Letter* 30, no. 6 (2015): 63–70, doi: 10.1097/01. BACK.0000466235.48757.02; David. J. Linden, *Touch: The Science of Hand, Heart, and Mind* (New York: Viking Press, 2015); and Ronald Siegel, *The Mindfulness Solution: Everyday Practices for Everyday Problems* (New York: Guilford Press, 2010).

204 The group environment also helps: The results of a 2010 study reported in *Biology Letters* showed that exercise performed in a synchronized manner in a group increased individuals' pain thresholds more than the same exercise performed alone. Researchers hypothesize that the group activity boosts the level of endogenous opioids, and may be the reason that in nearly every culture, people gather together in groups to dance, play music, and pray. See Emma E. A. Cohen et al., "Rowers' High: Behavioural Synchrony Is Correlated with Elevated Pain Thresholds," *Biology Letters* 6, no. 1 (2010): 106–8, doi: 10.1098/rsbl.2009.0670.

204 In boot camp, patients learn how to get through a tough day: Studies show that many chronic pain patients have been sexually, physically, or emotionally abused; there's a strong association between early life or long-standing abuse of any kind and the development of hypervigilance and catastrophizing, resulting in increased sensitivity to all physical stimuli and heightened reactivity to pain. Exposure to trauma alters patients' ability to cope with the stress of chronic pain, leaving them feeling out of control and certain that pain will persist and get worse.

Children who have consistently been exposed to emotional abuse, one study's authors wrote, "know from experience that bad things can happen, and that pain is associated with those bad things." There are strong links, notes Peter Przekop, director of pain management at Hazelden Betty Ford, between a high degree of chronic stress resulting from adverse experiences and the development of chronic pain. "It is not enough to simply focus on symptoms," says Przekop. "We must address the underlying foundation that is holding the chronic-pain patient hostage," including symptoms of depression, catastrophic thinking, and poor emotional self-care.

See Randy A. Sansone, Daron A. Watts, and Michael W. Wiederman, "Childhood Trauma and Pain and Pain Catastrophizing in Adulthood: A Cross-Sectional Survey Study," *Primary Care Companion for CNS Disorders* 15, no. 4 (2013): PCC.13m01506, doi: 10.4088/PCC.13m01506; B. E. Bailey et al., "Lifetime Physical and Sexual Abuse in Chronic Pain Patients: Psychosocial Correlates and Treatment Outcomes," *Disability and Rehabilitation* 25, no. 7 (2003): 331–42, doi: 10.1080/0963828021000056866; and Peter Przekop, "Can Past Trauma and Stinking Thinking Be Causing My Chronic Pain?" Hazelden Betty Ford, October 21, 2015, http://www.hazeldenbettyford.org/articles/can-past-trauma-and-stinking-thinking-be-causing-my-chronic-pain.

204 **How to have sex without getting hurt:** The particulars of how to manage sexual intimacy when you're in pain will be taken up again in chapter 10.

204 **qualified pain psychologists':** A pain psychologist is a doctoral-level clinical psychologist who has completed a board certified postdoctoral fellowship in pain psychology. Checking the American Psychological Association's psychologist locator, I found 1,715 therapists listed under "pain management," but very few even mentioned pain in the description of their practice. There are few formal programs in the country dedicated to training psychology graduates to become specialists in this field. You want someone who has specialized training and substantial experience in treating chronic pain. Ideally your pain psychologist will have a PhD in clinical psychology and specialized fellowship training in chronic pain. I recommend choosing a psychologist who uses a cognitive behavioral approach (CBT), as this is evidence-based treatment for chronic pain. Currently the most likely place to find a chronic pain psychologist is at an academic chronic pain rehab program.

204 **only 7 percent reported poor sleep:** Studies show that sleep deprivation for as few as three consecutive nights can precipitate depression, and those who sleep badly tend to be more anxious about their health. They report more pain, exhibit lower pain tolerance, and engage in pain catastrophizing. Because lack of sleep affects the HPA axis, which controls hypothalamic, pituitary, and adrenal gland function, it results in elevated levels of cortisol, as well as other hormonal imbalances. Sleep deprivation may also contribute to systemic inflammation and the development of obesity and diabetes. Muscles and bones suffer when patients don't experience the phases of deep sleep, during which blood pressure drops and breathing and brain activity slow down. The phases of deep sleep provide additional oxygen and nutrients to muscles and ligaments, enhancing tissue growth and repair. Insufficient sleep over extended periods may lead to osteoporosis and reduce the ability of spinal vertebrae to sustain the pounding they take all day. If antidepressants are part of the pharmaceutical cocktail, there may be even more trouble: In a study published in the journal *Bone in* 2012, patients who were prescribed SSRIs (selective serotonin reuptake inhibitors) like Lexapro, Zoloft, and Paxil showed decreased bone mineral density in the lumbar spine.

205 **Although they have side effects:** The serious side effects of zolpidem (Ambien) include memory loss; anxiety; and abnormal thoughts and behavior, such as aggressive behavior, confusion, hallucinations, depression, or suicidal thoughts. In some cases, people taking the drug have reported "sleep-driving" and doing other activities while not fully awake—cooking, eating, walking, or having sex—with no memory of their actions in the morning.

206 **In a neurosurgeon's waiting room at the Cleveland Clinic:** The Cleveland Clinic's own comprehensive chronic pain rehab program, an excellent one, is practically in Parseghian's backyard in Toledo, but because no physician, not even the neurosurgeon, ever mentioned it to her, she did not know of its existence.

208 the luxury of taking it easy: In a 2004 report written for the British National Health Service, the chief medical officer concluded that "physical activity is as effective in the treatment of clinical depression and can be as successful as psychotherapy or medication, especially in the longer term." Exercise has been shown to be more effective for moderate to severe depression than it is for mild to moderate depression, notes clinical psychologist Irving Kirsch in his excellent 2010 book, *The Emperor's New Drugs.* "The antidepressant benefits of exercise seem to be long-lasting, so long as the person continues to exercise regularly. In fact, the benefits of exercise seem to increase as time goes on. Twenty minutes of exercise three days a week seems to be enough to produce the antidepressant effect, and the kind of exercise that is practiced does not seem to matter much." In a comparison of SSRI treatment and aerobic exercise, initially those on antidepressants and the exercise group improved equally, but six months down the line, writes Kirsch, "significantly more exercise patients had recovered from depression, and more SSRI patients had relapsed." See Department of Health, Physical Activity, Health Improvement and Prevention, *At Least Five a Week* (London: UK Department of Health, 2004), 58, http://webarchive.nationalarchives.gov.uk/20130107105354/http://www.dh.gov.uk/prod_consum_dh/groups/dh_digitalassets/@dh/@en/documents/digitalasset/dh_4080981.pdf; and Irving Kirsch, *The Emperor's New Drugs: Exploding the Antidepressant Myth* (New York: Basic Books, 2010), 164.

209 "I knew the acetaminophen was going to ruin my liver": According to *Consumer Reports*, it's very easy to get too much acetaminophen: A person who takes the maximum dosages recommended for Tylenol Extra Strength, Nyquil Cold and Flu, and a sleep aid would get 6,600 milligrams; add Vicodin to the mix, and the dose far exceeds the 4,000 milligrams linked to liver damage. See "The Dangers of Painkillers: A Special Report," *Consumer Reports*, July 2014, http://www.consumerreports.org/cro/magazine/2014/09/the-dangers-of-painkillers/index.htm.

210 When Stanos switched Wilson: Melinda did not know that Steven Stanos's conflict-of-interest disclosure statement revealed his financial relationships with several opioid manufacturers. She also did not know that he was a key opinion leader who was an author of continuing education materials that endorsed chronic opioid therapy, or that RIC's research branch was funded by painkiller manufacturers and other pharmaceutical companies to pay for expenses incurred in research and clinical trials. She was unaware that the city of Chicago was preparing to pursue legal action against several painkiller manufacturers, and the doctors who advanced their causes, or that Steve Stanos, while ultimately not targeted, would be one of the doctors who were asked to answer questions about their relationship with opioid manufacturers.

See "Dollars for Docs: How Industry Dollars Reach Your Doctors," *ProPublica*, search results for Steven Stanos, accessed April 2, 2015, https://projects.propublica.org/docdollars/; Steven P. Stanos and Gagan Mahajan, "Appropriate Use of Opioids in Chronic Pain: Caring for Patients, Reducing

Risks," supplement to live symposium at the Internal Medicine 2011 Education Program, April 6, 2011, release date January 1, 2012; Office of the Mayor,
City of Chicago, "City of Chicago Sues Big Pharma for Deceptively Marketing
Highly Addictive Prescription Painkillers," news release, June 3, 2014, http://
www.cityofchicago.org/content/dam/city/depts/mayor/Press%20Room/
Press%20Releases/2014/June/06.03.14BigPharma.pdf; and Steven Stanos, DO,
in discussion with the author, February 7, 2014, and in correspondence with the
author, March 23, 2015, in which Stanos wrote, "I am still peripherally involved
in the City of Chicago case (not named, but asked to answer questions)."

210 **Fentanyl was a powerhouse of a drug:** In 2007, the Division of Public
Health Sciences at Wake Forest University School of Medicine and the Institute for Safe Medication Practices performed an Adverse Events Reporting
System Review of the FDA's most dangerous drugs. The study discovered
fentanyl to be the second most dangerous drug available on the market with
the second highest number of suspect drug deaths. Fentanyl was involved in
no fewer than thirty-five hundred suspect drug deaths during the eight-year
period of the study. See Thomas J. Moore et al., "Serious Adverse Drug Events
Reported to the Food and Drug Administration, 1998–2005," *Archives of Internal Medicine* 167, no. 16 (2007): 1752–59, doi: 10.1001/archinte.167.16.1752.

211 **RIC's protocol did not incorporate a drug treatment program:** The Las
Vegas Recovery Center, PRIDE, the Mayo Clinic, and Cleveland Clinic incorporate drug treatment programs in their offerings.

213 **As we entered the small sunny gym:** In November 2012, the Functional
Restoration Program moved into a twenty-five-hundred-square-foot dedicated
building on the Dartmouth-Hitchcock medical campus.

216 **fear-avoidant behavior and guarding had vanished:** How was it possible for people in so much pain to suddenly ignore it? Psychiatrist Stuart Brown,
who founded the National Institute for Play, has looked into this, and learned
that play—which by definition has no purpose and meets no biologic need—is
particularly good, because it provides freedom from worry and stress, and leads
to "a diminished consciousness of self." Play "generates optimism, seeks out
novelty, makes perseverance fun, leads to mastery, gives the immune system a
bounce, fosters empathy and promotes a sense of belonging and community,"
he says. "As a clinician, I've seen the negative effects of discontinuing playing
all too often. When adults don't play much, the consequences are rigidity, depression, lack of adaptability, the loss of irony, and such. When we're playing,
we cultivate all those talents that help us explore a demanding world, and we
roll with the punches life throws at us." See "What About 'Play' as a Treatment
for Back Pain? Could Fun and Games Be More Restorative Than Usual Care?"
Back Letter 28, no. 6 (2013): 63–71, doi: 10.1097/01.BACK.0000431456.87737.e6;
and "Discovering the Importance of Play Through Personal Histories and
Brain Images: An Interview with Stuart L. Brown," *American Journal of Play*,
Spring 2009, 405, http://www.journalofplay.org/sites/www.journalofplay
.org/files/pdf-articles/1-4-interview-importance-ofplay-stuart-brown.pdf.

Chapter 10: The Back Whisperers

222 National Commission for Certifying Agencies: Responsible for accrediting professions like psychotherapy.

222 American College of Sports Medicine: http://www.acsm.org.

222 National Strength and Conditioning Association: http://www.nsca.com/Membership/Member-Tools/Find-A-Trainer/.

225 If I stopped working out: When you stop exercising, you quickly sacrifice capillary density and the volume of mitochondria available to bring oxygen and nutrients to your muscles, and you lose the ground you've gained really fast. Sadly, it takes much longer to get fitness back than to destroy it.

234 *gua sha*: *Gua* means to scrape or scratch. *Sha* translates as sand, because the purple-and-red rash that arises after the treatment is sand-like in texture. *Gua sha* is a traditional Chinese medical treatment, commonly used in Vietnam and other parts of Asia.

235 In the in vivo lab: Using loading machines, an acceleration rack, sectioning equipment, and an X-ray suite meant to document progressive tissue damage.

237 "Core Myths": The origins of the "core" myth, writes Gretchen Reynolds, can be traced to an Australian study conducted in the mid-1990s in which scientists learned that patients with healthy backs tensed a muscle in the pelvis called the transverse abdominis before commencing a simple exercise. In patients with back pain, that muscle didn't fire as early, leading the researchers to postulate that increased abdominal strength would mitigate back pain. Remarkably quickly, that news reached gyms and Pilates classes, and trainers began to direct clients to "tighten the core," which was interpreted as a directive to suck in their bellies and to flatten their backs against the floor when doing crunches. Subsequently, the *British Journal of Sports Medicine* published an article indicating that tightening the transverse abdominis in preparation for exercise was not particularly helpful, especially for those with healthy backs. See Gretchen Reynolds, "Core Myths," *New York Times*, June 18, 2009, http://www.nytimes.com/2009/06/21/magazine/21FOB-physed-t.html?_r=0; and Garry T. Allison and S. L. Morris, "Transversus Abdominis and Core Stability: Has the Pendulum Swung?" *British Journal of Sports Medicine* 42 (2008): 930–31, doi: 10.1136/bjsm.2008.048637.

240 "Every time you do a traditional crunch": The traditional sit-up, Stuart McGill says, imposes 730 pounds of compression on the spine, and a torso extension on a Roman chair imposes over 890 pounds. Even worse, observes McGill, is the back extension task commonly prescribed in clinics, in which the patient lies prone and extends the legs and outstretched arms; this imposes 1,300 pounds of compression on a hyperextended spine. "After examining the lumbar compression that results from performing sit-ups with full flexion in the lumbar spine, it is clear that enough sit-ups will cause damage in most people," he has written. Each sit-up produces low back compression levels close to the National Institute of Occupational Safety and Health (NIOSH) action limit, and repeatedly compressing the spine to higher levels than NIOSH's action limit has been shown to increase the risk of back disorders. See Stuart McGill, *Low Back Disorders: Evidence-Based Prevention and Rehabilitation* (Champaign, IL: Human Kinetics, 2002), 104.

241 In a YouTube video posted on my website: http://cathrynjakobson ramin.com/?s=McGill&post_type=resources.

243 missionary position: In the missionary position, two postures were tested. In one, the male supported his upper body with his hands and the female bent her knees slightly. In the other, the male supported his upper body with his elbows and the female had knees and hip joints slightly bent.

243 "quadruped," or "doggy" position: The two variations of the quadruped position included one in which the female supported her upper body with her elbows, and the other where she supported her upper body with arms extended.

244 often disruptive-of-the-status-quo *Back Letter*: The *Back Letter* reviews all current literature in the back care field and well beyond. Granted that it's published by Lippincott Williams & Wilkins—and therefore kin to such peer-reviewed journals as *Pain* and *Spine*—Schoene's tone is skeptical, irreverent, and investigative rather than ponderously academic. An annual subscription costs $269, and can be obtained at https://www.lwwjournals.com/details?issn=0894-7376.

248 Jerome Groopman: His research at Beth Israel focuses on understanding how blood and vascular cells grow, communicate, and migrate.

254 If a person stays continually in a state of threatened arousal: Ronald Siegel conceded that, as John Sarno maintained, unacknowledged emotion could also trigger the tight muscles. "We're so frightened that those thoughts are going to slip into awareness that we have to block them constantly." That may explain why chronic pain is far more common in people with histories of physical or sexual abuse. But most pain patients are not victims of trauma.

254 flooding the body with the hormone cortisol: Cortisol in turn inhibits the activity of cells called fibroblasts, which are the source of connective tissue. In time, muscles become weakened and dysfunctional.

Chapter 11: The Right Kind of Hurt

276 it broke down the precious muscle you were trying to build: Further research showed me that this is a disputable hypothesis—some studies show that aerobic exercise and strength training can occur in the same session with no adverse consequences.

280 those who were malingering: "A failure to produce consistent results . . . during repeated tests is an indication of a noncooperative subject," Jones explained. "Experienced individuals have been unable to duplicate a faked abnormal strength test using MedX equipment. . . . It is easily possible to reproduce a zero level of torque, but repeating an exact level of submaximal effort is very difficult, if not impossible. Cooperative subjects will produce repeated test results that are so close to being identical that any difference is insignificant; a lack of such consistent results is an indication of a noncooperative subject."

281 pursue self-insured organizations: To self-insure means that rather than paying an insurance company to pay medical, dental, and vision claims, the company pays the claim itself, using a third-party administrator to process the claims on its behalf.

Chapter 12: The Posture Mavens

284 I yearned to stop a group of teenage girls: Spero Karas, orthopedic surgeon at Emory Sports Medicine Center, observes that carrying an extra-large bag depresses one shoulder, causing the other shoulder to hike up. This is turn tilts the spine, causing back spasms. In the midst of writing this book, I spotted a billboard on the side of a Manhattan bus shelter featuring a pair of shapely female legs and feet, decked out in sky-high heels. If the ad had been for Louboutin or Jimmy Choo, I'd have ignored it. But this was an ad for Tylenol. The pitch was perfectly clear: "Go ahead, darling, cripple yourself. And rely on us for help in dealing with this self-inflicted pain." A few weeks later, I observed that Motrin, not to be outdone by its competitor in the analgesic wars, offered the same help to mothers who wore slings to carry their infants.

286 sitting "straight": For more information on sitting postures and chair design, see A. C. Mandal, "Balanced Sitting Posture on Forward Sloping Seat," acmandal.com; Peter Opsvik, *Rethinking Sitting* (New York: W. W. Norton & Company, 2008); and Torsten Mandal, "Better Furniture Types for Work and Studies Reduce Bending and Pain," Association for Body Conscious Design, http://bodyconsciousdesign.com/uploads/mandal_article.pdf.

287 David Kahl: Watch a video of my interview with Kahl: https://vimeo.com/104790377.

287 Fully: www.fully.com.

290 inexpensive Feldenkrais programs: In Northern California, for instance, Kaiser-Permanente offers members six classes for $41—a bargain by back pain industry standards. The Feldenkrais Guild website includes an online directory (http://www.feldenkrais.com/AF_MemberDirectory.asp) where you can find certified teachers in practically every region of the United States.

290 physical therapist Marek Wyszynski: He also runs his private physical therapy practice out of the Feldenkrais Institute of New York.

291 *Learn to Learn:* *Learn to Learn* is available from Feldenkrais Resources: http://www.feldenkraisresources.com/Learn-to-Learn-Feldenkrais-Book let-p/1160.htm.

291 "heavy water": A form of water with a unique atomic structure. It contains two atoms of deuterium (an isotope of hydrogen) and one oxygen atom. A nuclear reactor that uses heavy water can use a form of uranium commonly found in nature rather than enriched uranium, which is costly to produce.

293 **we were to listen to his words:** Because nearly all Feldenkrais lessons are recorded for posterity, later I was able to look up what the teacher had said. "Hold your right knee in both hands over your body. Several times, bring your knee closer to and then further from your chest . . . then hold your knee still in space and lift your right foot up and down several times, partially straightening and bending the leg . . . then repeat, bringing the knee towards the chest . . . easier? Now take your knee a little to the right and left several times . . . is your foot going right and left with your knee? Following? Leading? Do the movement several times with the foot going right and left with the knee, and then several times with the foot staying more or less fixed in space as the knee moves . . . then make circles in space with the knee, first clockwise, then counter-clockwise . . . then stretch out and rest. Compare your legs and note the differences." See "Lesson of the Month #1: Gentle Twist," Flowing Body, Flexible Mind, accessed December 14, 2015, http://www.flowingbody .com/low1.htm.

297 **"Fasciae":** Singular, fascia, pronounced "faah-sha."

298 **When I called the Rolfing Structural Integration headquarters:** You can find Rolfers internationally on the Rolf Institute website at http://www .rolf.org.

301 **"mesentery":** When the mesentery is released, bowel function improves and long-standing back pain can disappear. Getting higher fiber and more water into one's diet is important, but when the mesentery is tied down, even eating a box of prunes won't provide sustained relief.

303 **professor James Harvey Robinson:** Robinson was also a future founder of the New School for Social Research.

305 **Judith Stern:** I would not discover until much later that her husband, neurosurgeon Jack Stern, had a booming spine surgery practice. I wondered how that worked. He sent patients to an affiliated practice called Spine Options, staffed by a physiatrist, acupuncturist, and biofeedback expert. However, despite his wife's reputation and convictions, there was no Alexander teacher on staff. Several times, I asked Stern to explain that omission, but he never did so.

308 **"yoga teacher mills":** In an effort to gain control over the "quickie" certification of instructors in yoga teacher mills, the Yoga Alliance was formed in 1999. The organization provides accreditation for schools that certify yoga teachers, insisting on a minimum standard of two hundred hours of training, generally accomplished in four to five weeks. Only a third of the seventy thousand yoga instructors in the United States have such a certification, and although two-hundred-hour yoga courses include basic education regarding anatomy and physiology, there's no guarantee of expertise in musculoskeletal conditions.

The Yoga Alliance's highest-level certification is "E-RYT 500," meaning that teachers have five hundred hours of training. If you use the Yoga Alliance's directory to search for an instructor (https://www.yogaalliance.org/Directory), filtering your search for "alignment-oriented yoga" and "therapeutic yoga," you will winnow the numbers considerably: in the entire city of Chicago, there are only six teachers with these qualifications.

See "Yoga Alliance Through the Years," Yoga Alliance website, last updated March 20, 2015, https://www.yogaalliance.org/About_Us/Our_History; William J. Broad, *The Science of Yoga* (New York: Simon & Schuster, 2012), 135; and Pamela Paul, "When Yoga Hurts," *Time*, October 4, 2007.

308 "yoga therapists": Although the title "yoga therapist" sounds impressive, there are no industry-wide standards—anyone can hang out that shingle. There's a promising-sounding International Association of Yoga Therapists in Little Rock, Arkansas, but that turned out to be primarily a trade association rather than a certifying body.

309 a Viniyoga therapist: There's a search function on the American Viniyoga Institute's website at http://www.viniyoga.com/learn-experience/vini yoga-teachers-and-yoga-therapists.

311 B. K. S. Iyengar: The young Iyengar got a place in a maharaja's entourage. The teenager, basically hired to entertain, twisted himself into complicated poses for the amusement of visiting dignitaries, injuring his joints in the effort. Later Iyengar developed his own sequences of poses, emphasizing precise structural alignment and the use of props.

In 1952, after a decade of anonymous teaching in Pune, which is about a hundred miles south of Mumbai, Iyengar met American-born violinist Yehudi Menuhin. What was scheduled to be a five-minute conversation with the musician became a three-hour practice session. That year, Menuhin introduced Iyengar to his friends in Switzerland, where the yogi attracted quite a following. In 1958, Iyengar traveled to New York.

To get things rolling, Menuhin, who called Iyengar "my best violin teacher," and would write the introduction to *Light on Yoga*, introduced the thirty-eight-year-old yogi to Rebekah Harkness, the fiftyish widow of William Hale Harkness, the Standard Oil heir. Harkness, who by all accounts played by her own rules, was one of the richest women in America. She invited the strikingly attractive Iyengar to spend the summer at Holiday House, her Watch Hill, Rhode Island, waterfront mansion. Then she invited all her society friends to participate in the guru's group yoga classes. In a photo spread in *Life* magazine's August 1956 issue titled "A New Twist for Society," Harkness is portrayed in a shoulder stand, her backside sheathed in a bathing suit. She had "her society neighbors doing yoga, and plans to go to India for advanced lessons from Iyengar," the author observed.

For Harkness, the visit might have been a summer's lark. But Iyengar, with his lion's mane of hair and wild eyebrows, was deadly serious. His teaching style was fiery; he gave strong verbal commands. He was adamant about alignment; only that way could he ensure his students' safety. He believed in tough love: He would slap any body part that did not follow his directive.

In 2004, *Time* magazine included him on its global list of the world's hundred most influential people.

See Ellen Barry, "B. K. S. Iyengar, Who Helped Bring Yoga to the West, Dies at 95," *New York Times,* August 20, 2014, http://www.nytimes.com/2014/08/21/world/asia/bks-iyengar-who-helped-bring-yoga-to-west-dies-at-95.html; Craig Unger, *Blue Blood* (New York: William Morrow & Company, 1988); "A New Twist for Society," *Life,* August 20, 1956, 53, https://books.google.com/books?id=eEgEAAAAMBAJ&lpg=PA53&dq=iyengar%20william%20harkness&pg=PA53#v=onepage&q&f=false; Judy Landecker, Iyengar Yoga Association of the Northwest, "Regional Condolences," *Yoga Samachar* 18, no. 2 (Fall 2014/Winter 2015): 31; and Michael Richards, "B. K. S. Iyengar," in "The 2004 Time 100," *Time,* April 26, 2004, http://content.time.com/time/specials/packages/article/0,28804,1970858_1970910_1972051,00.html.

311 **I quickly agreed:** Before class, I read B. K. S. Iyengar's book, *Light on Yoga.* Translated into seventeen languages, it has sold more than three million copies. (By comparison, John Sarno's successful *Healing Back Pain* sold just over a million copies.) "Mr. Iyengar," or "Guruji," as his admirers refer to him, could hold a headstand for six minutes when he was in his eighties. He taught around the world, traveling to Moscow and Guangzhou, China, when he was well into his nineties, and practiced yoga daily until his death at ninety-four. He created a unique form of orthopedic yoga, setting up yoga institutes in more than seventy-five countries. See B. K. S. Iyengar, *Light on Yoga* (New York: Schocken Books, 1979); and Ellen Barry, "B. K. S. Iyengar, Who Helped Bring Yoga to the West, Dies at 95," *New York Times,* August 20, 2014, http://www.nytimes.com/2014/08/21/world/asia/bks-iyengar-who-helped-bring-yoga-to-west-dies-at-95.html.

314 **he was sent to a string of internment camps:** Pilates, interned with other German nationals, taught other inmates the concepts and exercises he'd absorbed over two decades of self-study and apprenticeship in yoga, Zen, and ancient Greek and Roman physical regimens. See "An Exercise in Balance: The Pilates Phenomenon," Pilates Method Alliance, accessed September 2, 2015, http://www.pilatesmethodalliance.org/i4a/pages/index.cfm?pageid=3277.

315 **Pilates Method Alliance-Certified Personal Trainer:** At least four Pilates organizations in the United States provide rehabilitation training programs for instructors: Polestar Pilates, Stott Pilates, Phi Pilates, and APPI (Australian Physiotherapy and Pilates Institute), an Australian organization that has begun to train teachers in the United States. Brent Anderson, the head of Polestar Pilates, told me in November 2015 that although the organization's website was in the process of being overhauled, a new search engine would list more than six thousand graduates of Polestar's program, more than half of whom are physical therapists who have trained in Pilates.

316 **Gyrotonic Expansion System:** To find a Gyrotonic Expansion System class, visit https://gyrotonic.com/studios_classes_and_courses.aspx. For more specific information on Level Two trainers, contact Gyrotonic International Headquarters: call (570) 828–0003 or e-mail info@gyrotonic.com.

317 **Gyrotonic is beautiful to watch:** I tried Gyrotonic for the first time under

something short of the best circumstances. My son had landed in the hospital with a horrible case of stomach flu, and I'd been sitting on the edge of his hospital bed until I was groaning right along with him. On a whim, I made an appointment to see a trainer at a Gyrotonic studio, Body Evolution, deep in Manhattan's East Village. My young instructor, a dancer who had used Gyrotonic to recover from a serious injury, told me to have faith: No matter how fragile I thought my spine was, it would surprise me with its resilience. And in fact there was something mesmerizing and liberating about soaring forward with my arms extended in front of me, in full extension, and then circling back into flexion, as if I were doing the breaststroke. With each grand swoop of my arms, I imagined my tense muscles relaxing and my vertebrae separating, sending fluids and nutrients to the perpetually cramped intervertebral discs. Walking home, I observed something new: With every step, my trunk moved up and away from my hips and legs, the crown of my head reaching for the sky. I wasn't quite flying, but there was ease in my body I hadn't experienced for a long time. Before I knew it, I had covered five long crosstown blocks to the Astor Place subway station, without the slightest hint of pain.

318 **Fit, younger clients often participate:** Research published in the *Journal of Physical Therapy Science* in 2014 demonstrated that, compared with stretching, regular Tai Chi classes reduced symptoms of acute lower back pain in young men in their twenties. See YongHo Cho, "Effects of Tai Chi on Pain and Muscle Activity in Young Males with Acute Low Back Pain," *Journal of Physical Therapy Science,* no. 5 (2014): 679–81, doi: 10.1589/jpts.26.679.

318 **especially suitable for older back pain patients:** Yang and Sun styles are used therapeutically, to improve balance and decrease the risk of falling. Sun style, which incorporates small steps rather than leaps, involves less knee flexion than some other versions and is less burdensome to the knee and ankle joints. See Amanda Hall et al., "The Effectiveness of Tai Chi for Chronic Musculoskeletal Pain Conditions: A Systematic Review and Meta-Analysis," *Arthritis Care & Research* 61, no. 6 (2009): 717–24, doi: 10.1002/art.24515.

318 **Beyond improving back pain:** According to the Cochrane Collaboration, Tai Chi has been shown to reduce the prevalence of falls in elderly people. See Lesley D. Gillespie et al., "Interventions for Preventing Falls in Older People Living in the Community," *Cochrane Database of Systematic Reviews* 9 (2012), doi: 10.1002/14651858.CD007146.pub3.

318 **A 2015 study showed:** The study showed that both cognitive behavioral therapy and Tai Chi were very helpful. Among older adults with insomnia, cognitive behavioral therapy reduced systemic inflammation, Tai Chi reduced cellular inflammatory responses, and both treatments reduced expression of genes encoding pro-inflammatory mediators. See Michael R. Irwin, "Cognitive Behavioral Therapy and Tai Chi Reverse Cellular and Genomic Markers of Inflammation in Late-Life Insomnia: A Randomized Controlled Trial," *Biological Psychiatry* 78, no. 10 (2015): 721–29, http://dx.doi.org/10.1016/j.biopsych.2015.01.010.

318 **the Hands of the Eighteen Luohan:** The next level beyond Luohan is to become a Buddha. The Eighteen Luohan were Buddha's main disciples. See "What Is the Luohan Gong?" Embrace the Moon website, accessed December 14, 2015, http://www.embracethemoon.com/luohan.htm.

319 **Qigong in China remains strictly regulated:** In China, Qigong is regulated by the Chinese Health Qigong Association, which was established in 2000. It places limits on public gatherings, requires state-approved training and certification of instructors, and restricts the practice to state-approved forms.

322 **the relief of psychological stress:** There is a clear link between body position and mood; slouching can generate bad feelings. Johannes Michalak, a clinical psychologist at Germany's University of Hildesheim, studied the subject after observing that Qigong had helped boost his own sense of well-being. See Johannes Michalak, Judith Mischnat, and Tobias Teismann, "Sitting Posture Makes a Difference—Embodiment Effects on Depressive Memory Bias," *Clinical Psychology and Psychotherapy* 21, no. 6 (2014): 519–24, doi: 10.1002/cpp.1890.

322 **The Arthritis Foundation:** The Arthritis Foundation (www.arthritis.org; 800–283–7800, toll-free) can tell you whether its Tai Chi program, a twelve-movement, easy-to-learn sequence, is offered in your area.

323 **In Chinese martial arts:** There is no shortage of Chinese martial arts websites, many of them packed with useful information. Almost every instructor has one. On Paul Lam's website, you can filter results for instructors he has trained in arthritis therapy and back care. One hitch: Although e-mail addresses are listed state by state for teachers, physical addresses are not. Therefore, one Google search will lead to several more, as you try to track down a teacher near you. See "Instructors," Tai Chi for Health Institute, accessed August 20, 2015, http://taichiforhealthinstitute.org/instructors/.

Bibliography

Aldridge, Susan. *Magic Molecules: How Drugs Work*. Cambridge: Cambridge University Press, 1998.

Alexander, Frederick M. *The Use of the Self*. London: Orion, 2001.

Benedetti, Paul, and Wayne MacPhail. *Spin Doctors: The Chiropractic Industry Under Examination*. Ontario, Canada: Dundern Press, 2002.

Benson, Herbert, and Miriam Z. Clipper. *The Relaxation Response*. New York: HarperTorch, 1976.

Beringer, Elizabeth, ed. *Embodied Wisdom: The Collected Papers of Moshé Feldenkrais*. Berkeley, CA: North Atlantic Books, 2010.

Black, Jonathan. *Making the American Body: The Remarkable Saga of the Men and Women Whose Feats, Feuds, and Passions Shaped Fitness History*. Lincoln: University of Nebraska Press, 2013.

Bourke, Joanna. *The Story of Pain: From Prayer to Painkillers*. Oxford: Oxford University Press, 2014.

Brady, Scott. *Pain-Free for Life: The 6-Week Cure for Chronic Pain Without Surgery or Drugs*. New York: Center Street, 2006.

Broad, William J. *The Science of Yoga: The Risks and Rewards*. New York: Simon & Schuster, 2012.

Brownlee, Shannon. *Overtreated: Why Too Much Medicine Is Making Us Sicker and Poorer*. New York: Bloomsbury USA, 2007.

Caplan, Deborah. *Back Trouble: A New Approach to Prevention and Recovery*. Gainesville, FL: Triad Publishing, 2000.

Chapman-Smith, David. *The Chiropractic Profession: Its Education, Practice, Research, and Future Directions*. Des Moines, IA: NCMIC Group, 2000.

Clippinger, Karen Sue. *Dance Anatomy and Kinesiology*. Champaign, IL: Human Kinetics, 2006.

Cranz, Galen. *The Chair: Rethinking Culture, Body, and Design*. New York: W. W. Norton & Company, 2000.

Darnall, Beth. *Less Pain, Fewer Pills: Avoid the Dangers of Prescription Opioids and Gain Control over Chronic Pain*. Boulder, CO: Bull Publishing Company, 2014.

Deyo, Richard A. *Hope or Hype: The Obsession with Medical Advances and the High Cost of False Promises.* New York: AMACOM, 2005.

_____. *Watch Your Back! How the Back Pain Industry Is Costing Us More and Giving Us Less.* Ithaca, NY: ILR Press, 2014.

Duhigg, Charles. *The Power of Habit: Why We Do What We Do in Life and Business.* New York: Random House, 2012.

Feitis, Rosemary, ed. *Ida Rolf Talks About Rolfing and Physical Reality.* New York: Harper & Row, 1978.

Feldenkrais, Moshé. *Awareness Through Movement: Easy-to-Do Health Exercises to Improve Your Posture, Vision, Imagination, and Personal Awareness.* New York: HarperOne, 1972.

_____. *Learn to Learn.* San Diego, CA: Feldenkrais Resources, 1980.

Fessler, Richard G. *Endoscopic Spine Surgery and Instrumentation.* New York: Thieme Medical Publishers, 2004.

Filler, Aaron G. *The Upright Ape: A New Origin of the Species.* Franklin Lakes, NJ: Career Press, 2007.

Fishman, Loren, and Carol Ardman. *Sciatica Solutions: Diagnosis, Treatment, and Cure of Spinal and Piriformis Problems.* New York and London: W. W. Norton & Company, 2006.

Fletcher, Anne M. *Inside Rehab: The Surprising Truth About Addiction Treatment—and How to Get Help That Works.* New York: Penguin Books, 2013.

Fordyce, Wilbert E. *Back Pain in the Workplace: Management of Disability in Nonspecific Conditions: A Report of the Task Force on Pain in the Workplace of the International Association for the Study of Pain.* Seattle, WA: IASP Press, 1995.

Foreman, Judy. *A Nation in Pain: Healing Our Biggest Health Problem.* Oxford: Oxford University Press, 2014.

Gawande, Atul. *Complications: A Surgeon's Notes on an Imperfect Science.* New York: Picador, 2002.

Gelb, Michael. *Body Learning: An Introduction to the Alexander Technique.* New York: Holt Paperbacks, 1996.

Gokhale, Esther. *8 Steps to a Pain-Free Back: Natural Posture Solutions for Pain in the Back, Neck, Shoulder, Hip, Knee, and Foot (Remember When It Didn't Hurt).* Stanford, CA: Pendo Press, 2008.

Gonzalez, Erwin G., and Richard S. Materson. *The Nonsurgical Management of Acute Low Back Pain: Cutting Through the AHCPR Guidelines.* New York: Demos Medical Publishing, 1997.

Groopman, Jerome. *The Anatomy of Hope.* New York: Random House, 2004.

_____. *How Doctors Think.* New York: Houghton Mifflin, 2007.

Hadler, Nortin M. *The Last Well Person: How to Stay Well Despite the Health-Care System.* Montreal, Quebec, Canada: McGill–Queen's University Press, 2004.

_____. *Stabbed in the Back: Confronting Back Pain in an Overtreated Society.* Chapel Hill: University of North Carolina Press, 2009.

Hanna, Thomas. *Somatics: Reawakening the Mind's Control of Movement, Flexibility, and Health.* Cambridge, MA: Da Capo Press, 1988.

Harer, John B., and Sharon Munden. *The Alexander Technique and Resource Book.* Lanham, MD: Scarecrow Press, 2009.

Harrington, Anne. *The Cure Within: A History of Mind-Body Medicine.* New York: W. W. Norton & Company, 2009.

Herbert, Lauren. *Sex and Back Pain.* 3rd ed. Greenville, ME: Impacc USA, 1997.

Herkowitz, Harry, et al. *The Lumbar Spine.* 3rd ed. Philadelphia: Lippincott Williams & Wilkins, 2004.

Homola, Samuel. *Inside Chiropractic: A Patient's Guide.* New York: Prometheus Books, 1999.

Hyman, Mark. *Until It Hurts: America's Obsession with Youth Sports and How It Harms Our Kids.* Boston: Beacon Press, 2009.

Illich, Ivan. *Medical Nemesis.* London: Calder & Boyars, 1974.

Iyengar, B. K. S. *Light on Yoga.* New York: Schocken Books, 1979.

Jones, Frank Pierce. *Body Awareness in Action: A Study of the Alexander Technique.* Berlin: Schocken, 1987.

Juhan, Deane. *Job's Body: A Handbook for Bodywork.* New York: Barrytown, Ltd., 1998.

Kabat-Zinn, Jon. *Full Catastrophe Living: Using the Wisdom of Your Body and Mind to Face Stress, Pain, and Illness.* New York: Bantam Books, 1990.

Kahneman, Daniel. *Thinking, Fast and Slow.* New York: Farrar, Straus and Giroux, 2011.

Katz, Jeffrey. *Heal Your Aching Back: What a Harvard Doctor Wants You to Know About Finding Relief and Keeping Your Back Strong (Harvard Medical School Guides).* New York: McGraw-Hill, 2007.

Keer, Rosemary, and Rodney Grahame. *Hypermobility Syndrome: Recognition and Management for Physiotherapists.* London: Butterworth Heinemann, 2003.

Keleman, Stanley. *Emotional Anatomy: The Structure of Experience.* Berkeley, CA: Center Press, 1986.

Kirsch, Irving. *The Emperor's New Drugs: Exploding the Antidepressant Myth.* New York: Basic Books, 2010.

Knaster, Mirka. *Discovering the Body's Wisdom.* New York: Bantam, 1996.

Kraus, Hans. *Backache, Stress and Tension (Their Cause, Prevention and Treatment).* New York: Simon & Schuster, 1978.

LeDoux, Joseph. *The Emotional Brain: The Mysterious Underpinnings of Emotional Life.* New York: Touchstone, 1996.

Lewin, Philip. *Backache and Sciatic Neuritis.* Philadelphia: Lea & Febiger, 1943.

Liebenson, Craig. *Functional Training Handbook.* Philadelphia: Wolters Kluwer Health, 2014.

———, ed. *Rehabilitation of the Spine: A Practitioner's Manual.* Baltimore: Lippincott Williams & Wilkins, 1996.

Lieberman, Daniel. *The Story of the Human Body: Evolution, Health, and Disease.* New York: Random House, 2013.

Linden, David J. *Touch: The Science of Hand, Heart, and Mind.* New York: Viking Press, 2015.

Long, Preston H. *Chiropractic Abuse: An Insider's Lament*. New York: American Council on Science and Health, 2013.

Macdonald, Glynn. *Natural Ways to Health: Alexander Technique—A Practical Programme for Health, Poise, and Fitness*. Alexandria, VA: Time-Life Books, 1998.

Magner, George J., III. *Chiropractic: The Victim's Perspective*. Edited by Steven Barrett, MD. Amherst, NY: Prometheus Books, 1995.

Mahar, Maggie. *Money Driven Medicine: The Real Reason Health Care Costs So Much*. New York: HarperCollins, 2006.

Marcus, Norman. *Freedom from Pain: The Breakthrough Program That Brings Relief to Chronic Sufferers*. New York: Fireside, 1995.

Marras, William S. *The Working Back: A Systems View*. Hoboken, NJ: Wiley, 2008.

McGill, Stuart. *Low Back Disorders: Evidence-Based Prevention and Rehabilitation*. Champaign, IL: Human Kinetics, 2002.

_____. *Ultimate Back Fitness and Performance*. Ontario, Canada: Wabuno Publishers, 2004.

McKenzie, Robin. *Against the Tide: Back Pain Treatment—The Breakthrough*. Wellington, NZ: Dunmore Publishing, 2009.

_____. *Treat Your Own Back*. Raumati Beach, NZ: Spinal Publications of New Zealand Ltd., 2006.

Meier, Barry. *Pain Killer: A "Wonder" Drug's Trail of Addiction and Death*. Emmaus, PA: Rodale, 2003.

_____. *A World of Hurt*. New York: New York Times Company, 2013.

Miller, Alice. *The Body Never Lies: The Lingering Effects of Hurtful Parenting*. New York: W. W. Norton, 2004.

Mooney, Vert. *The Unguarded Moment: A Surgeon's Discovery of the Barriers to Prescription of Inexpensive, Effective Healthcare in the Form of Therapeutic Exercise*. New York: Vantage Press, 2007.

Myers, Thomas W. *Anatomy Trains: Myofascial Meridians for Manual and Movement Therapists*. 3rd ed. Edinburgh: Churchill Livingstone, 2014.

Neal, Joseph, and James P. Rathmell. *Complications in Regional Anesthesia and Pain Medicine*. Philadelphia: Lippincott Williams & Wilkins, 2012.

Obermark, Sherri A. *Back Story: Breaking the Cycle of Chronic Pain*. Cincinnati: Four Zone Media, 2015

Olivares, Jonathan. *A Taxonomy of Office Chairs*. London: Phaidon Press, 2011.

Opsvik, Peter. *Rethinking Sitting*. New York: W. W. Norton & Company, 2008.

Reid, T. R. *The Healing of America: A Global Quest for Better, Cheaper, and Fairer Health Care*. New York: Penguin Press, 2009.

Royal College of General Practitioners. *The Back Book: The Best Way to Deal with Back Pain—Get Back Active*. Norwich, UK: Stationery Office Books, 2002.

Sarno, John E. *The Divided Mind: The Epidemic of Mindbody Disorders*. New York: HarperCollins, 2006.

_____. *Healing Back Pain: The Mind-Body Connection*. New York: Warner, 1991.

_____. *Mind over Back Pain*. New York: Berkley Books, 1982.

_____. *The Mindbody Prescription: Healing the Body, Healing the Pain.* New York: Warner Books, 1998.

Schubiner, Howard, and Michael Betzold. *Unlearn Your Pain: A 28-Day Process to Reprogram Your Brain.* Pleasant Ridge, MI: Mind-Body Publishing, 2010.

Schuenke, Michael, et al. *Thieme Atlas of Anatomy: General Anatomy and Musculoskeletal System.* Stuttgart and New York: Georg Thieme Verlag, 2006.

Schwartz, Susan E. B. *JFK's Secret Doctor.* New York: Skyhorse Publishing, 2012.

Sennett, Richard. *Flesh and Stone: The Body and the City in Western Civilization.* New York: W. W. Norton & Company, 1996.

Seppala, Marvin D., and David P. Martin. *Pain-Free Living for Drug-Free People: A Guide to Pain Management in Recovery.* St. Paul, MN: Hazelden Publishing, 2005.

Seppala, Marvin D., and Mark E. Rose. *Prescription Painkillers: History, Pharmacology, and Treatment.* St. Paul, MN: Hazelden Publishing, 2010.

Shafran, Roz. *Overcoming Perfectionism: A Self-Help Guide Using Cognitive Behavioral Techniques.* London: Robinson Publishing, 2010.

Shorter, Edward. *From Paralysis to Fatigue: A History of Psychosomatic Illness in the Modern Era.* New York: Free Press, 1992.

Siegel, Ronald D. *Back Sense: A Revolutionary Approach to Halting the Cycle of Chronic Back Pain.* New York: Broadway Books, 2001.

_____. *The Mindfulness Solution: Everyday Practices for Everyday Problems.* New York: Guilford Press, 2010.

Singh, Simon, and Edzard Ernst. *Trick or Treatment: The Undeniable Facts About Alternative Medicine.* New York and London: W. W. Norton & Company, 2008.

Stanford, Craig. *Upright: The Evolutionary Key to Becoming Human.* New York: Houghton Mifflin, 2003.

Stephens, Jackson T. *Golf Forever: The Spine and More—A Health Guide to Playing the Game.* Las Vegas, NV: Stephens Media Group, 2003.

Stern, Jack. *Ending Back Pain: 5 Powerful Steps to Diagnose, Understand and Treat Your Ailing Back.* New York: Avery, 2014.

Todd, Edwin M. *The Neuroanatomy of Leonardo da Vinci.* Santa Barbara, CA: Capra Press, 1983.

Trager, Milton, and Cathy Guadagno-Hammond. *Trager Mentastics: Movement as a Way to Agelessness.* Barrytown, NY: Station Hill Press, 1989.

Vad, Vijay. *Back Rx: A 15-Minute-a-Day Yoga-& Pilates-Based Program to End Low Back Pain.* New York: Gotham Books, 2004.

_____. *Stop Pain: Inflammation Relief for an Active Life.* New York: Hay House, 2010.

Waddell, Gordon. *The Back Pain Revolution.* 2nd ed. London: Churchill Livingstone, 2004.

Waddell, Gordon, et al. *The Back Book.* Norwich, UK: TSO, 2009.

Wayne, Peter, and Mark Fuerst. *The Harvard Medical School Guide to Tai Chi: 12 Weeks to a Healthy Body, Strong Heart, and Sharp Mind.* Boston: Shambhala, 2013.

Webster's New World Medical Dictionary. 2nd ed. New York: Wiley, 2003.

Williams, Frances. *Inside Guides: Human Body.* New York: DK Publishing, 1997.

Index

NOTE: Page numbers followed by an "*n*" indicate an endnote on that page or pages; "*nn*" indicates multiple endnotes.

practice-building consultants, 338n
Prague School of Rehabilitation
  and Manual Medicine, Czech
  Republic, 36, 340n
Prather, Heidi, 38–39, 326
PRECISION trial (Pfizer), 185–86
pregabalin and gabapentin, 184
prescription drug compounders,
  59–62, 344n
prescriptions
  Ambien (zolpidem), 205, 367n
  benzodiazepines, 170–71
  buprenorphine "bupe," 172–73, 211,
    361–62n, 364n
  concurrent with opioids, 13
  COX-2 inhibitors, 159, 185–86, 360n
  Duragesic transdermal patch with
    fentanyl, 210, 211, 369n
  for emotional and physiological pain
    or distress, 155–57
  for exercise, 39–44
  FDA initiating state-run prescription
    drug registries, 166–67
  gabapentin and pregabalin, 184
  methadone, 164–65
  Miltown, 195, 363n
  MS Contin, 156
  NMDA antagonists, 184
  OxyContin, 156–61
  for physical therapy, 36, 38–39
  Sativex, 187
  See also opioid painkillers;
    pharmaceutical companies
"President-Elect in Magazine Article
  Says, 'Flabbiness' Menaces U.S.
  Security" (*New York Times*), 337n
primary care doctor, 7–8, 12, 160, 335n
Primary Care Musculoskeletal
  Research Centre (U.K.), 336n
ProDisc-L Total Disc Replacement
  prosthesis
  cognitive behavioral therapy
    compared to, 150

demise of, 150–51
and FDA, 137
procedure description, 149
recovery process, 149–50, 151
Rosen and Cunningham fighting
  back, 151–52
and surgeons' conflicts of interest,
  145–46
proprioception, 40, 341n
prostaglandins, 184
prosthesis. *See* disc replacement
provocative discography test, 78–79
Przekop, Peter, 366n
pseudo-addiction, 167
psoas muscles, 233–34
psychological support, 252–55
pulverized bone fill for interbody
  fusion cage, 83, 86, 87, 92
Purdue Frederick pharmaceutical firm
  overview, 155–56
  creating and promoting OxyContin,
    156–59
  sales reps and website, 159–60
  training physicians and hospital
    personnel, 160, 360n
Pure Healthy Back (PHB), 279–82
Putzier, Michael, 134

Q

Qigong and Tai Chi, 289–90, 317–23,
  365n, 376–77nn
Quackbusters, 338n
quacks, success of, 3

R

radiation, 8, 335n, 342n
radiology clinics, 10
Rainville, James, 221, 244–48, 250–52,
  254–55
Rashbaum, Ira, 193–94
Rathmell, James, 56

About the Author

CATHRYN JAKOBSON RAMIN is an investigative journalist and the author of the *New York Times* bestseller *Carved in Sand: When Attention Fails and Memory Fades in Midlife*. She's written for many national magazines on topics such as health care, neuroscience, business, public policy, travel, art, design, and culture. Cathryn is married to Ron Ramin, a composer. They have two adult sons, Avery and Oliver, and a Jack Russell–Daschund cross named Dasch, after the punctuation mark, which he resembles. She divides her time between Northern California and New York City.